Part B OSCE

Anatomy

MRCS Part B OSCE

Anatomy

Jeremy Lynch MBChB MRCS (Eng)
Specialist Registrar in General Surgery,
Royal Sussex County Hospital,
Brighton, UK

Susan Shelmerdine MBBS BSc (Hons) MRCS (Eng)
Specialty Registrar in Clinical Radiology,
St. George's Hospital, London, UK

Vishy Mahadevan MBBS PhD FRCS (Ed & Eng)
Professor of Surgical Anatomy and
Barbers' Company Professor of Anatomy,
The Royal College of Surgeons of England,
London, UK

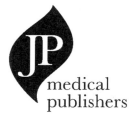

JP
medical
publishers

London • St Louis • Panama City • New Delhi

© 2013 JP Medical Ltd.
Published by JP Medical Ltd,
83 Victoria Street, London, SW1H 0HW, UK
Tel: +44 (0)20 3170 8910   Fax: +44 (0)20 3008 6180
Email: info@jpmedpub.com   Web: www.jpmedpub.com

ISBN: 978-1-907816-34-5

British Library Cataloguing in Publication Data
A catalogue record for this book is available from the British Library

Library of Congress Cataloging in Publication Data
A catalog record for this book is available from the Library of Congress

JP Medical Ltd is a subsidiary of Jaypee Brothers Medical Publishers (P) Ltd, New Delhi, India

Publisher:	Richard Furn
Commissioning Editor:	Hannah Applin
Senior Editorial Assistant:	Katrina Rimmer
Design:	Designers Collective Ltd
Indexer:	Liz Granger

Typeset, printed and bound in India.

Preface

The MRCS Part B OSCE Examination is a highly structured, standardised and comprehensive assessment of a surgical trainee's competence in a wide variety of surgical subjects and skills. These include the applied basic sciences, verbal communication, history taking, clinical examination of patients and manual procedures.

The anatomy component of the exam is often the most feared, due to the seeming magnitude of the knowledge required. Whilst there are many excellent anatomy textbooks, it can be a difficult subject to learn by reading alone. The purpose of this book is to provide a more stimulating method of learning and consolidating anatomical knowledge. It is more than just a few practice stations to be attempted in the remaining few days before the exam (although it can be used as such). It aims to be wide-ranging and can be dipped into during stolen moments in the working day and evening. This is a key advantage, since study leave is usually limited to a short period of time.

The exam is not designed to trick candidates and the knowledge required for the anatomy component is not arcane. It is anatomy that is encountered in the operating theatre and the emergency department. To mirror the anatomy component of the MRCS exam, the majority of specimens, radiological images, and surface anatomy pictures in this book depict normal anatomy. We have based each station around a specific anatomical region so that trainees can develop knowledge of these parts of the body in depth. All stations in the exam are manned by examiners, and working through this book with a colleague (preferably one due to sit the same exam) will make revision more realistic, rewarding and enjoyable.

We have aimed to cover the entire MRCS anatomy syllabus in depth. At times, the questions may seem harder than those likely to be encountered in the exam and this is because we feel that it is better for you to be stretched during revision, not during the exam. For this reason, do not be disheartened if some of the questions seem beyond your reach – we have made every effort to include detailed explanations to prepare you for the real thing.

Good luck!

Jeremy Lynch
Susan Shelmerdine
Vishy Mahadevan
October 2012

Contents

About the exam

The aim of the MRCS Part B OSCE Examination is to determine whether or not trainees have acquired the knowledge, skills and attributes commensurate with the completion of core training in surgery.

Structure of the exam

As of February 2013, the nature, format, and marking scheme will be significantly different from that employed in previous diets of the MRCS OSCE examination. This book is written in keeping with the new changes. There are 18 examined stations in the OSCE circuit and candidates must complete each station within nine minutes. The 18 stations cover applied basic surgical sciences, clinical and procedural skills, communication skills, and history taking.

To summarise, out of a total of 18 stations, three shall be anatomy stations, two will be pathology stations, three will be given to applied surgical sciences and critical care, four will be devoted to communication skills and history taking, and finally, two stations will assess procedural skills and four stations clinical examination technique.

Each station is scored out of 20 marks.

For more details on the marking and further information regarding the MRCS Part B OSCE, we recommend that you read the Candidate Instructions and Guidance Notes provided on the MRCS exam website.

Tips and tricks

We have come up with a few tips and hope this knowledge will help you achieve success.

1. In the weeks before the exam, try to gauge those areas in anatomy in which you feel your knowledge is inadequate, and attempt to rectify this. For example, if you find radiological images confusing then arrange an afternoon sitting in with a radiologist. Candidates in the UK may consider visiting the Wellcome Museum of Anatomy and Pathology at the Royal College of Surgeons of England, where various specimens and prosections are on display. Alternatively your nearest medical school may let you visit their dissection laboratory.

2. Arrive early for the exam and remember to carry all the necessary identification documents.

3. Dress appropriately and bring the right equipment. Be smart, bare below the elbows, with hair tied back if it is long. You may bring your own stethoscope and other similar equipment. **Do not under any circumstance carry your mobile phone to the OSCE circuit as this will certainly disqualify you from the exam.**

4. Whilst waiting outside the anatomy station in the exam, read the instruction sheet carefully. Although the questions that will be asked will not be listed on this sheet, it will give you a clue about the anatomical theme in which you will be examined. This will prevent you rushing into the station feeling completely in the dark.

5. Listen to the question! Answer each question clearly, concisely and confidently, making eye contact with your examiner. Do ensure that your answers are well structured and presented in a systematic manner. Feel free to ask for the question to be repeated if you do not understand or hear the question the first time.

6. If the answer to a particular question escapes you at the time, do not panic. Instead ask the examiner whether you can return to the question later. This will be allowed and you can save time and perhaps gain confidence by answering other questions you are more familiar with than wasting time on a question you do not know. If there is time at the end of the station, you will be able to have another go at answering the missed question.

7. Many of the prosections used in the exam will have been carefully prepared and arranged for the candidates to inspect. Do not disturb the specimens, unless asked by the examiner to point out relevant anatomy.

8. If asked to point out anatomical features on a prosection, ensure gloves are worn and use a pointer (these are provided in the station). Do not touch the specimens with bare hands. This sounds like common sense but it can be easily forgotten in the heat of the moment.

9. It is an oft-observed phenomenon that a candidate who does poorly in a station proceeds to perform sub-optimally in subsequent stations too, presumably owing to a loss of confidence. Remember that each new station is a chance to start afresh, so move on and give yourself a chance to prove what you really know.

Acknowledgements

The authors gratefully acknowledge the generosity of the trustees of the Royal College of Surgeons of England for allowing the use of anatomical specimen images from the Wellcome Museum of Anatomy and Pathology.

We are deeply indebted to John Carr of the Photography Department at the Royal College of Surgeons for his outstanding and immensely skilful help with many of the images in the book.

We would also like to thank Mandeep Gill Sagoo, Anatomist at St George's, University of London, for allowing us to photograph the prosections of the inguinal canal and right iliac fossa.

We would like to thank our parents, families and friends for their support and encouragement.

JL, SS, VM
October 2012

Image sources

The Anatomical Department of the Royal College of Surgeons of England.
- Chapter 1: Stations 1, 6, 8, 13, 21, 24, 25, 26, 27, 31, 30, 31, 39
- Chapter 2: Stations 5, 6, 7, 12, 13, 14, 21, 22, 23, 24, 27, 28, 30, 31, 32, 35, 37, 44
- Chapter 3: Stations 1, 6, 8, 9, 10, 11, 12, 16, 22, 27, 32, 33, 34
- Chapter 4: Stations 3, 4, 5, 9, 10, 13, 14, 19, 21

By permission from The Visible Human Project of the US National Library of Medicine, Bethesda, MD, USA.
- Chapter 1: Stations 9, 18, 19, 34, 36, 38
- Chapter 2: Stations 11, 20 (prosection), 25
- Chapter 3: Stations 17, 20, 23

Surface anatomy images were originally published in *Pocket Tutor Surface Anatomy* (©2012 JP Medical Ltd) and are reproduced courtesy of Sam Scott-Hunter, London.
- Chapter 1: Stations 2, 5, 11, 23
- Chapter 2: Stations 1, 3, 36, 39, 40, 45

The Anatomical Department of St George's, University of London and reproduced courtesy of Mandeep Gill Sagoo.
- Chapter 1: Stations 14, 17, 37

The Otolaryngology Department of the Royal Sussex County Hospital, Brighton and reproduced courtesy of Ketan Desai.
- Chapter 3: Station 30

Chapter 1

Thorax and trunk

Syllabus topics

The following topics are listed within the Intercollegiate MRCS examination syllabus for trunk and thorax anatomy. Tick them off as you revise these topics to ensure you have covered the syllabus.

Thorax

Development:

- ❑ Heart and great vessels
- ❑ Fetal circulation
- ❑ Oesophagus
- ❑ Diaphragm

Wall:

- ❑ Thoracic wall
- ❑ Mechanics of breathing

Thoracic cavity and viscera:

- ❑ Superior and inferior mediastinum
- ❑ Heart and pericardium
- ❑ Lungs
- ❑ Pleurae

Surface and imaging anatomy:

- ❑ Heart & heart valves
- ❑ Auscultation sites
- ❑ Lungs and pleurae
- ❑ Surface plane of sternal angle
- ❑ Dermatomes
- ❑ Chest drains
- ❑ Incisions
- ❑ Chest X-ray
- ❑ CT/MRI

Abdomen and pelvis

Development:

- ❑ Foregut/midgut/hindgut
- ❑ Gut rotation
- ❑ Anal canal
- ❑ Kidneys and ureters
- ❑ Bladder and urethra
- ❑ Testis

Walls and spaces and associated structures:

- ❑ Anterior abdominal wall
- ❑ Posterior abdominal wall
- ❑ Inguinal canal, spermatic cord, Inguinal hernia
- ❑ Pelvic floor and wall
- ❑ Lumbar plexus
- ❑ Sacral plexus
- ❑ Peritoneal cavity
- ❑ Intra-abdominal spaces

Abdominal viscera:

- ❑ Oesophagus
- ❑ Stomach
- ❑ Small and large intestine
- ❑ Appendix
- ❑ Liver

- ☐ Gall bladder
- ☐ Bile ducts
- ☐ Pancreas
- ☐ Spleen
- ☐ Kidney and ureter
- ☐ Adrenal gland

Pelvic viscera:

- ☐ Rectum
- ☐ Bladder
- ☐ Prostate
- ☐ Seminal vesicles
- ☐ Uterus
- ☐ Uterine tubes
- ☐ Ovaries
- ☐ Vagina

Perineum:

- ☐ Anal triangle: anal canal and ischioanal fossa

- ☐ Male urogenital triangle: scrotum, Testis and epididymis, penis and urethra
- ☐ Female urogenital triangle: vulva

Surface and imaging anatomy:

- ☐ Quadrants/nine regions
- ☐ Planes: subcostal, transpyloric, transtubercular
- ☐ Dermatomes
- ☐ Abdominal incisions
- ☐ Rectal and vaginal examinations
- ☐ Imaging appearances of abdomen/ gastrointestinal/biliary/urinary tracts,
- ☐ Arteriography
- ☐ CT/MRI/Ultrasound

Station 1

A 66-year-old man is struck in the chest by a winch whilst attempting to repair his car. In the emergency department he is diagnosed with multiple right-sided rib fractures.

Image (a) below shows the inferior aspect of a right rib (demonstrating normal anatomy):

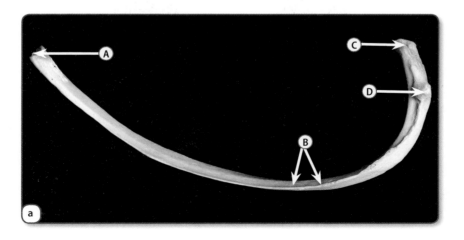

1.1 Identify the bony landmarks labelled B, C and D.

1.2 What does A articulate with?

1.3 What runs in the groove indicated by B?

1.4 What is the arterial supply of the intercostal muscles of the second and tenth intercostal spaces?

1.5 Where do the intercostal veins drain?

1.6 What is meant by the term 'flail chest'?

1.7 What type of joint is the first costochondral joint?

Image (b) below shows the anterior aspect of the sternum:

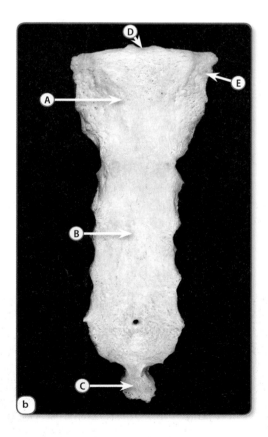

1.8 Identify the parts labelled A, B, C, and D.

1.9 Name the structure that articulates with the sternum at E.

Station 2

A 54-year old woman attends the preoperative clinic in preparation for abdominal surgery. History taking reveals that she has had haemoptysis on and off for a couple of weeks. On clinical examination there is dullness to percussion over her left lower chest.

The images below are of the anterior (a) and posterior (b) aspects of the chest:

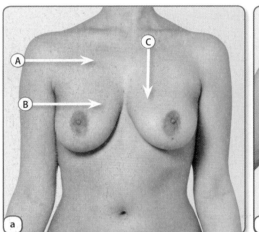 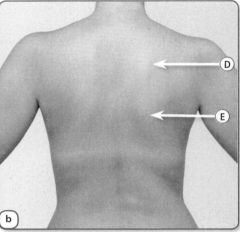

2.1 Which lung lobes are auscultated at sites labelled A to E?

2.2 Describe the surface marking of the pleural edges in terms of their relations to the thoracic skeleton.

2.3 Describe the surface marking of the lung edges in terms of their relations to the thoracic skeleton.

2.4 What are the surface markings for:

    2.4a the oblique fissure of the lungs?

    2.4b the transverse fissure of the lungs?

2.5 Which costal cartilage attaches to the sternum at the sternal angle?

2.6 At which vertebral level is the suprasternal notch?

2.7 At which vertebral level is the xiphisternal joint?

2.8 What are the boundaries of the superior mediastinum?

2.9 What are the contents of the superior mediastinum?

Station 3

A 22-year-old man is brought to the emergency department after being hit by a car. He is intubated by the paramedics at the scene of the accident. On arrival in the emergency department it is noted that he has extensive bruising over his lower chest. Review your knowledge of intrathoracic anatomy using the following image.

This is a contrast-enhanced axial computed tomography (CT) scan of a normal thorax:

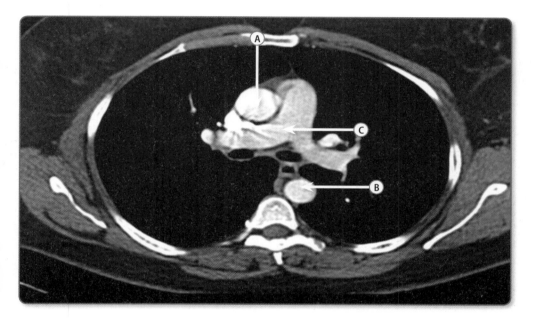

3.1 Identify the structures labelled A, B, C.

3.2 Classify the divisions of the mediastinum.

3.3 Through which division of the mediastinum is this slice taken?

3.4 What are the boundaries of this division of the mediastinum?

3.5 What is the innervation of the parietal and visceral pleura?

3.6 Name some of the important functions of the thoracic sympathetic chain, and state which spinal cord segments contribute to the sympathetic chain?

3.7 Define thoracic outlet syndrome.

3.8 Define subclavian steal syndrome.

Station 4

A 55-year-old male banker experiences a crushing type of retrosternal chest pain of sudden onset whilst climbing the stairs in his office. An echocardiogram shows severe aortic stenosis.

The image below is of an axial cardiac CT taken at the level of the aortic root (demonstrating normal anatomy):

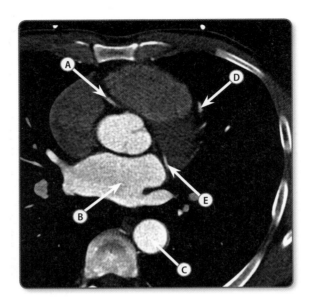

4.1 Identify the structures labelled A to E.

4.2 What is the origin of the right coronary artery? Name the branches of the right coronary artery.

4.3 What is the origin of the left coronary artery? Name the branches of the left coronary artery.

4.4 Which coronary artery most commonly supplies:

    4.4a the sinoatrial node?

    4.4b the atrioventricular node?

4.5 Describe the venous drainage of the heart.

4.6 Describe the conducting system of the heart.

4.7 Describe the efferent nerve supply to the heart.

4.8 Why is the pain of ischaemic heart disease referred to the chest wall?

Station 5

A 29-year-old woman is involved in a head-on collision with another car. She is brought to the emergency department where it is noted that she is restless, tachypnoeic and tachycardic. Clinical examination reveals she has a large right-sided tension pneumothorax and you are asked to perform emergency decompression.

This image displays the anterior aspect of the female chest:

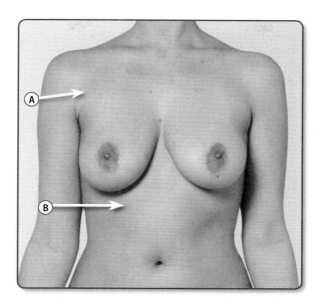

5.1 Where would you insert a cannula for emergency decompression of tension pneumothorax? What layers does this needle pass through?

5.2 What is the 'safe triangle' of chest drain insertion?

5.3 The point marked B is located within which dermatome?

5.4 What is the direction of relaxed skin tension lines at point A?

5.5 What is the surface marking for:

    5.5a the entry point of the needle for subclavian vein catheterisation?

    5.5b the entry point of the needle for internal jugular vein catheterisation?

    5.5c a posterolateral thoracotomy incision for exposure of upper thoracic structures?

5.6 At which vertebral level is:

    5.6a the sternal angle (plane of Louis)?

    5.6b the bifurcation of the trachea?

5.7 What are the surface markings for auscultation of the aortic and pulmonary valves?

5.8 What are the surface markings for the borders of the heart?

Station 6

Two days post-nephrectomy, a 59-year-old man is noted by the ward staff to have become suddenly very breathless. An emergency chest radiograph is requested and while you are waiting for the radiographs you wish to view a normal chest film to revise your knowledge of thoracic anatomy.

This is an anteroposterior plain radiograph of the chest (demonstrating normal anatomy):

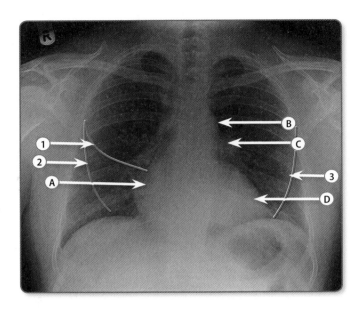

6.1 Identify the structures labelled A to D.

6.2 Which fissures do lines 1–3 indicate?

6.3 At what vertebral level do the bronchi enter the lungs?

6.4 Name the lobes of the right and left lungs.

6.5 Define the term 'bronchopulmonary segment'.

6.6 How many bronchopulmonary segments are there in each lung?

6.7 What is the blood supply to the lungs?

6.8 What is the lymphatic drainage of the lungs?

6.9 Describe the nerve supply to the lungs? What effect does stimulation of the sympathetic and parasympathetic system have on the lungs?

6.10 In which bronchus (right or left) are inadvertently aspirated foreign bodies most likely to lodge and why?

Station 7

A 72-year-old man is hit by a car. He is noted to be in haemodynamic shock when reviewed in the emergency department. There is suspicion of intrathoracic bleeding and the man is taken to theatre.

The image below is a dissection of the thorax and mediastinum viewed from the right:

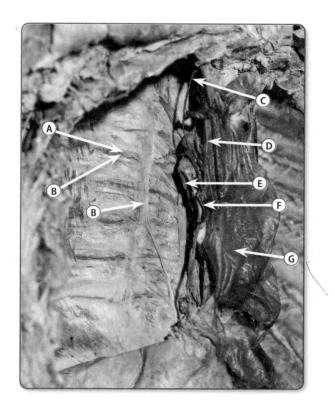

7.1 Identify the structures labelled A to G.

7.2 What are the contents of the pulmonary hilum?

7.3 How many pulmonary veins drain each lung?

7.4 How many embryonic pharyngeal arches are there and which numbered arch disappears without giving rise to any specific structures?

7.5 From which embryonic pharyngeal arch are the internal carotid arteries derived?

7.6 From which embryonic pharyngeal arch is the right subclavian artery derived?

Station 8

During the preoperative assessment of a 65-year-old man due to have general anaesthesia, a systolic murmur is detected. The man undergoes an echocardiogram which reveals severe tricuspid regurgitation. You discuss the patient with the cardiothoracic surgeons.

This is a prosection of the heart, displaying the inside of the right ventricle (demonstrating normal anatomy):

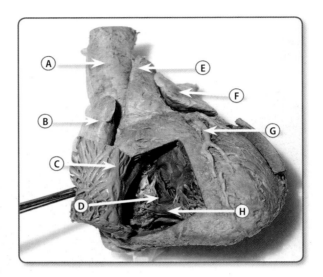

8.1 Identify the structures labelled A to G.

8.2 Identify the structure labelled H? What is its function?

8.3 Name the layers of pericardium.

8.4 Where is the pericardial space and what does it normally contain? What layers, from skin downwards, does a needle pass through to perform pericardiocentesis?

8.5 What structures are at risk of damage during pericardiocentesis?

8.6 What is the function and composition of the foramen ovale? What percentage of adults has an anatomically patent foramen ovale?

8.7 What structures do the ductus arteriosus connect in the fetus?

8.8 Where is the commonest site for coarctation of the aorta?

8.9 What do the bulbus cordis and truncus arteriosus give rise to in the adult?

Station 9

A 45-year-old man is involved in a high-speed road collision. He is intubated at the scene of the accident by the paramedic team, and bilateral chest drains are inserted. On arrival in the emergency department the man remains very hypoxic and the chest drains are continuing to drain large volumes of blood. You assist with a thoracotomy performed in the resuscitation room to identify the source of bleeding.

The following image is an axial dissection of the thorax at the level of T9 (demonstrating normal anatomy), viewed from below:

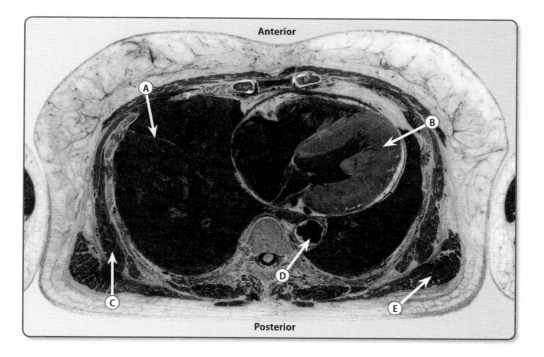

9.1 Identify the structures labelled A to E.

9.2 List the successive elements of the airway, starting with the trachea and leading on to the alveolus.

9.3 State the origin and termination of the azygos vein.

9.4 What tributaries do the hemiazygos and accessory veins receive, and where do they drain to?

9.5 Describe the arrangement of muscles in the intercostal spaces.

9.6 Which muscles contract to produce inspiration?

9.7 Name the accessory muscles of respiration.

Station 10

A 52-year-old man presents to the surgical clinic with progressive dysphagia for both liquids and solids over the last few months. He confesses to have lost a significant amount of weight recently and admits to being a heavy drinker and smoker.

He undergoes the following investigation (demonstrating normal anatomy):

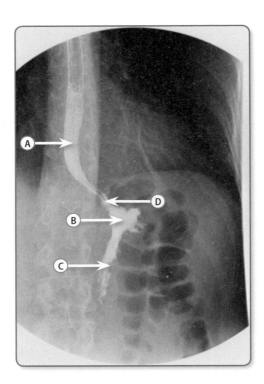

10.1 What type of radiological investigation is this?

10.2 Name the parts of the gastrointestinal tract indicated by A, B and C.

10.3 Comment on the narrowing at point D.

10.4 Oesophogastroduodenoscopy (OGD) is performed. State in centimetres the distance from the incisor teeth:

    10.4a at which the oesophagus commences.

    10.4b at which the oesophagus is crossed by the left bronchus.

    10.4c at which the oesophagus terminates.

10.5 Name the layers an endoscope must pass through to perforate the oesophagus.

10.6 What type of muscle fibre lies in the oesophageal wall, and what cell type lines the oesophageal mucosa?

10.7 What is the blood supply of the oesophagus?

10.8 What is meant by the term 'Barrett's oesophagus'?

10.9 What is the lymphatic drainage of the oesophagus?

10.10 What is 'Virchow's node' and why does it commonly present on the left side?

10.11 Where is the cisterna chyli and what is its function?

10.12 What is the embryological origin of the trachea?

Station 11

A 63-year-old woman presents acutely with generalised abdominal pain and constipation. On examination the abdomen is distended and a mass is felt in the right lower quadrant.

This image demonstrates some features of the anterior aspect of the abdomen:

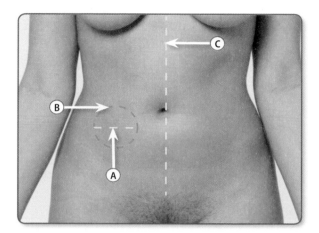

11.1 With your knowledge of anatomy, give a differential diagnosis of a mass located in the region indicated by circle B.

11.2 Define McBurney's point.

11.3 In which dermatome is the umbilicus located?

11.4 Name the sequence of layers you would pass through whilst incising through lines A and C to enter the abdomen?

11.5 What is the surface marking of the transpyloric plane and what structures are present at this level?

11.6 At what vertebral level is the subcostal plane and what structures are present at this level?

11.7 At what vertebral level does the aorta bifurcate? What is the surface marking for this point?

11.8 What are the surface markings for:

    11.8a the inferior border of the liver?

    11.8b the spleen?

    11.8c the fundus of the gallbladder?

11.9 Describe the location of these abdominal incisions:

    11.9a Gridiron

11.9b Kocher

11.9c Mercedes Benz

11.9d Pfannenstiel

Station 12

A 49-year-old woman presents with epigastric pain and weight loss over a period of 4 months. At the last clinic attendance an abdominal CT scan was requested. Before you review her scans you wish to familiarise yourself with the features of a normal abdominal scan.

This is an axial CT scan of the upper abdomen (a) (demonstrating normal anatomy):

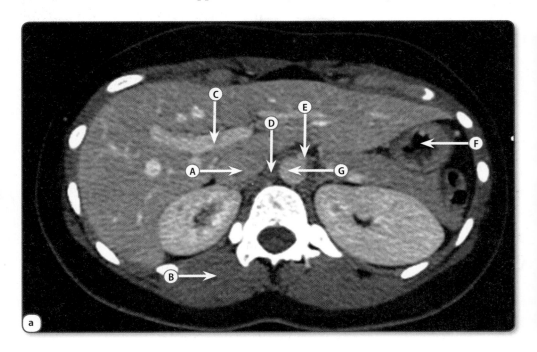

12.1 Identify the structures labelled A to G.

12.2 At what vertebral level is the above CT slice taken?

12.3 What is C and what are its tributaries?

12.4 What proportion of blood does C supply to the liver?

The image on the next page (b) is another axial CT scan of the same patient:

12.5 Identify the structures labelled A to E.

12.6 What are the functions of organ E?

12.7 Name the different parts of organ E.

12.8 Define the term 'pseudocyst'? Describe its pathogenesis.

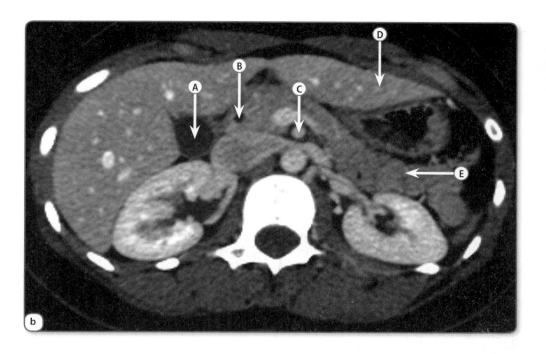

b

Station 13

A 23-year-old woman undergoes laparoscopy for investigation of abdominal pain. You assist the consultant who is performing the operation. On the fourth postoperative day you examine her wounds and note that there is an abscess developing in the umbilical wound.

This is a dissection of the anterior abdominal wall:

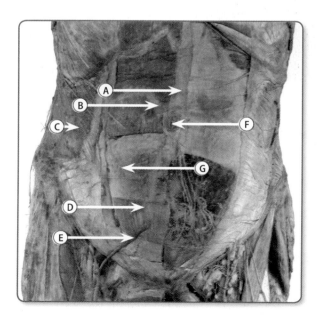

13.1 Identify the structure labelled A? What gives rise to its colour?

13.2 Identify the structures labelled B to G.

13.3 Name in sequence the layer of the abdominal wall traversed by the umbilical port.

13.4 In which direction do the fibres of the internal oblique, external oblique, and transversus abdominis fibres run at the level of the umbilicus?

13.5 What are the contents of the rectus sheath?

13.6 What is the surface marking of the arcuate line and what is its significance?

13.7 What is the distal limit of Scarpa's fascia?

13.8 What is the continuation of Scarpa's fascia in the perineum called?

13.9 Where is the median umbilical ligament located and what does it contain?

13.10 Where are the medial umbilical ligaments located and what do they contain?

Station 14

A 22-year-old woman presenting with right iliac fossa pain undergoes laparoscopy for suspected appendicitis. You assist the consultant performing the operation.

This is a dissection of the appendix and lower abdominal structures in a normal subject:

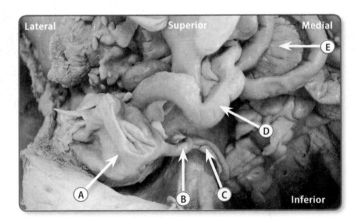

14.1 Identify the structures labelled A, B, D and E.

14.2 Identify the structure labelled C. What structures run in this tissue?

14.3 Explain on the basis of anatomical principles why infection of the appendix may result in necrosis whilst infection of the gallbladder usually does not.

14.4 Name four common positions assumed by the appendix.

14.5 Using embryological principles explain the changing nature and location of pain in appendicitis.

14.6 Which nerves may be damaged when performing an open appendicectomy?

14.7 What are taeniae coli and where do they converge?

14.8 What are appendices epiploicae?

Station 15

A 63-year-old woman gives a history of urinary incontinence a couple of weeks following an abdominoperineal resection for rectal cancer. At the last clinic attendance an abdominal CT was booked. Before you review her scans you wish to familiarise yourself with the features of a normal female subject.

Image (a) is a contrast-enhanced axial CT through the pelvis (demonstrating normal anatomy):

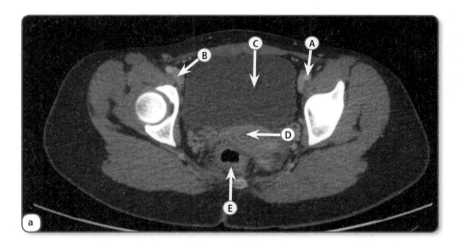

15.1 Identify the structures labelled A to E.

15.2 At what vertebral level does the structure labelled A divide?

15.3 What bony landmark in the pelvis defines this division?

15.4 Does the ureter pass anterior or posterior to this division?

Image (b) on the next page is an axial CT scan through the pelvis of the same patient:

15.5 Identify the structures labelled A to D

15.6 Name the parts of the levator ani.

15.7 What are the boundaries of the pelvic outlet?

15.8 What attaches to the perineal body?

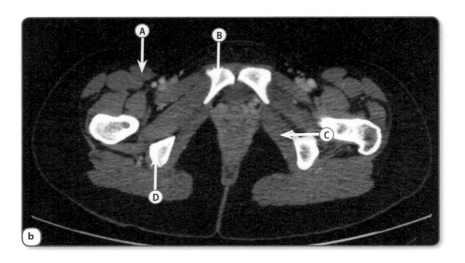

b

Station 16

A 79-year-old man presents to his general practitioner with a 3-month history of weight loss and change in bowel habit. He is referred to the colorectal clinic where he undergoes investigations to rule out colorectal malignancy.

This is a contrast study of the large bowel (demonstrating normal anatomy):

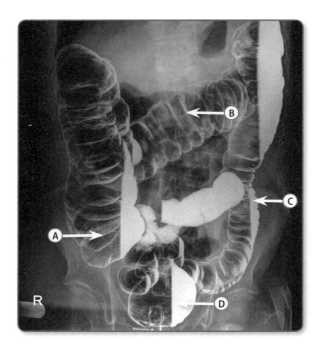

16.1 How does the small bowel differ in appearance from the large bowel on an abdominal plain film?

16.2 What type of radiological study is shown? Comment on the diameter of the bowel.

16.3 What name is given to the lines labelled B?

16.4 Name the segments of the colon labelled A and C. What is the blood supply to these structures?

16.5 What is the marginal artery of Drummond?

16.6 What are the topographical relations of structure D?

16.7 How does the peritoneum relate to structure D?

16.8 What parts of the large bowel are particularly susceptible to injury in blunt abdominal trauma?

16.9 What muscles make up the posterior abdominal wall?

Station 17

A 52-year-old man presents with a swelling in the left groin and is diagnosed with an inguinal hernia. You are assisting your consultant in theatre during the inguinal hernia repair, and he asks you to identify some of the anatomical structures.

This is a dissection of the left groin (demonstrating normal anatomy):

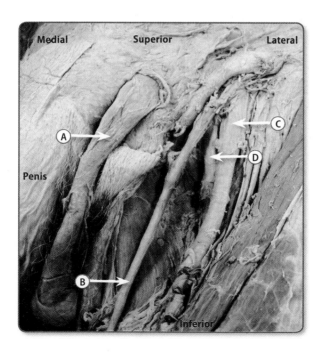

17.1 Identify the structures labelled A to D.

17.2 What are the contents of A?

17.3 What is the inguinal ligament? What are the medial and lateral attachments of the inguinal ligament?

17.4 What is the surface marking for the deep inguinal ring? Intraoperatively, what anatomical structure may be found that helps define this point?

17.5 How may an inguinal hernia be clinically distinguished from a femoral hernia?

17.6 What are the boundaries of the inguinal canal?

17.7 What is the embryological origin of the cremasteric fascia?

17.8 Describe the significance and boundaries of Hesselbach's triangle.

17.9 Why is one cautioned against taking deep bites when suturing the inferior border of a mesh to the inguinal ligament?

Station 18

A 52-year-old man presents to the colorectal clinic with rectal bleeding. On proctoscopy you identify first degree haemorrhoids and proceed to perform banding.

The image below is a normal axial dissection of the male pelvis viewed from below:

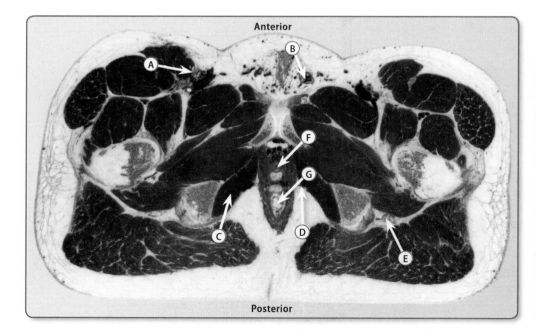

18.1 Identify the structures labelled A to G

18.2 Regarding the structure labelled G:

     18.2a what communication exists between the portal and systemic venous circulation in this region?

     18.2b Name other regions in the body where similar portosystemic communications exist.

18.3 Describe the boundaries of the anal triangle of the perineum.

18.4 What are the topographical relations of the prostate?

18.5 What are the contents and boundaries of the ischioanal fossae?

18.6 Where is the commonest site for an anal fissure?

18.7 Anatomically speaking, what is a haemorrhoid?

18.8 What is Goodsall's rule?

18.9 What are the lengths of the normal adult anal canal and rectum?

18.10 What are the topographical relations of the anal canal?

Station 19

A 45-year-old man known to have ulcerative colitis presents with acute abdominal pain. An abdominal radiograph is requested and reveals toxic megacolon. You assist your consultant in performing a subtotal colectomy.

This image is an axial dissection of the abdomen at the level L2 (demonstrating normal anatomy) viewed from below:

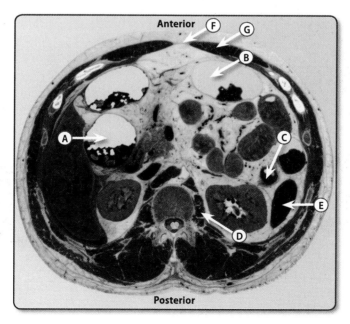

19.1 Identify the parts of the bowel labelled A, B and C.

19.2 What muscle is present at D?

19.3 Identify the structures labelled E, F, and G.

19.4 What are the posterior topographical relations of the ascending colon?

19.5 What are the posterior topographical relations of the descending colon?

19.6 Which circumferential positions in the colonic wall are susceptible to acquired diverticular disease?

19.7 What does the transverse mesocolon attach to on the posterior abdominal wall?

19.8 What structures run within the transverse mesocolon?

19.9 Of what clinical significance is the ileocaecal valve in a patient with large bowel obstruction?

19.10 Which part of the bowel most commonly undergoes volvulus?

Station 20

A 75-year-old man with a history of hypertension and hypercholesterolaemia presents with post-prandial abdominal pain. Ultrasound and OGD do not reveal any abnormalities. Chronic mesenteric ischaemia is suspected and an angiogram is requested.

Image (a) is a digital subtraction angiogram of the coeliac plexus and its branches (demonstrating normal anatomy):

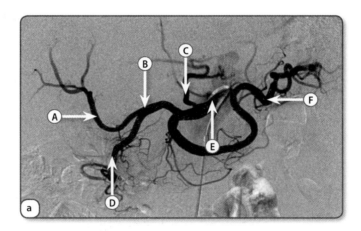

20.1 Identify the arteries labelled A to F.

20.2 At what vertebral level does the coeliac artery (coeliac axis) leave the aorta?

20.3 What organs does D supply?

20.4 Within what peritoneal structure does A run, and what topographical relationship does it have to the bile duct and portal vein?

Image (b) on the next page is a digital subtraction angiogram of the superior mesenteric artery and its branches (demonstrating normal anatomy).

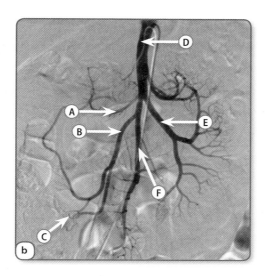

20.5 Identify the arteries labelled A to F.

20.6 At what vertebral level does the superior mesenteric artery leave the aorta?

20.7 At what vertebral level does the inferior mesenteric artery leave the aorta?

20.8 Over what structures does the superior mesenteric artery pass before entering the root of the small intestinal mesentery.

20.9 Which part of the large intestine is particularly susceptible to ischaemia?

Station 21

A 72-year-old man with a known abdominal aortic aneurysm is admitted with acute, severe abdominal and back pain. A diagnosis of leaking aneurysm is made and he is taken to theatre for an emergency operation.

This is a dissection of the retroperitoneal region of a normal subject:

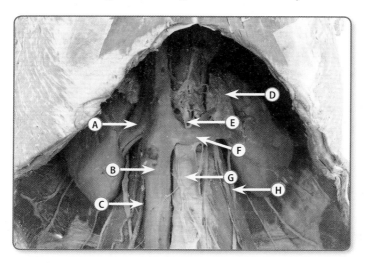

21.1 Identify the structures labelled A to H.

21.2 What is the ligament of Treitz?

21.3 What are the lateral branches of the aorta?

21.4 What is the arterial supply of the adrenal glands?

21.5 What is the venous drainage of the adrenal glands?

21.6 At operation the inferior mesenteric artery can often be ligated without serious consequence. What is the anatomical explanation for this?

21.7 Regarding structure B:

    21.7a at what vertebral level does it commence?

    21.7b as it ascends, what are its successive anterior topographical relations?

    21.7c name the tributaries.

Station 22

An obese 55-year-old woman presents with long standing intermittent, colicky right upper quadrant pain. An abdominal ultrasound scan proves inconclusive and she is referred for magnetic resonance cholangiopancreatography (MRCP). You are due to review her in the outpatient clinic and wish to familiarise yourself with normal biliary anatomy as seen on a MRCP.

The image below is a MRCP demonstrating the normal anatomy of the biliary system:

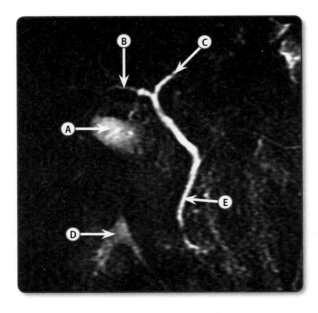

22.1 Identify the structures labelled A to E.

22.2 What route does bile take to enter the intestinal tract? In gallstone ileus, what route does a gallstone usually travel to enter the intestinal tract?

22.3 What is the narrowest part of the extrahepatic biliary system?

22.4 What is the function and composition of bile?

22.5 Which hormone stimulates the release of bile? What is the trigger for this hormone and where is the hormone synthesised.

22.6 What epithelium lines the extrahepatic biliary ducts?

22.7 What is Pringle's manoeuvre?

22.8 What is Mirizzi's syndrome?

Station 23

A 23-year-old female bank official presents as an emergency after being shot during a bank raid. There is a bullet wound in her right loin with extensive bleeding from a superficial vessel. She is taken to theatre for exploration of the wound.

This photograph demonstrates some features of the surface anatomy of the anterior aspect of the abdomen:

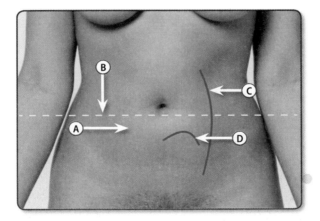

23.1 What anatomical lines are indicated by C and D?

23.2 What plane is indicated by dotted yellow line B? What anatomical structures can be found at this level?

23.3 Which vessels in the anterior abdominal wall, indicated by point A, may have been punctured by the bullet?

23.4 What are the origins of these vessels?

23.5 Define the linea semilunaris.

23.6 What is the innervation and action of the internal oblique?

23.7 List the functions of the muscles of the abdominal wall.

Station 24

A 70-year-old man presents in shock with a rigid abdomen. He is taken to theatre and found to have a perforated duodenal ulcer, which is repaired with an omental patch.

This is a prosection showing the stomach and other upper abdominal viscera in a normal subject:

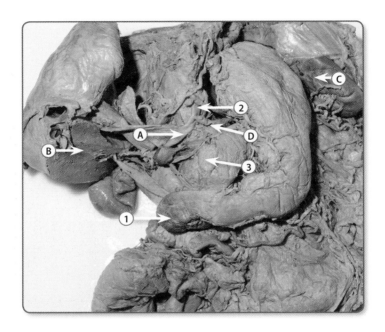

24.1 Identify the structure labelled 1? What are its parts? Which of these parts are mobile?

24.2 Identify the structure labelled 2? What are its branches?

24.3 Identify the structure labelled 3? Describe its blood supply.

24.4 Identify the structures labelled A to D.

24.5 What is the name of the fold of peritoneum that hangs from the greater curvature of the stomach? What blood vessels run in this tissue?

24.6 What is the epiploic foramen (foramen of Winslow)? Define its boundaries.

24.7 What are the topographical relations of the second part of the duodenum?

24.8 What is the definition and contents of the supracolic compartment?

24.9 What are the contents of the splenorenal (lienorenal) ligament?

24.10 What vessels are carried within the gastrosplenic ligament?

24.11 Where is the root of the small bowel mesentery attached?

Station 25

A 45-year-old woman with recurrent bouts of epigastric pain is noted to have gallstones on ultrasound scanning. She attends for laparoscopic cholecystectomy. You are assisting the consultant who is performing the procedure.

This is a prosection displaying the inferior surface of the liver (demonstrating normal anatomy):

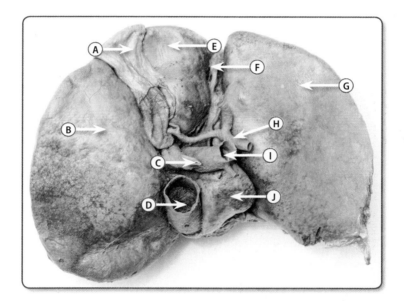

25.1 Identify structures labelled A to J.

25.2 State the blood supply, lymphatic drainage, and nerve supply of structure A?

25.3 What epithelium lines structure A?

25.4 What are the boundaries of Calot's triangle and what does the triangle contain?

25.5 What is the upper limit of the normal diameter of the common bile duct on ultrasound in a 20-year-old?

25.6 What is the embryological origin of the ligamentum teres hepatis?

25.7 What is the embryological origin of the liver?

Station 26

A 64-year-old man is diagnosed with rectal adenocarcinoma and is admitted for an anterior resection of the rectum. You are assisting your consultant who is performing the procedure.

This is a sagittal prosection of the left hemipelvis of a normal adult male:

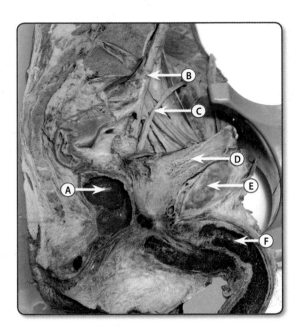

26.1 Identify the structures labelled A to F.

26.2 Name the segments of the gastrointestinal tract that are immobile.

26.3 What are the branches of the inferior mesenteric artery?

26.4 What epithelium lines the anal canal?

26.5 Where in the adult gut are the junctions between the embryological foregut and midgut, and the embryological midgut and hindgut?

26.6 What is the superior boundary of the left paracolic gutter?

26.7 What is the most dependent part of the peritoneal cavity in the supine position?

26.8 List the routes via which rectal adenocarcinoma spreads.

Station 27

A 45-year-old male builder sustains a heavy blow to the thorax and abdomen by a reversing truck. On arrival at the emergency department, the trauma series of radiographs reveals a fractured pelvis and diaphragmatic rupture.

The image on the next page is a dissection of the superior surface of the normal diaphragm, showing the structures that traverse it.

27.1 What structure passes through the opening labelled A? At what vertebral level does this structure traverse the diaphragm and what accompanies it through this opening?

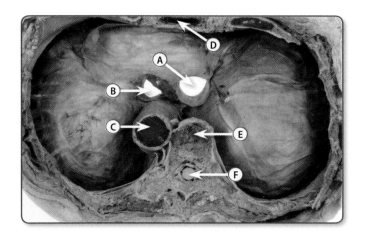

27.2 What structure passes through the opening labelled B?

27.3 Identify the structure labelled C. At what vertebral level does it traverse the diaphragm and what accompanies it through this opening?

27.4 Identify the structures labelled D to F

27.5 At what vertebral levels do the following traverse the diaphragm:

   27.5a the vagus nerves?

   27.5b the right phrenic nerve?

   27.5c the left gastric artery?

27.6 Where, respectively, do the splanchnic nerves and sympathetic chain traverse the diaphragm?

27.7 What nerves provide the motor innervation of the diaphragm?

27.8 Describe the course of these nerves.

27.9 What four components contribute to the embryological origin of the diaphragm?

27.10 Name two common types of acquired diaphragmatic hernias.

27.11 Name two common types of congenital diaphragmatic hernias.

Station 28

A 24-year-old man presents with severe colicky pain in the left renal angle radiating to the groin. He undergoes an intravenous urogram. Before reviewing the scan, you familiarise yourself with some of the normal features of this type of scan.

On the next page is a normal intravenous urogram.

28.1 At what vertebral levels do the kidneys lie?

28.2 Identify the structures labelled A, B and C.

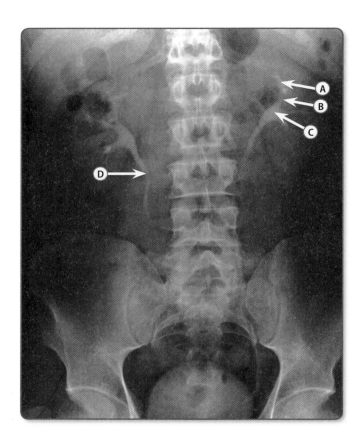

28.3 What are the three natural narrowings in D?

28.4 What is the blood supply to D?

28.5 What is the topographical relationship between the renal artery and the renal vein?

28.6 Can you ligate the left renal vein without serious consequences and if so, why?

28.7 Name the retroperitoneal structures of the abdomen.

28.8 From what embryological structures are the kidneys and ureters derived?

28.9 What arrests the ascent of a horseshoe kidney from the pelvis during development?

Station 29

A 37-year-old woman is referred to the surgical team with abdominal pain. However, soon after arriving in the emergency department she collapses, shocked. A urine test is positive for β-hCG and she is suspected to have a ruptured ectopic pregnancy.

This is a sagittal view of a normal female left hemipelvis:

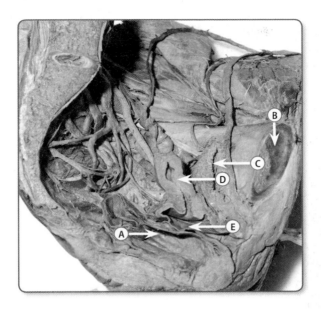

29.1 Identify the structures labelled A, B, C.

29.2 Regarding structure D:

    29.2a what is it?

    29.2b name the various parts of structure D.

    29.2c what is the blood supply to structure D?

    29.2d what are different positions in which it can lie?

29.3 Regarding structure E:

    29.3a what is it?

    29.3b what are its topographical relations?

    29.3c what is the blood supply?

    29.3d what epithelium lines it?

29.4 Name the parts of the fallopian tube.

29.5 Where are the Bartholin's glands and what is their function?

29.6 What are the broad ligaments of the uterus?

29.7 What is the round ligament of the uterus?

29.8 Name three other ligaments that support the uterus and vagina.

Station 30

A 63-year-old man is diagnosed with bladder cancer and undergoes a radical cystectomy and ileal conduit formation. You are assisting the consultant who is performing the operation.

This is a dissection of the male pelvis (demonstrating normal anatomy):

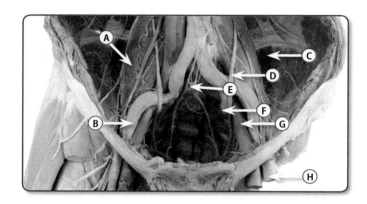

30.1 Identify the structures labelled A to H.

30.2 What are the boundaries of the urogenital triangle? What are its contents in the male?

30.3 What is the blood supply of the bladder?

30.4 Describe the innervation of the bladder.

30.5 What layers, from skin inwards, does a needle pass through when aspirating a hydrocele?

30.6 What is the lymphatic drainage of the testes?

30.7 What is the origin of the left testicular artery?

30.8 Name the parts of the male urethra. What is its approximate length in the adult male?

30.9 Is ejaculation mediated by the sympathetic or parasympathetic nervous system?

30.10 Which epithelium lines the prostatic urethra?

Station 31

A 75-year-old woman presents to the surgical clinic with rectal prolapse that occurs during defecation. You assess her using your knowledge of the anatomy of the pelvis and rectum.

The image on the next page is a sagittal prosection of the left hemipelvis of a normal subject.

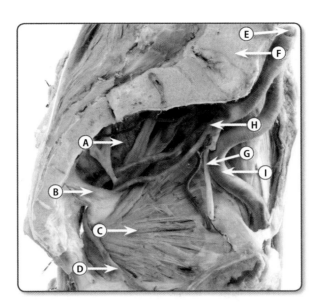

31.1 Identify the structures labelled A to I.

31.2 What is the origin and insertion of the muscle labelled A?

31.3 What are the origin, insertion, action and nerve supply of C?

31.4 From which nerve roots does the lumbar plexus arise?

31.5 What branches of the lumbar plexus emerge from the lateral border of the psoas?

31.6 What are the root values for the femoral nerve?

31.7 What are the root values for the sacral plexus?

31.8 Describe the course and relations of the right and left lumbar sympathetic chains.

31.9 What are the indications for lumbar sympathectomy?

31.10 From where does the parasympathetic supply of the abdomen originate?

Station 32

A 45-year-old male sushi chef presents with weight loss and epigastric pain. He has a family history of stomach cancer and is worried that this might be the diagnosis. You request urgent outpatient radiological investigations.

The image on the next page is a contrast study of a normal stomach:

32.1 What type of study is this?

32.2 Identify the parts of the stomach labelled A, B, C, D, F and G.

32.3 What do the vertical lines at point E indicate?

32.4 Describe the arterial supply of the stomach.

32.5 Describe the innervation of the stomach.

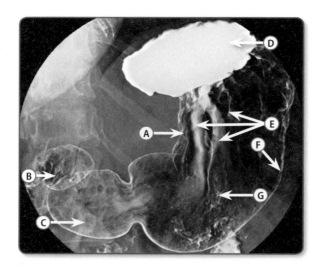

32.6 What are the consequences of highly selective vagotomy?

32.7 What are the anterior and posterior relations of the stomach?

32.8 What anatomical landmarks demarcate the duodenum from the stomach?

32.9 Describe the cardiac sphincter of the stomach.

32.10 Describe the lymphatic drainage of the stomach.

Station 33

A 35-year-old man presents to the hospital with left upper quadrant pain following a game of rugby, where he thinks he may have been elbowed in the stomach. On questioning he admits to having had a sore throat for the past week. You assess him and request a CT scan as you think he may have ruptured his spleen.

The images below are contrast-enhanced axial CT slices taken at the level of the spleen in two different normal subjects. Both images demonstrate normal anatomy. Image (a) has been acquired during the venous phase and image (b) has been acquired during the arterial phase.

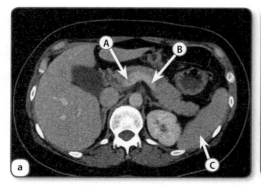
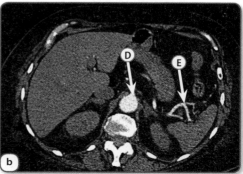

33.1 Identify the structures labelled A to E.

33.2 Which pathogen causes upper respiratory tract infection and also predisposes the individual to splenic rupture?

33.3 In what direction does a spleen enlarge and why?

33.4 What organs are in direct contact with the spleen?

33.5 Is the spleen intraperitoneal or retroperitoneal?

33.6 What splenic ligaments must be cut during splenectomy?

33.7 What are the branches of the splenic artery?

33.8 Describe the functions of the spleen.

33.9 What embryological structure does the spleen develop from?

33.10 What is the innervation of the adrenal glands?

33.11 Name the different macroscopic regions of the adrenal gland and their respective functions.

Station 34

A 47-year-old man undergoes a liver biopsy for investigation of jaundice. Twenty-four hours later he presents to the emergency department in shock, complaining of right upper quadrant pain. You suspect that he may be bleeding from his biopsy site.

The following image is an axial dissection obtained at the level of the hepatic hilum (demonstrating normal anatomy):

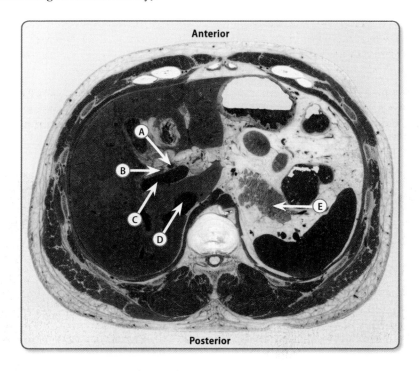

34.1 Identify the structures labelled A to E.

34.2 What anatomical layer, related to the liver, may help contain hepatic bleeding?

34.3 Describe the functional divisions of the liver.

34.4 Describe the innervation of the liver.

34.5 What are the contents and attachments of the falciform ligament?

34.6 What is the ligamentum venosum?

34.7 How are the portal vein, hepatic artery, and bile duct related to each other in the free edge of the lesser omentum?

Station 35

A 57-year-old male builder is struck by a falling metal girder on a building site. In the emergency department he is complaining of severe pain in the left pelvis, and there is significant bruising in this area.

This is a plain anteroposterior radiograph of the pelvis (demonstrating normal anatomy):

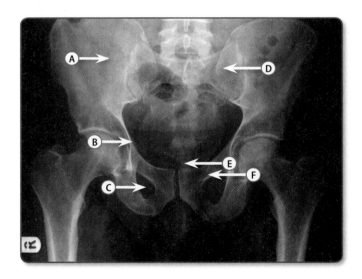

35.1 Identify the structures labelled A, B, D, E and F.

35.2 Name the foramen indicated by C. What structures pass through here?

35.3 What type of joint is the sacroiliac joint?

35.4 What type of joint is the sacrococcygeal joint?

35.5 What are the boundaries of the pelvic inlet?

35.6 Define the false pelvis.

35.7 What are contents of the pudendal (Alcock's) canal?

35.8 What lies medial to the pudendal canal, and what lies laterally?

35.9 What are the clinical consequences of superior hypogastric plexus damage?

35.10 What are the branches of the pudendal nerve?

Station 36

A 78-year-old man presents to the urology clinic with a swollen left testicle. On palpation the testicle feels firm, non-tender and enlarged.

Test your knowledge of the regional axial anatomy on the following axial cadaveric dissection done at the level of the testes and penis (note, in this specimen this subject has only one testis).

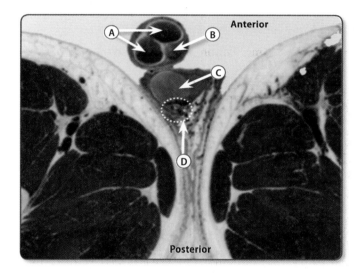

36.1 Identify the structures labelled A to D.

36.2 Trace the pathway of semen from the seminferous tubules to the terminal urethra.

36.3 What is the blood supply to the testis?

36.4 What are the functions of the Leydig and Sertoli cells of the testis?

36.5 List the possible locations for an undescended or incompletely descended testis.

36.6 What is a varicocele? On which side are they most common?

36.7 What is a hydrocele? How may peritoneal fluid enter the scrotum in some individuals?

36.8 What is the clinical significance and embryological origin of the appendix testis (hydatid of Morgagni)?

36.9 What is Fournier's gangrene?

Station 37

A 72-year-old man presents with frequency of micturition and nocturia. On rectal examination the left lobe of his prostate is enlarged and hard. He has a prostate specific antigen of 20 ng/mL. You suspect prostate cancer and request an MRI.

This is a sagittal MRI of a normal male pelvis:

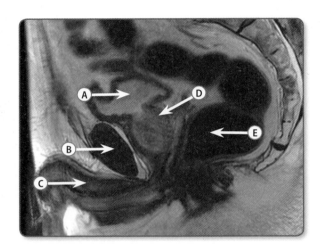

37.1 Identify the structures labelled A to E.

37.2 What does 'BPH' stand for?

37.3 Which zone of the prostate becomes enlarged in BPH?

37.4 In which zone of the prostate does cancer most commonly occur?

37.5 What is the arterial supply to the prostate?

37.6 By what route may prostatic metastases travel to the spine?

37.7 What is the seminal colliculus (verumontanum)?

37.8 What is the prostatic utricle? What is its embryological origin?

37.9 Describe the structure of the body of the penis. In which part does the urethra run?

37.10 What is the arterial supply to the penis?

Station 38

A 25-year-old woman suffers from acute right iliac fossa pain and undergoes laparoscopy. The appendix is seen to be normal. However there is a large haemorrhagic ovarian cyst on the right side.

The image below is an axial dissection through a normal adult female pelvis:

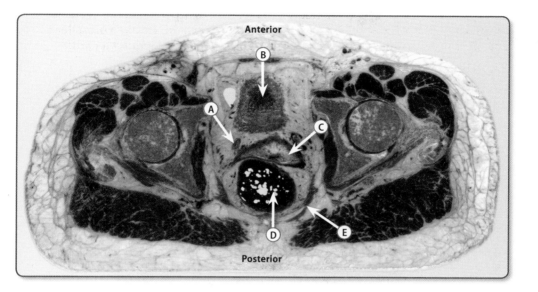

38.1 Identify the structures labelled A to E.

38.2 What is the blood supply to the ovaries?

38.3 What is the lymphatic drainage of the ovaries?

38.4 In which structure do the vessels and nerves of the ovary run?

38.5 Which ligaments are connected to the ovary?

38.6 What is the name of the layer which envelopes the ovary?

38.7 Which tumour marker rises in ovarian cancer?

Station 39

A 47-year-old man presents with pain in the left upper medial thigh 6 months after undergoing an inguinal hernia repair. The consultant suspects that the ilioinguinal nerve was damaged during the operation.

The prosection on the next page displays abdominal contents and branches of the lumbar plexus in a normal subject.

39.1 Identify structures A to D.

39.2 Where is the lumbar plexus located?

39.3 What does the genitofemoral nerve supply?

39.4 What does the ilioinguinal nerve supply?

39.5 Describe the cremasteric reflex.

39.6 Where does the sympathetic trunk enter the abdomen?

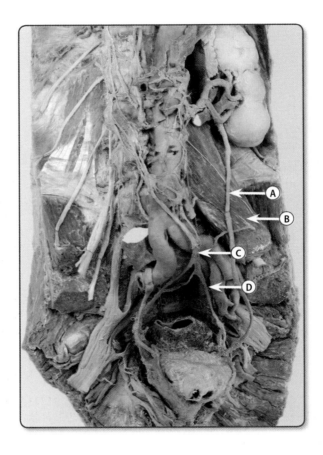

Answers

Station 1

1.1 B Costal groove

   C Head

   D Tubercle

1.2 The costal cartilages.

1.3 The neurovascular bundle accompanying the ribs runs in the subcostal groove in-between the internal and innermost intercostal muscles (the order of **V**eins, **A**rteries and **N**erves from superior to inferior can be remembered by the mnemonic **VAN**).

1.4 The muscles of rib spaces 1–9 are supplied by the posterior and anterior intercostal arteries, whereas those of rib spaces 10 and 11 have only posterior arteries. The posterior intercostal arteries of the first two rib spaces come from the superior intercostal branch of the costocervical trunk, whereas the posterior intercostal arteries of the bottom nine come directly off the aorta (there are only 11 rib spaces). The anterior intercostal arteries are branches of the internal thoracic arteries and its branches.

1.5 The anterior intercostal veins drain into the internal thoracic and musculophrenic veins. The drainage of the posterior intercostal veins is more complicated. These drain into the azygos, hemiazygos or accessory hemiazygos veins with the following exceptions: the 1st posterior vein (the supreme intercostal vein) drains into the ipsilateral brachiocephalic or vertebral veins; the left 2nd, 3rd and 4th veins join to form a superior intercostal vein, which drains into the left brachiocephalic vein.

1.6 The term 'flail chest' describes a scenario in which a section of chest wall is disconnected from its surrounding bony skeleton by multiple rib fractures. This can occur unilaterally (where the ribs often fracture both at the angle and near the costochondral junction), or bilaterally (where the sternum itself can be flail).

1.7 A costochondral joint is a primary cartilaginous joint, with the costal hyaline cartilage connecting directly with the rib without any intervening fibrous tissue. As with all primary cartilaginous joints virtually no movement occurs at the costochondral joint.

1.8 A Manubrium

   B Body

   C Xiphisternum

   D Jugular notch

1.9 1st rib

Station 2

2.1 See **Figure 1.1**.

    A Upper lobe

    B Middle lobe

    C Upper lobe

    D Upper lobe

    E Lower lobe

2.2 The pleural edge extends from the junction between the middle and medial thirds of the clavicle, to an apex about 2.5 cm above the medial end of the clavicle, and

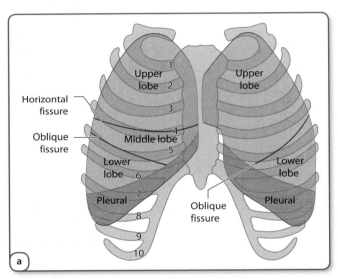

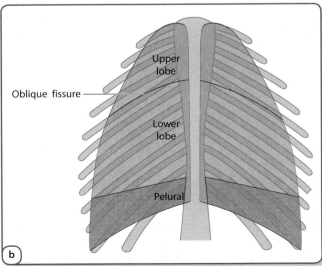

Figure 1.1 (a) Anterior thoracic wall and lobes of the lung. (b) Posterior thoracic wall and lobes of the lung.

then down to the sternoclavicular joint. It then meets the pleura of the contralateral side in the midline at the level of the 2nd costal cartilage. The right pleural edge extends down to the level of the 6th costal cartilage. It then turns laterally crossing the 8th rib in the midclavicular line and the 10th rib in the midaxillary line; it then meets the 12th rib at the lateral border of erector spinae. On the left side the heart, at the level of the 4th costal cartilage, reflects the pleura laterally but otherwise the pleural reflexion follows a similar course to that on the right side.

2.3 The apex of the lung follows the pleura. The lower border of the lung is parallel to the line of pleural reflexion but two ribs above: thus the lower border of the lung crosses the 6th rib in midclavicular line, the 8th rib in the midaxillary line, and the 10th rib adjacent to the vertebral column posteriorly.

2.4a The oblique fissure divides the upper and lower lobes. For the most part, it corresponds to the line of the 5th rib. It may be indicated on the surface as a line running obliquely downwards and outwards from just lateral to the spine of the 3rd thoracic vertebra to the 6th costal cartilage 4 cm from the midline. With the shoulders abducted fully this line corresponds to the medial border of the scapula.

2.4b The horizontal (transverse) fissure divides the middle from the upper lobe of the right lung. It follows a line along the 4th costal cartilage to meet the oblique fissure where it crosses the 5th rib near the midaxillary line.

2.5 The 2nd costal cartilage articulates with the lateral aspect of the manubriosternal junction.

2.6 The suprasternal notch lies at the level of the T2/T3 intervertebral disc.

2.7 The xiphisternal joint lies at the level of T9.

2.8 The superior mediastinum is bounded anteriorly by the manubrium, laterally by the pleurae, posteriorly by the T1–T4 vertebral bodies, superiorly by the superior thoracic aperture, and inferiorly by the plane of Louis (transverse thoracic plane at the T4/T5 intervertebral disc).

2.9 The superior mediastinum contains the great vessels (aortic arch, brachiocephalic artery and veins, left common carotid and subclavian arteries, superior vena cava), trachea, oesophagus, remains of the thymus, thoracic duct, right and left vagi, left recurrent laryngeal nerve and right and left phrenic nerves, and very importantly, lymph nodes.

Station 3

3.1 A Ascending aorta

B Descending aorta

C Pulmonary trunk

3.2 The mediastinum is the space in the thoracic cavity between the right and left pleural sacs. It is conventionally divided into a superior mediastinum and inferior mediastinum by an imaginary plane plotted perpendicular to the sternum at the plane of Louis (**Figure 1.2**). The inferior mediastinum is further subdivided into anterior, middle, and posterior mediastina by the fibrous pericardium.

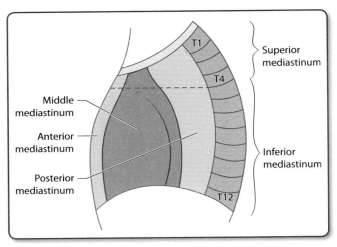

Figure 1.2 Divisions of the mediastinum.

In figure labels:
- T1
- Superior mediastinum
- T4
- Middle mediastinum
- Anterior mediastinum
- Inferior mediastinum
- Posterior mediastinum
- T12

3.3 It shows the inferior mediastinum. This requires knowledge of the contents of each division of the mediastinum.

- The superior mediastinum contains the great vessels (aortic arch, brachiocephalic artery and veins, left common carotid and subclavian arteries, superior vena cava), lymph nodes, trachea, oesophagus, remains of the thymus, thoracic duct, vagi, left recurrent laryngeal nerve and phrenic nerves.
- The anterior mediastinum contains the remains of the thymus and branches of the right and left internal thoracic arteries.
- The middle mediastinum contains the heart inside the pericardium, the ascending aorta, the superior vena cavae, the bifurcation of the trachea, the pulmonary arteries and veins, the phrenic nerves and pericardiophrenic vessels.
- The posterior mediastinum contains the descending thoracic aorta and its branches, the azygos/hemiazygos/accessory hemiazygos veins, the right and left vagus nerves, the right and left splanchnic nerves, the oesophagus, and the thoracic duct. The ganglionated thoracic sympathetic chains may also be regarded as contents of the posterior mediastinum.

3.4 This, the inferior mediastinum, is bounded anteriorly by the body of the sternum (mesosternum), laterally by the pleurae, posteriorly by the T5–T12 vertebral bodies, inferiorly by the diaphragm, and superiorly by the plane of Louis.

3.5 The *parietal* pleura are sensitive to pain, temperature, touch and pressure. Its innervation depends on region: intercostal nerves supply the costal pleura; the phrenic nerve supplies the mediastinal pleura; and the phrenic nerve and lower six intercostal nerves supply the diaphragmatic pleura. The *visceral* pleura are sensitive to stretch and receive their sensory innervation from the autonomic pulmonary plexus (formed from branches of the thoracic sympathetic trunk and vagus nerve).

3.6 The thoracic sympathetic chain has three main branches. It supplies sympathetic fibres to the skin, postganglionic fibres from T1–T5 to the thoracic viscera, and mostly preganglionic fibres from T5–T12 to supply the abdominal viscera (in the form of the greater splanchnic, lesser splanchnic and least splanchnic nerves). The chain receives preganglionic white ramus communicans from each spinal nerve to a corresponding ganglion, and gives back a grey ramus containing postganglionic fibres.

3.7 Thoracic outlet syndrome is caused by compression at the superior thoracic aperture of neurovascular structures passing above the first rib, either between the anterior and middle scalene muscles or in front of scalenus anterior. It can affect the brachial plexus (most commonly, lower trunk of the brachial plexus) or subclavian artery/vein. A rare cause of thoracic outlet syndrome is a cervical rib or a cervical band of fibrous tissue. The syndrome manifests most commonly in the hands with pain, weakness, and coldness. Note that the superior thoracic aperture is usually referred to by clinicians as the thoracic outlet but by anatomists as the thoracic inlet!

3.8 Subclavian steal occurs when blood flows in a retrograde direction in the vertebral artery in association with proximal ipsilateral subclavian artery stenosis or occlusion. This blood is 'stolen' from the circle of Willis via the ipsilateral vertebral artery. Patients with retrograde flow are usually asymptomatic but they may develop dizziness, vertigo, syncope, dysarthria, and visual symptoms. There is usually a drop in blood pressure in the ipsilateral arm distal to the stenosis.

Station 4

4.1 A Right coronary artery

   B Left atrium

   C Descending thoracic aorta

   D Left anterior descending artery (anterior interventricular artery)

   E Left circumflex artery

4.2 The right coronary artery (**Figure 1.3**) originates from the anterior aortic sinus of the ascending aorta. It has the following branches:

- The *anterior ventricular branches* supply the anterior surface of the right ventricle.

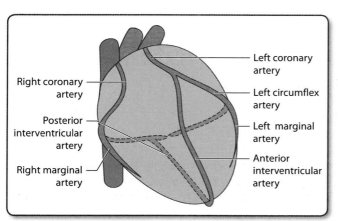

Figure 1.3 Arterial supply of the heart.

- The *marginal artery* is a branch of the anterior ventricular and runs towards the apex.
- The *posterior ventricular branches* supply the diaphragmatic surfaces of the right ventricle.
- The *posterior interventricular artery* supplies the right and left ventricles and runs in the posterior interventricular groove.
- The *atrial branches* supply the right atrium.

4.3 The left coronary artery originates from the left posterior aortic sinus of the ascending aorta. Its branches are:

- The *anterior interventricular artery* (also known as *left anterior descending artery*). This is the major branch of the left coronary artery and supplies the anterior aspect of both ventricles and the anterior half of the interventricular septum before proceeding to anastomose with the posterior interventricular branch of the right coronary artery.
- The *circumflex artery* is the continuation of the left coronary artery after the anterior interventricular is given off. It winds around the left margin of the heart in the atrioventricular groove.
- The *left marginal artery* is a branch of the circumflex.
- The *anterior/posterior ventricular arteries* are branches of the circumflex.
- The *atrial* branches are also branches of the circumflex.

4.4a The sinoatrial node is supplied by the right coronary artery in about two-thirds of people, and by the left in approximately one-third.

4.4b The atrioventricular node is supplied by the posterior interventricular branch of the right coronary artery in over 90% of individuals and less commonly by the left coronary artery via its circumflex branch.

4.5 The coronary veins drain in to the coronary sinus, which is located in the posterior atrioventricular groove. The coronary sinus drains into the right atrium. The major veins it receives are the great cardiac vein (in the anterior interventricular groove), the middle cardiac vein (in the posterior interventricular groove), the small cardiac vein (running along the lower border of the heart), and the cardiac oblique vein (on the posterior surface of the left atrium). The anterior cardiac veins drain the anterior surface of the heart and empty anteriorly into the right atrium directly. There are numerous much smaller veins emptying directly into the chambers that they overlie.

4.6 The sinoatrial node is located in the wall of the right atrium, to the right of the opening of the superior vena cava. It generates rhythmic electrical impulses that radiate out throughout the atrial muscle, causing contraction. The atrioventricular node is in the ventricular end of the atrial septum and conducts the atrial impulse to the ventricles, via the atrioventricular bundle of His. The time that it takes for this conduction (about one tenth of a second) allows the atria to empty their blood into the ventricles. The bundle of His divides into two branches, one for each ventricle. The right bundle travels down on the right side of the interventricular septum to reach the anterior wall of the right ventricle and becomes continuous with the Purkinje plexus of the right ventricle. The left bundle divides into anterior and posterior branches, and these fibres are continuous with the Purkinje plexus of the left ventricle. These fibres induce contraction of the ventricles.

4.7 The parasympathetic supply of the heart is the vagus nerve. The heart's sympathetic supply is the cervical and upper thoracic sympathetic trunk. The cardiac plexuses are located below the arch of the aorta and transmit all of the heart's autonomic fibres. Sympathetic stimulation increases the force and rate of contraction and dilates the coronary arteries. Parasympathetic stimulation decreases the force and rate of contraction and constricts the coronary arteries.

4.8 Afferent fibres from the heart run with sympathetic fibres and enter the spinal cord through the posterior roots of T1–T4. The pain of ischaemia is referred to the skin areas of the skin supplied by the corresponding spinal nerves, i.e. the upper four intercostal nerves and the intercostobrachial nerve. This territory is the left chest wall and the upper part of the left arm.

Station 5

5.1 Tension pneumothorax requires emergency decompression with a 14–16 gauge needle in the 2nd intercostal space in the midclavicular line. The needle passes through skin, superficial fascia and fat, pectoralis major, external intercostal, internal intercostal, innermost intercostal, and parietal pleura.

5.2 The safe triangle is made up of the lateral border of the pectoralis major, the anterior border of latissimus dorsi, and the upper border of the 6th rib (about the level of the nipple), with the apex slightly below the axilla.

5.3 T6 or T7 (**Figure 1.4**)

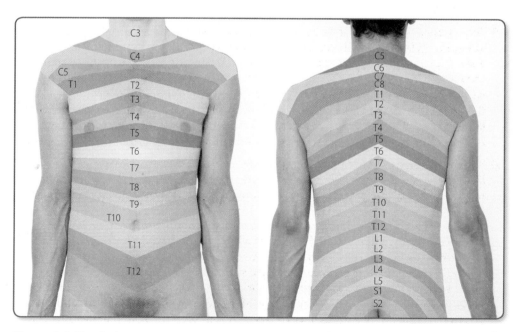

Figure 1.4 Trunk dermatomes.

5.4 At this point the lines are not horizontal, but are actually directed towards the axillary skin crease.

5.5a The target is 1 cm inferior to the junction of the middle and distal third of the clavicle. The tip should be directed towards the sternal notch.

5.5b With the patient's head turned away from the insertion site, the target is the apex of the triangle formed by the sternal and clavicular heads of the sternocleidomastoid muscle. The needle should be inserted at a 30° angle to the skin directed towards the ipsilateral nipple.

5.5c The site is somewhat dependent on what access is necessary, but the incision usually lies at the level of the 5th rib for upper thoracic structures (for exposure of lower structures the incision is at the 6th or 7th rib). The incision is started at a point midway between the medial border of the scapula and the thoracic spine. The incision curves about 3 cm below the inferior angle of the scapula and turns to run parallel with the rib.

5.6a The intervertebral disc between T4 and T5.

5.6b The normal level is the plane of Louis, but in full inspiration the level is the T6 vertebra.

5.7 The aortic valve is auscultated at the 2nd intercostal space, right upper sternal border (**Figure 1.5**). The pulmonary valve is heard at the 2nd intercostal space, left upper sternal border. The mitral valve is heard at the 5th intercostal space, left midclavicular line. The tricuspid valve is heard at the 4th intercostal space, lower left sternal border. Note that these sites do not actually overlie the valves themselves.

5.8 The left border of the heart is from the 2nd costal cartilage, left of the sternum, to the 5th left intercostal space, midclavicular line (**Figure 1.5**). The right border of the heart is from the 3rd right costal cartilage, right of the sternum, to the 6th right costal cartilage, right of the sternum.

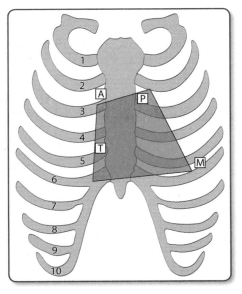

Figure 1.5 Borders and auscultation areas of the heart. A, aortic valve; P, pulmonary valve; T, tricuspid valve; M, mitral valve.

Table 1.1 Surface anatomy landmarks of the thorax

Landmark	Location and significance
Midaxillary line	Vertical line intersecting a point midway between the anterior and posterior axillary folds
Midclavicular line	Vertical line passing through the midshaft of the clavicle
Nipple	Superficial to the 4th intercostal space in the male and prepuberal female Usually within the T4 dermatome
Sternal angle	Junction of the manubrium and body of the sternum Attachment of the 2nd costal cartilage rib to the sternum, the T4/T5 intervertebral disc, the inferior boundary of the superior mediastinum
Suprasternal notch	Curved superior border of the manubrium

Station 6

6.1 A Right atrium

B Arch of aorta

C Left lung hilum

D Left ventricle

6.2 1 Right horizontal or transverse

2 Right oblique

3 Left oblique

6.3 The right main bronchus is about 2.5 cm long and enters the hilum of the lung at T5. It gives off an upper lobe branch before reaching the hilum. The left main bronchus is about 5 cm, and passes downwards and laterally below the arch of the aorta, anterior to the oesophagus and descending aorta. It enters the hilum of the lung at T6.

6.4 The right lung is divided by the oblique and horizontal fissures in to upper, middle, and lower lobes. The left lung is divided by an oblique fissure into upper and lower lobes. The lingula (Latin: 'little tongue') of the left upper lobe is composed of two bronchopulmonary segments that are analogous to the right middle lobe.

6.5 A bronchopulmonary segment is a discrete anatomical and functional unit of the lung that can be removed without disturbing the function of the other segments. They are pyramid shaped with their apices at the hilum. Each is served by its own tertiary bronchi, vein, artery, and lymph and has its own autonomic nerve supply.

6.6 Each lung has 10 bronchopulmonary segments. It would be unlikely that you would need to recite them in the exam, but they are listed here for reference purposes (**Table 1.2**):

Table 1.2 Bronchopulmonary segments of the lung

Right	Left
Upper lobe	**Upper lobe**
1. Apical	1. Apical
2. Posterior	2. Posterior
3. Anterior	3. Anterior
Middle lobe	**Lingula**
4. Lateral	4. Superior
5. Medial	5. Inferior
Lower lobe	**Lower lobe**
6. Superior (apical)	6. Superior (apical)
7. Medial basal (cardiac)	7. Medial basal
8. Anterior basal	8. Anterior basal
9. Lateral basal	9. Lateral basal
10. Posterior basal	10. Posterior basal

6.7 The bronchial arteries supply oxygenated blood to the bronchial and connective tissue of the lungs. The left superior and inferior bronchial arteries arise from the thoracic aorta, whereas the single right bronchial artery has a variable origin (either the aorta, the left superior bronchial artery, or the right intercostal arteries). The bronchial veins drain into the azygous and hemiazygos veins. The pulmonary arteries supply deoxygenated blood to the alveoli via their terminal branches, and the superior and inferior pulmonary veins drain oxygenated blood to the left atrium.

6.8 The superficial lymphatic plexus lies under the visceral pleura and drains the surface of the lungs towards the hilum, whereas the deep plexus drains along the blood vessels towards the hilum. Lymph passes from the bronchopulmonary lymph nodes at the hilum to the tracheobronchial nodes at the bifurcation of the trachea, and thence to bronchomediastinal lymph trunks.

6.9 The pulmonary plexus at the hilum of the lung receives afferent autonomic nerve fibres from the mucous membranes of the bronchioles and alveoli stretch receptors, and serves efferent fibres to the bronchial musculature. Sympathetic fibres cause bronchodilatation and vasoconstriction, whereas parasympathetic fibres cause bronchoconstriction, vasodilatation, and glandular secretion.

6.10 Foreign objects are aspirated more commonly in the right bronchus because it is wider and has a steeper angle than the left.

Station 7

7.1 A A right intercostal artery and vein

   B Right sympathetic chain

   C Right phrenic nerve

   D Superior vena cava

   E Right principal bronchus

   F Right pulmonary vein

   G Pericardial sac (over right atrium)

7.2 The pulmonary hilum contains: the pulmonary artery, the pulmonary vein, the main bronchus, the bronchial arteries and veins, lymph nodes, and autonomic nerves.

7.3 Two veins drain each lung (so there are four in total).

7.4 There are six but the fifth exists only transiently, and no human structures are derived from it.

7.5 The 3rd arch.

7.6 The 4th arch.

Station 8

8.1 A Ascending aorta

   B Auricle of right atrium

   C Pectinate muscles on right ventricular wall

   D Chordae tendineae

   E Pulmonary trunk

   F Auricle of left atrium

   G Anterior interventricular branch of left coronary artery

8.2 H Papillary muscles. These attach to the cusps of the atrioventricular valves (in this case the tricuspid valve) to prevent prolapse.

8.3 The pericardium is divided in to fibrous and serous layers, the latter of which is subdivided into parietal and visceral layers. The fibrous pericardium is a tough layer fused with the central tendon of the diaphragm and the outer coats of the great vessels. It is attached to the sternum via the sternopericardial ligaments. The parietal pericardium lines the inner surface of the fibrous pericardium and is reflected around the great vessels to become continuous with the visceral pericardium that lines the heart.

8.4 The pericardial space exists between the parietal and visceral layers, and is filled with about 50 mL of pericardial fluid.

   In the *subcostal* approach the needle is positioned left of the xiphoid process with the needle angulated upwards at 45° to the skin. The needle passes through skin, superficial/deep fascia, the anterior layer of the rectus sheath, rectus abdominis, the posterior layer of the rectus sheath, diaphragm, endothoracic fascia, fibrous pericardium, and the parietal layer of serous pericardium.

In the *parasternal* approach the needle is placed at the 5th intercostal space near the left sternal margin. The needle passes through skin, superficial/deep fascia, pectoralis major muscle, intercostal muscles, transversus thoracis muscle, endothoracic fascia, fibrous pericardium, and the parietal layer of serous pericardium.

8.5 In the subcostal approach, the main risk is of puncturing the liver if the needle is angulated too inferiorly. In the parasternal approach, the main risk is of puncturing the lungs. In both approaches, there is the risk of damage to the coronary arteries and atrial/ventricular walls.

8.6 In the fetus, the foramen ovale allows oxygenated blood from the umbilical vein (via the inferior vena cava) to flow from the right to left atrium. It is composed of the septum primum and septum secundum. These are forced together at birth due to pressure changes resulting from expansion of the lungs, and usually fuse at about 3 months. In 10% of people fusion is incomplete.

8.7 The ductus arteriosus is a vascular shunt in the fetus connecting the pulmonary artery to the descending thoracic aorta, allowing blood from the right ventricle to bypass the lungs (which are non-functioning at this stage).

8.8 Aortic coarctation is associated with a patent ductus arteriosus, and occurs in the area where the ductus arteriosus inserts. Narrowing can be preductal, ductal, or postductal. It usually occurs distal to the origin of the left subclavian artery.

8.9 The bulbus cordis and the primitive ventricle give rise to the ventricles of the heart. The cranial end of bulbus cordis and the truncus arteriosus give rise to the aorta and pulmonary trunk.

Station 9

9.1 A Right oblique fissure of the right lung

    B Left ventricle

    C Right latissimus dorsi muscle

    D Descending thoracic aorta

    E Left trapezius

9.2 The trachea splits into the left and right principle bronchi and thence to lobar (secondary bronchi), and segmentary (tertiary) bronchi. After entering the bronchopulmonary segment the bronchi undergoes successive branching into smaller and smaller tubes until they give rise to bronchioles. These are less than 1 mm in diameter and contain no cartilage. Bronchioles divide into terminal bronchioles, which give rise to respiratory bronchioles in their walls. These structures end in alveolar ducts that lead to alveolar sacs, across which gas exchange takes place with the surrounding capillaries.

9.3 The azygos vein forms about the level of the right renal vein from either a posterior tributary of the inferior vena cava or from the junction of the right ascending lumbar and right subcostal veins. It traverses the aortic opening of the diaphragm and lies to the right of the vertebra, behind the oesophagus. The vein ends by running anteriorly over the hilum of the right lung to enter the superior vena cava at T4. The azygos vein has tributaries of: the lower eight right posterior intercostal veins, the right superior intercostal vein, bronchial and oesophageal veins, and the accessory azygos/hemiazygos veins.

9.4 The hemiazygos vein drains the four lower left posterior intercostal veins. It arises from the left ascending lumbar, the left subcostal, and often the left renal veins.

The accessory hemiazygos vein drains the 5–8th left posterior intercostal veins, and has tributaries from the bronchial and mid-oesophageal veins.

9.5 There are three layers of muscle in the intercostal space (**Figure 1.6**). The *external intercostal* muscle forms the outermost layer; its fibres are directed forwards and downwards from the inferior border of the rib above to the superior border of the rib below. The *internal intercostal* muscle is the intermediate layer; its fibres are directed downwards and backwards from the subcostal groove of the rib above to the upper border of the rib below. The deepest layer is the *innermost intercostal* muscle (really composed of a group of three muscles). These muscles cross more than one intercostal space.

9.6 The external intercostal muscles aid in forced and passive inspiration. The internal intercostal muscles aid in forced expiration. Passive expiration is achieved by relaxation of the muscles and the elastic recoil of the lungs.

9.7 The accessory muscles of respiration help to increase the thoracic capacity in deep inspiration. They are the sternocleidomastoid, scalenus anterior and medius, serratus anterior and pectoralis major and minor.

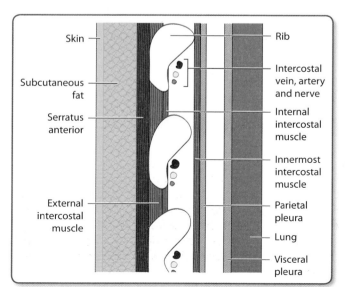

Figure 1.6 The layers of the chest wall.

Station 10

10.1 Barium swallow

10.2 A Lower oesophagus

  B Stomach

  C Also stomach

10.3 D This narrowing represents the site of the lower oesophageal sphincter.

10.4a 17 cm

10.4b 28 cm

10.4c 43 cm

10.5 To perforate the oesophagus one must pass through first mucosa, submucosa, a muscular layer (the composition of which depends on level), and an outer connective tissue layer (areolar tissue). The thoracic oesophagus has no serosa.

10.6 The oesophagus has outer longitudinal and internal circular muscular layers. The muscle fibres of the upper two-thirds of the oesophagus are striated (and hence under voluntary control), and the lower one-third is smooth. In health, it is lined by squamous epithelium.

10.7 The blood supply to the oesophagus, like most long tubes, is segmental. The upper third is supplied by the inferior thyroid artery and vein, the middle third by descending aortic branches and veins to the azygos, and the lower third by the left gastric artery and vein (portal system). Note that there is anastomosis between the portal and systemic systems; in portal hypertension these veins distend in to oesophageal varices that can cause life-threatening haemorrhage.

10.8 Barrett's oesophagus is metaplasia of the squamous epithelium of the lower oesophagus into columnar epithelium. It is thought to be an adaption to chronic acid exposure from gastro-oesophageal reflux. There is a strong association with adenocarcinoma of the oesophagus.

10.9 Lymph drainage follows arterial supply. The upper third of the oesophagus drains into the deep cervical nodes, the middle third into the superior and posterior mediastinal nodes, and the lower third in to coeliac nodes.

10.10 Virchow's node is an enlarged lymph node in the left supraclavicular fossa (the associated sign is called Troisier's sign). It is associated with gastric and other intra-abdominal cancer. The lymph node is on the left side because the majority of lymph drains via the thoracic duct in to the left subclavian vein. Metastases block the thoracic duct causing reflux in to the surrounding nodes.

10.11 The cisterna chyli is a dilated sac at the lower end of the thoracic duct that is the common pathway of drainage of lymph and chyle from the abdomen and lower limbs. It is usually positioned between the abdominal aorta and right crus of the diaphragm. Its position and existence are, however, inconsistent.

10.12 The trachea develops from the floor of the foregut. Initially the laryngotracheal groove appears, which later becomes a tube. Buds appear on either side of the tube and develop into the lungs. The shared origin of the trachea and oesophagus explains the association of tracheoesophageal fistula with oesophageal atresia.

Station 11

11.1 Skin/soft tissue: sebaceous cyst, lipoma

Muscle: sarcoma, psoas abscess

Bowel: appendix abscess/mass, Crohn's, carcinoma, tuberculosis

Gynaecological: ovarian tumour, fibroids

Urological: pelvic kidney, bladder diverticulum

Vascular: aneurysm of the external or common iliac artery, enlarged iliac lymph node

11.2 McBurney's point (**Figure 1.7**) is the typical location of the appendix, and is located at a point two thirds from the umbilicus to the anterior superior iliac spine.

11.3 T10 (see **Figure 1.4**).

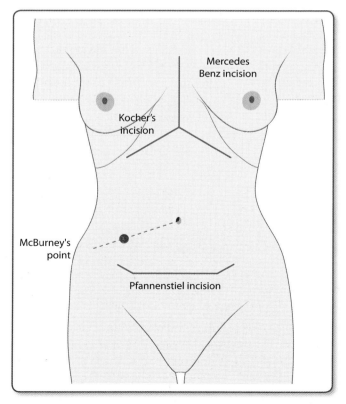

Figure 1.7 Abdominal incisions.

11.4 A Skin, subcutaneous fat, Scarpa's fascia, external oblique muscle, internal oblique muscle, transversalis fascia, extraperitoneal fat, parietal peritoneum.

C Skin, subcutaneous fat, Scarpa's fascia, linea alba, transversalis fascia, extraperitoneal fat, parietal peritoneum.

11.5 The transpyloric plane (**Figure 1.8**) is located halfway between the suprasternal notch and the pubic symphysis, at the level of the L1 vertebral body. At this level lie the following structures: the pylorus of stomach, fundus of gallbladder, pancreatic neck, duodenojejunal flexure (and first part of duodenum), spinal cord termination, line of attachment of transverse mesocolon, left renal hilum, origin of the superior mesenteric artery, origin of portal vein.

11.6 The subcostal plane (**Figure 1.8**) is the line parallel to the lowest part of the thoracic cage. The inferior mesenteric artery and L3 vertebra are present at this level.

11.7 The aorta bifurcates at the L4 vertebral level, which is usually about the level of the umbilicus. This is also the level of the supracristal plane (**Figure 1.8**), which is a line joining the most superior parts of the iliac crests.

11.8a The inferior border of the liver extends from the tip of the right 10th rib to the left 5th intercostal space medial to the midclavicular line. The superior border is at the level of the 5th intercostal space.

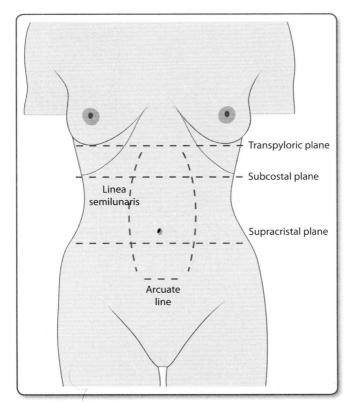

Figure 1.8 Lines and planes of the abdomen.

11.8b The spleen lies under the 9–11th ribs on the left side. The long axis of the spleen lies along the 10th rib, the posterior pole being just to the left of the vertebral column, and the anterior pole is in the midaxillary line.

11.8c The fundus of the gallbladder is at the point at which the rectus abdominis intersects the costal margin, at the tip of the 9th costal cartilage.

11.9 See **Figure 1.7** and **Table 1.3**.

Table 1.3 Abdominal surface anatomy landmarks

Landmark	Location	Significance
Arcuate line (Douglas' line)	Approximately one-third of the distance from the umbilicus to the pubic symphysis	Lower limit of the posterior sheath
Deep inguinal ring	Midway between anterior superior iliac spine and pubic tubercle	Opening in the transversalis fascia for the vas deferens and gonadal vessels (or round ligament in the female)
Linea alba	Midline aponeurotic band extending from xiphoid process to the pubic symphysis	Formed by the combined abdominal muscle aponeuroses.
McBurney's point	Two-thirds from the umbilicus to the anterior superior iliac spine	Typical location of the appendix
Mid-inguinal point	Midway between the anterior superior iliac spine and the pubic symphysis	Location of the femoral artery
Semilunar line	The lateral edge of the rectus abdominis muscle	Formed by the combined aponeuroses of the abdominal wall muscles at the lateral margin of the rectus sheath.
Subcostal plane	Line parallel to the lowest part of the thoracic cage	Origin of inferior mesenteric artery
Supracristal plane	Horizontal plane at the upper margin of the iliac crests	L4 Bifurcation of the aorta
Transpyloric line	Half the distance between the jugular notch and the pubic crest	Pylorus of stomach Fundus of gallbladder Pancreatic neck Duodenojejunal flexure (and first part of duodenum) Spinal cord termination Line of attachment of transverse mesocolon Left renal hilum Origin of the superior mesenteric artery Origin of portal vein
Umbilicus		Within T10, approximately at level of L4 vertebra

11.9a Gridiron: A 2.5–5 cm oblique incision at McBurney's point, perpendicular to a line running from the anterior superior iliac spine to the umbilicus. Used for appendicectomy.

11.9b Kocher: an oblique incision below and parallel to the right costal margin (starting below the xiphoid process). Used for access to biliary structures.

11.9c Mercedes Benz: bilateral low Kocher's incisions with an upper midline limb up and through the xiphisternum. For access to upper abdominal viscera. Also known as a roof-top incision.

11.9d Pfannenstiel: A transverse lower abdominal incision centered above the pubic symphysis, slightly upturned at the ends (a 'smile' incision).

Station 12

12.1 A Inferior vena cava

B Erector spinae muscle

C Portal vein

D Right crus of diaphragm

E Superior mesenteric artery

F Fundus of the stomach

G Aorta (abdominal)

12.2 At the level of the superior mesenteric artery, below the level of the spleen.

12.3 The portal vein (C) drains the gastrointestinal tract and associated viscera. It is formed from the splenic and superior mesenteric veins as they unite behind the neck of the pancreas. The splenic vein receives the short gastric, left gastroepiploic, inferior mesenteric, and pancreatic veins. The superior mesenteric vein receives the jejunal, ilial, ileocolic, right colic, middle colic, inferior pancreaticoduodenal and right gastroepiploic veins. There are three other direct tributaries of the portal vein: the left gastric, right gastric, and cystic veins.

12.4 The portal vein supplies about 70% of the blood to the liver. The remaining 30% is oxygenated blood from the hepatic arteries.

12.5 A Gallbladder

B Biliary tract

C Superior mesenteric artery

D Left lobe of the liver

E Tail of the pancreas

12.6 The pancreas (E) has exocrine and endocrine functions. The pancreatic islets (Islets of Langerhans) produce insulin and glucagon. The pancreas also secretes enzymes capable of hydrolysing proteins, fats, and carbohydrates.

12.7 The pancreas is divided in to a head, uncinate process, neck, body, and tail. The head lies within the concavity of the duodenum, with its uncinate process extending to the left behind the superior mesenteric vessels. The neck is positioned anterior to the portal vein and superior mesenteric artery origins. The body runs upwards and to the left and the tail abuts the hilum of the spleen.

12.8 The lesser sac separates the stomach from the pancreas. If fluid leaks from the pancreas during acute pancreatitis this can become trapped within the lesser sac forming a pseudocyst.

Station 13

13.1 A Linea alba ('white line'). The whiteness indicates that it is a relatively avascular structure and hence ideal for incision without bleeding.

13.2 B Tendinous insertion

   C External oblique muscle

   D Rectus abdominis

   E Superficial epigastric vessels

   F Umbilicus

   G Posterior layer of rectus sheath

13.3 Skin, subcutaneous fat, Scarpa's fascia, umbilical cicatrix pillar, extraperitoneal fat, parietal peritoneum.

13.4 External oblique fibres run inferiorly and anteriorly. Internal oblique fibres run perpendicular to the external oblique muscle, directed superiorly and anteriorly. Transversus abdominis fibres run transversely.

13.5 The rectus sheath contains the large rectus abdominis muscle (extending from the pubic symphysis to the xiphisternum/lower costal cartilages), the pyramidalis muscle, the superior and inferior epigastric vessels, ventral primary rami of T7–T12, and lymphatics.

13.6 The arcuate line (Douglas' line) demarcates the lower limit of the posterior sheath. It is located about one-third of the distance from the umbilicus to the pubic crest. Above the level of this line, the internal oblique aponeurosis splits to envelope the rectus abdominis muscle, and the transversus abdominis aponeurosis runs under the rectus abdominis. Below the arcuate line, the internal oblique and transversus abdominis aponeuroses merge and pass superficial to the rectus muscle. Hence, below the arcuate line the only layers deep to the rectus abdominis are the transversalis fascia, extraperitoneal fat, and parietal peritoneum.

13.7 Scarpa's fascia extends in to the thigh and fuses with the fascia lata at the flexure of the skin crease of the hip joint (about 1 cm below the inguinal ligament).

13.8 It fuses with Colles' fascia in the perineum.

13.9 The median umbilical ligament extends from the bladder to the umbilicus, on the deep surface of the anterior abdominal wall. It can be seen easily during laparoscopy by pointing the laparoscope towards the anterior abdominal wall in the median plane. It contains the urachus, which is the remnant of the allantois, a canal that drains the urinary bladder of the fetus that joins and runs through the umbilical cord. If the allantois fails to close then urine continues to leak through the umbilicus after birth.

13.10 The medial umbilical ligaments are lateral to the median umbilical ligament on the deep surface of the anterior abdominal wall. They contain the remnant of the fetal umbilical arteries.

Station 14

14.1 A Caecum

B Appendix

D Ileum

E Mesentery of small bowel

14.2 C Mesoappendix. The most important structures are the appendicular artery and vein, which may bleed if not ligated carefully. There are also autonomic nerves, lymphatic vessels, and sometimes a lymph node.

14.3 A small non-anastomosing single artery, the appendicular artery, supplies the appendix (**Figure 1.9**). When the appendix becomes inflamed, oedema of the wall compresses the artery causing thrombosis. This leads to necrosis and perforation of the blind ending tip of the appendix. In contrast, in addition to the cystic artery, the gallbladder has collateral supply from the liver bed, ensuring that adequate blood supply is preserved.

14.4 Common positions include: retrocolic/retrocaecal, pelvic/subcaecal, retroileal/preileal. The order of frequency is disputed but the commonest two are probably

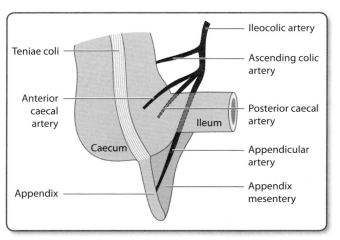

Figure 1.9 Appendix and arterial supply.

pelvic and retrocaecal. This variability of the appendix position can make diagnosis sometimes difficult and removal technically difficult.

14.5 Visceral pain from the appendix is triggered by distension of the lumen or muscle spasm. Afferent pain fibres travel to the T10 spinal level, and a midline periumbilical pain is felt. As the appendix becomes more inflamed it can cause localised inflammation of the peritoneum, and pain is referred to the right iliac fossa.

14.6 The ilioinguinal and iliohypogastric nerves. To avoid these nerves incision should not be closer than 3 cm from the anterior superior iliac spine.

14.7 The teniae coli are three bands of smooth muscle running longitudinally along the caecum, ascending, transverse and descending and sigmoid colon (**Figure 1.9**). They contract to form haustra, which are sacculations of the large bowel that can be seen on radiographs. The teniae coli converge at the vermiform appendix and the rectum.

14.8 Appendices epiploicae are small fat-filled peritoneal pouches along the teniae coli. They can sometimes become inflamed (epiploic appendagitis) mimicking appendicitis and other intra-abdominal conditions.

Station 15

15.1 **A** Right external iliac artery

  B Right external iliac vein

  C Urinary bladder

  D Uterus

  E Rectum

15.2 L5/S1.

15.3 The sacroiliac joints.

15.4 The ureter passes anteriorly over the bifurcation of the iliac arteries.

15.5 **A** Sartorius

  B Superior pubic ramus

  C Obturator internus

  D Ischium

15.6 The levator ani originates from the body of the pubis, the ischial spine, and the fascia of obturator internus. It inserts in to the perineal body, the anococcygeal body, and the walls of the pelvic organs below the bladder (the prostate, vagina, rectum and anal canal). As well as the functions listed in **Table 1.4** it also increases intra-abdominal pressure during defecation, micturition, and parturition. The parts are outlined in **Table 1.4**.

15.7 The pelvic outlet is bounded posteriorly by the coccyx, laterally by the ischial tuberosities, and anteriorly by symphysis pubis (see **Figure 1.11**).

Table 1.4 The parts and functions of levator ani

Part	Name	Functional anatomy
Anterior	Levator prostatae Sphincter vaginae	Forms a sling around the prostate/vagina and inserts in to the perineal body, helping to stabilise it
Intermediate	Puborectalis Pubococcygeus	Forms a sling around the junction of the rectum/anal canal
Posterior	Iliococcygeus	Inserted into the anococcygeal body and the coccyx

15.8 The perineal body is a pyramidal fibromuscular mass of tissue at the junction of the urogenital triangle and the anal triangle. It has attachments to: the external anal sphincter, bulbospongiosus muscle, superficial and deep transverse perineal muscles, anterior fibres of levator ani, and the external urinary sphincter.

Station 16

16.1 The large bowel is peripheral and less coiled. It has haustra (which on an abdominal radiograph do not traverse the entire diameter of the colon). The lumen of large bowel is greater than the small bowel.

16.2 Double contrast barium enema. The bowel has been inflated by air pumped through the rectum.

16.3 **B** Haustra

16.4 **A** Caecum/ascending colon. This is supplied by the colic branch of the ileocolic artery, and the right colic artery (both branches of the superior mesenteric artery).

C Descending colon. This is supplied by the left colic artery (a branch of the inferior mesenteric artery).

The blood supply to the rest of the large bowel is illustrated in **Figures 1.13** and **1.18** (see pp. 69 and 77). The proximal two-thirds of the transverse colon is perfused by the middle colic artery (superior mesenteric), and the latter one-third by the inferior mesenteric. The sigmoid arteries supply the sigmoid colon. The rectum is supplied by the superior rectal artery (inferior mesenteric), middle rectal artery (internal iliac), and inferior rectal artery (internal iliac).

16.5 There is a continuous vascular arcade throughout the length of the gastrointestinal tract, due to anastomosis of branches of the superior and inferior mesenteric arteries along the marginal artery of Drummond.

16.6 D Rectum. The rectovesical fascia of Denonvilliers separates the rectum from anterior structures and is dissected in rectal dissection for carcinoma. Anteriorly in the upper two-thirds are coils of small intestine that lie in the space between the rectum and bladder in men, or rectum and uterus in women (the pouch of Douglas). In the lower two-thirds anteriorly are the prostate, bladder, vas deferens, and seminal vesicles in males, and vagina in the female. Posteriorly are the sacrum, coccyx, median sacral and rectal vessels, sympathetic trunk, pelvic splanchnic nerves, and piriformis. Laterally lies levator ani, coccygeus and obturator internus muscles, fat, lymph nodes, ischioanal fossa, and the lateral ligaments of the rectum.

16.7 D The upper third of the rectum has peritoneum on its anterior and lateral surfaces, the middle third has peritoneum on its anterior surface only, and the lower third is beneath the rectal floor and has no peritoneal attachments.

16.8 Injuries occur at the junctions of where mobile parts of the colon (the transverse and sigmoid) join the fixed parts (ascending and descending).

16.9 From medial to lateral are the psoas major, quadratus lumborum (above the iliac crest), or iliacus (below the iliac crest), transversus abdominis and internal oblique (**Figure 1.10**). The posterior part of the diaphragm also contributes to the upper posterior wall of the abdomen.

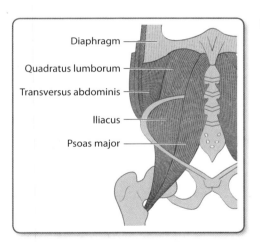

Figure 1.10 Posterior abdominal wall.

Station 17

17.1 A Spermatic cord

B Long saphenous vein

C Common femoral artery

D Common femoral vein

17.2 The most well-known mnemonic for the contents of the spermatic cord (A) is the 'rule of threes' (**Table 1.5**).

Table 1.5 The 'rule of threes' for contents of the spermatic cord

Layers of fascia	External spermatic
	Cremasteric
	Internal spermatic
Arteries	Testicular
	Cremasteric
	Artery of the vas
Veins	Pampiniform plexus
	Cremasteric
	Vein of the vas
Nerves	Nerve to the cremaster
	Sympathetic fibres (T10–T11)
	Ilioinguinal nerve (this is actually on, not in, the cord)
Other structures	Vas deferens
	Lymphatics
	Processes vaginalis (pathologically, in patients with an indirect inguinal hernia)

17.3 The inguinal ligament is formed from the rolled over aponeurosis of the external oblique. It runs from the pubic tubercle to the anterior superior iliac spine.

17.4 The deep inguinal ring is an opening in the fascia transversalis at the mid-point of the inguinal ligament. Medially run the inferior epigastric vessels.

17.5 The opening of an inguinal hernia is above and medial to the pubic tubercle whereas a femoral hernia is below and lateral.

17.6 The boundaries of the inguinal canal:
- anterior: external oblique aponeurosis, reinforced at its lateral one-third by the origin of the internal oblique
- posterior: conjoint tendon medially (the fused insertion of the internal oblique and transversus abdominis), transversals fascia laterally
- roof: arching fibres of the internal oblique and transversus abdominis
- floor: the inguinal ligament, and the lacunar ligament medially.

17.7 As the processus vaginalis descends into the scrotum during development it brings with it layers of the abdominal wall. The external spermatic fascia is derived from the external oblique aponeurosis. The cremasteric fascia is derived from the internal oblique. The internal spermatic fascia is derived from the fascia transversalis.

17.8 Direct inguinal hernias pass through Hesselbach's triangle, a defect in the transversalis fascia, whereas indirect hernias must traverse the deep inguinal ring. The boundaries of Hesselbach's triangle are:

- medially – the lateral border of rectus abdominis
- superolaterally – the inferior epigastric vessels
- inferolaterally – the inguinal ligament.

17.9 Because the femoral vessels run just under this ligament, and may bleed profusely! The femoral vein is more difficult to control than the femoral artery.

Station 18

18.1 **A** Right superficial femoral artery

B Right vas deferens and spermatic cord

C Right obturator internus

D Alcock's canal, internal pudendal vessels, pudendal nerve

E Left sciatic nerve

F Membranous urethra

G Anus

18.2a There is communication between the superior rectal vein (portal system), and the inferior rectal veins (draining to the internal iliac vein via the internal pudendal veins, systemic circulation).

18.2b The other communications are shown in **Table 1.6**.

18.3 This is formed by the two ischial tuberosities and the coccyx (**Figure 1.11**). The anterior border is the posterior border of the perineal membrane, and the sacrotuberous ligaments form the two sides.

18.4 Anterior: the pubic symphysis (separated by extraperitoneal fat), and the prostatic plexus of veins.

Posterior: the rectum separated by the fascia of Denonvilliers.

Superior: the bladder.

Inferior: the external sphincter of the bladder.

Table 1.6 Portal-systemic communications	
Lower oesophagus	Between the oesophageal branch of the left gastric vein (portal system), and the oesophageal vein (azygos system)
Abdominal wall	Between portal branches in the liver and the veins passing to the abdominal wall (forming a caput medusae)
Bare area of liver	Between portal veins in the liver and veins of the diaphragm (across the bare area)
Retroperitoneum	Between the portal tributaries in the mesentery and retroperitoneal veins

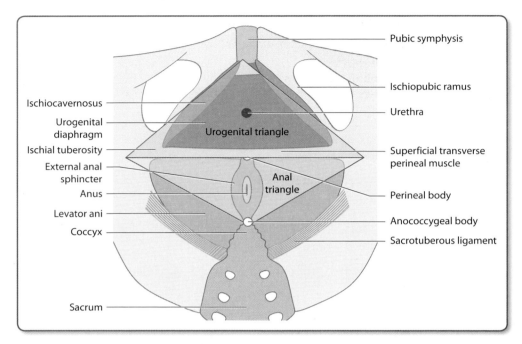

Figure 1.11 Anal and urogenital triangles.

18.5 The ischioanal fossae (or ischiorectal fossae, an old term) are wedge shaped spaces on either side of the anal canal. Their boundaries are:
- laterally: obturator internus muscle and fascia
- medially: levator ani and pelvic fascia, external anal sphincter
- anteriorly: the urogenital perineum
- posteriorly: sacrotuberous ligament and gluteus maximus
- inferiorly: skin and subcutaneous fat
- superiorly: levator ani

The space contains fat (which is particularly prone to infection and abscess formation) and the inferior rectal nerve and vessels. The lateral walls contain Alcock's canal, which has in it the pudendal nerve and vessels.

18.6 Anal fissures occur most commonly in the posterior midline. Fissures develop in the anal valves (the lower ends of the anal columns) as hard faecal matter catches during defecation. This area may be susceptible due to a lack of support from the superficial part of the external sphincter.

18.7 A haemorrhoid is fold of mucosa and submucosa containing a varicosed tributary of the superior rectal vein and a terminal branch of the superior rectal artery.

18.8 Goodsall's rule states that the external opening of a fistula situated behind the transverse anal line will open in to the anal canal in the posterior midline, but a fistula that opens anterior to this line is associated with a direct tract.

18.9 The anal canal is approximately 4 cm long and the rectum is about 13 cm long.

18.10 The topographical relations of the anal canal are:
- posteriorly: the anococcygeal body
- laterally: the ischiorectal fossae
- anteriorly in men: the perineal body, the urogenital diaphragm, and the membranous part of the urethra
- anteriorly in women: the lower part of the vagina.

Station 19

19.1 A Hepatic flexure or ascending colon

B Transverse colon

C Small bowel

19.2 D Left psoas major muscle

19.3 E Spleen

F Linea alba

G Rectus abdominis muscle

19.4 Posterior to the ascending colon lies:
- musculoskeletal: iliac crest, iliacus, quadratus lumborum, transversus abdominis, and the right psoas.
- organs: lower pole of the right kidney.
- nerves: iliohypogastric and ilioinguinal nerves.

19.5 Posterior to the descending colon lies:
- musculoskeletal: iliac crest, iliacus, quadratus lumborum, transversus abdominis, and the left psoas.
- organs: lateral border of left kidney
- nerves: iliohypogastric, ilioinguinal, femoral nerves and the lateral cutaneous nerve of the thigh.

19.6 Diverticula are herniations of the mucosa through the circular muscle at points where the blood vessels pierce the muscle (natural points of weakness).

19.7 The transverse mesocolon attaches the transverse colon to the posterior wall of the abdomen and the pancreas. It is continuous with the two posterior layers of the greater omentum (**Figure 1.15**).

19.8 The transverse mesocolon contains the transverse colon (in its free edge), the middle colic vessels and their branches, lymphatics, autonomic nerves, and extraperitoneal fatty tissue.

19.9 An incompetent ileocaecal valve allows decompression of the large intestine in patients with large bowel obstruction and thereby reduces the risk of perforation.

19.10 The sigmoid colon has a long mesentery and may rotate upon it, causing an obstructed, often massively distended, loop of bowel. Volvulus of the caecum and transverse colon may also occur less commonly.

Station 20

20.1 See **Figure 1.12**.

    A Proper hepatic artery

    B Common hepatic artery

    C Left gastric artery

    D Gastroduodenal artery

    E Coeliac trunk

    F Splenic artery

20.2 Upper part of L1 (not T12, although many textbooks claim this).

20.3 The gastroduodenal artery (D) supplies the stomach, the duodenum, and, indirectly, the pancreatic head and neck (via the anterior and posterior superior pancreaticoduodenal arteries).

20.4 The hepatic artery (A) runs in the free border of the lesser omentum, anterior to the portal vein and left of the bile duct.

20.5 See **Figure 1.13**.

    A Right colic artery

    B Ileocolic artery

    C Appendicular artery

    D Superior mesenteric artery

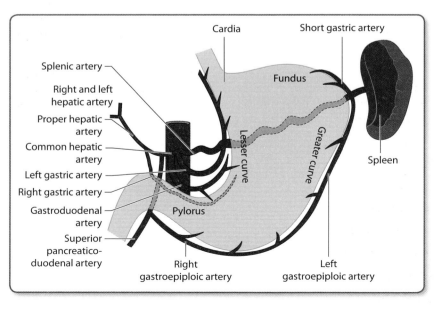

Figure 1.12 The coeliac axis.

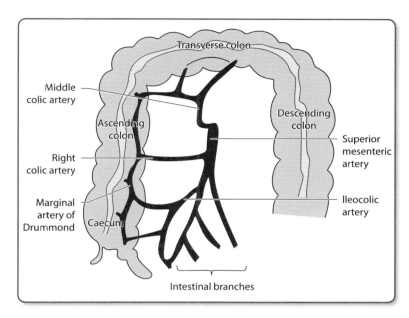

Figure 1.13 Branches of the superior mesenteric artery.

E Main stem of jejunal arteries

F Main stem of ileal arteries

20.6 L1

20.7 L3

20.8 After leaving the aorta, the superior mesenteric artery passes over the left renal vein, beneath the splenic vein and neck of the pancreas. It then passes over the uncinate process of the pancreas and the junction of the third and fourth parts of the duodenum, before entering the mesentery of the small and large bowel to give off its terminal branches.

20.9 The distal third of the transverse colon/splenic flexure is termed a 'watershed' area, as there is a change in blood supply from the superior mesenteric to the inferior mesenteric artery. Watershed areas are vulnerable to ischaemia as they do not have good collateral supply.

Station 21

21.1 A Right renal vein

B Inferior vena cava

C Testicular vein (right)

D Left suprarenal organ

E Superior mesenteric artery

F Left renal vein

      G Abdominal aorta

      H Left ureter

21.2 The ligament of Treitz connects the duodenojejunal junction to the diaphragm (this 'ligament' actually contains muscular fibres that on contraction widen the angle of the duodenojejunal flexure assisting movement of intestinal contents). The ligament is commonly cut to access the aorta.

21.3 The branches of the aorta are outlined in **Table 1.7**.

Table 1.7 Branches of the abdominal aorta	
Three anterior visceral branches	Coeliac
	Superior mesenteric
	Inferior mesenteric
Three lateral visceral branches	Suprarenal
	Renal
	Testicular or ovarian
Five lateral abdominal wall branches	Inferior phrenic
	Four lumbar branches
Three terminal branches	Two common iliac branches
	Median sacral

21.4 The adrenal glands are supplied by the superior adrenal artery (from the inferior phrenic), middle adrenal artery (abdominal aorta), and inferior adrenal artery (renal artery).

21.5 The adrenal vein (the right adrenal vein drains into the inferior vena cava, the left adrenal vein drains in to the left renal vein).

21.6 Due to collateral supply via the marginal artery of Drummond. It is sometimes ligated in operations such as open aortic aneurysm repair.

21.7a Commences at L5 behind the common iliac arteries.

21.7b It is initially related anteriorly to the small intestine, the third part of the duodenum, the head of the pancreas, and the first part of the duodenum. It passes behind the epiploic foramen (in front of which is the portal vein, common bile duct and hepatic artery); it then ascends in a groove in the liver before traversing the diaphragm.

21.7c This can be remembered by the mnemonic: **I** **L**ike **T**o **R**ise **S**o **H**igh: **I**liac, **L**umbar, **T**esticular, **R**enal, **S**uprarenal, **H**epatic.

Station 22

22.1 A Gallbladder

B Right hepatic duct

C Left hepatic duct

D Right renal pelvis

E Common bile duct

22.2 Bile is stored in the gallbladder. It passes in to the cystic duct, which joins the common hepatic duct to form the common bile duct (**Figure 1.14**). This travels in the free edge of the lesser omentum (with the hepatic artery and portal vein). The duct is joined by the main pancreatic duct (of Wirsung) at the ampulla of Vater, which enters the second part of the duodenum past the sphincter of Oddi.

Gallstone ileus is the condition of a gallstone causing mechanical intestinal obstruction (hence the condition is not really ileus at all). Instead of travelling through bile ducts, gallstones usually erode through the wall of the gallbladder over a period of time. They often get lodged in the distal ileum.

22.3 Its opening in to the second part of the duodenum.

22.4 Bile is produced by hepatocytes in the liver. It is composed mainly of water (85%), bile salts, mucous, pigments, fats, inorganic salts, and cholesterol. Bile acts as a surfactant, emulsifying fats. The increased surface area allows for more efficient action of enzymes such as pancreatic lipase. Its other functions include: being the route of excretion for the haemoglobin breakdown product bilirubin, and neutralising excess stomach acid before it enters the ileum.

22.5 Cholecystokinin is a peptide hormone that stimulates the contraction of the gallbladder and the relaxation of the sphincter of Oddi. It is synthesised by the

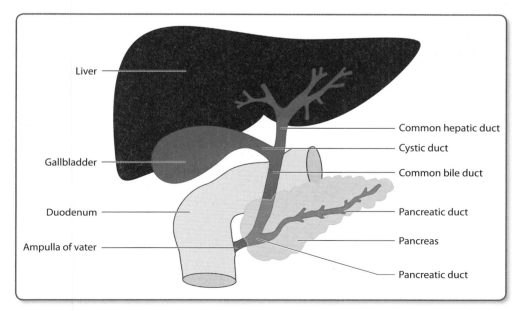

Figure 1.14 The biliary system.

'I-cells' of the mucosal epithelium of the small intestine, and secreted in response to Chyme entering the duodenum. Its other functions include: increasing the production of bile in the liver; stimulation of the release of digestive enzymes in the pancreas; causing relaxation of the stomach musculature.

22.6 Extra-hepatic ducts are lined by tall columnar cells interspersed with mucous glands.

22.7 Pringle's manoeuvre temporarily prevents blood from entering the liver by compressing the hepatic artery and portal vein. Intraoperatively it can be performed by placing a finger within the foramen of Winslow and another on its anterior wall and squeezing.

22.8 Mirizzi's syndrome is a cause of obstructive jaundice caused by one or more gallstones becoming impacted in Hartmann's pouch. The biliary obstruction can be caused by either external compression of the common hepatic duct by the gallstone, or fistulisation of the gallstone in to the common hepatic duct.

Station 23

23.1 See **Figure 1.8**.

   C Linea semilunaris

   D Arcuate line

23.2 B The supracristal plane (**Table 1.3**). This is a transverse plane through the uppermost part of the iliac crest, at the level of the L4 vertebra. It usually passes close to the umbilicus. The plane divides the lower and upper quadrants of the abdomen. At this level the abdominal aorta bifurcates.

23.3 The inferior epigastric artery is a branch of the external iliac artery, and enters the rectus sheath anterior to the arcuate line by piercing the transversalis fascia. It runs in the sheath posterior to the rectus abdominis muscle and supplies the anterior abdominal wall. It ends by anastomosing with the superior epigastric branch of the internal thoracic artery. The inferior epigastric vein follows a similar course and drains in to the external iliac vein.

23.4 The external iliac artery and vein.

23.5 The linea semilunaris (**Figure 1.8** and **Table 1.3**) is a tendinous line lateral to the rectus abdominis, extending from the cartilage of the ninth rib to the pubic tubercle. It demarcates the lateral fusion of the anterior and posterior rectus sheath layers.

23.6 The internal oblique is supplied by the lower six thoracic nerves, the iliohypogastric nerve, and the ilioinguinal nerve (also true for the external oblique and the transversus abdominis). It assists in flexion and rotation of the trunk.

23.7 The muscles of the anterior and lateral walls have a number of functions. They assist during forced expiration by pulling down the ribs and sternum. During inspiration they aid the diaphragm by relaxing. They protect the abdominal contents from trauma. They can increase abdominal pressure during micturition, defecation, vomiting and parturition by contracting simultaneously with the diaphragm with a closed glottis.

Station 24

24.1 **1** The duodenum

The first part of the duodenum begins at the pylorus and runs up and backwards (at the transpyloric plane). The second part of the duodenum runs vertically downward in front of the hilum of the right kidney. The bile duct and pancreatic duct enter the duodenum at the ampulla of Vater, with the accessory pancreatic duct nearby. The third part of the duodenum runs horizontally to the left on the subcostal plane, following the lower margin of the head of the pancreas. The fourth part of the duodenum runs up and to the left and ends at the duodenojejunal flexure, which is indicated by the suspensory ligament of Treitz.

Only the first few centimetres of the first part of the duodenum are intraperitoneal (mobile), the rest of the duodenum is retroperitoneal.

24.2 **2** Coeliac axis

The branches of the coeliac axis are the left gastric artery, the splenic artery, and the common hepatic artery (**Figure 1.12**).

24.3 **3** Pancreas

The splenic and superior/inferior pancreaticoduodenal arteries supply the pancreas. The veins are named after the arteries and drain in to the portal system.

24.4 **A** Common hepatic artery

B Right lobe of the liver

C The spleen

D The splenic artery

24.5 The greater omentum is a fold of parietal peritoneum that is suspended from the greater curvature of the stomach (**Figure 1.15**). Its anterior fold hangs over the small intestines before being reflecting back up on itself to reach the transverse colon, and then to the posterior abdominal wall. The right and left gastroepiploic vessels run in and supply the greater omentum. It also carries lymphatics (to the stomach) and autonomic nerves.

24.6 The epiploic foramen (foramen of Winslow) is the entrance to the lesser sac:
- anteriorly: border of lesser omentum carrying the bile duct, hepatic artery, and portal vein
- posteriorly: inferior vena cava
- superiorly: caudate process of the liver
- inferiorly: first part of the duodenum.

24.7 The topographical relations of the second part of the duodenum:
- anteriorly: gallbladder, right lobe of the liver, transverse colon, and small intestine

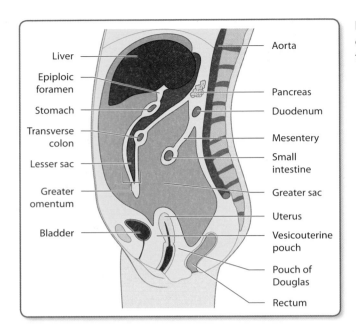

Figure 1.15 The compartments of the abdomen.

- posteriorly: right renal pelvis
- superiorly: head of the pancreas, bile ducts draining in to the duodenum
- inferiorly: ascending colon, right colic flexure, and right lobe of the liver.

24.8 The supracolic compartment is the division of the abdomen above the transverse mesocolon, and the infracolic compartment is the division below this level. The supracolic compartment contains the oesophagus, stomach, first part of duodenum, lesser omentum, spleen, liver, and gallbladder.

24.9 The splenic vessels and the tail of the pancreas.

24.10 The short gastric and left gastroepiploic vessels.

24.11 The left L2 transverse process to the right sacroiliac joint.

Station 25

25.1 See **Figure 1.16**.

   A Gallbladder

   B Right lobe of liver

   C Bile duct

   D Inferior vena cava

   E Quadrate lobe of liver

   F Ligamentum teres hepatis and falciform ligament

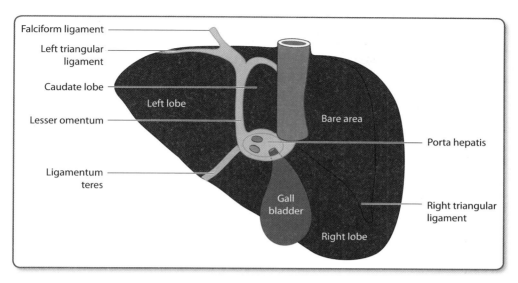

Figure 1.16 The posterior surface of the liver.

   G Left lobe of liver

   H Common hepatic artery

   I Portal vein

   J Caudate lobe of liver

25.2 The cystic artery is the main blood supply to the gallbladder (A). This is usually a branch of the right hepatic, but there are several anatomic variants. There are also small vessels that run from the gallbladder to the liver in the gallbladder bed. Lymph drains via a cystic lymph node near the neck of the gallbladder to the hepatic then coeliac nodes. The gallbladder receives sympathetic and parasympathetic supply via the coeliac plexus.

25.3 The gallbladder (A) is lined by tall columnar epithelium. This epithelium does not secrete mucous.

25.4 Calot's triangle is now conventionally defined as the cystic duct, the common hepatic duct, and the inferior surface of the liver (**Figure 1.17**) (although the original description in 1891 described the triangle as formed by the cystic duct, the bile duct and the cystic artery). The cystic artery is constantly found in this triangle. Visualising the ducts and arteries is essential before removing the gallbladder to ensure that they are not inadvertently injured. Common bile duct injury, especially those injuries unrecognised at time of surgery, can be disastrous.

25.5 The upper limit of the common bile duct diameter on ultrasound in adults is conventionally about 7 mm. In the elderly, and after cholecystectomy, the diameter increases.

25.6 The ligamentum teres hepatis is the remnant of the left fetal umbilical vein.

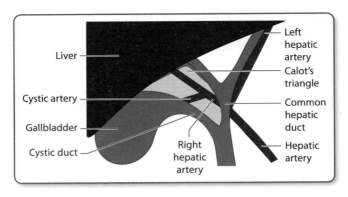

Figure 1.17 Calot's triangle.

25.7   The liver and biliary tree appear in the third/fourth week as hepatic diverticula from the ventral wall of the distal foregut endoderm.

Station 26

26.1 **A** Rectum

    B Internal iliac artery

    C Ductus deferens

    D Bladder

    E Pubic symphysis

    F Penis

26.2 Immobile implies retroperitoneal. This includes most of the duodenum, the ascending and descending colon, and the distal two thirds of the rectum.

26.3 Branches of the inferior mesenteric are: the left colic artery, branches to the sigmoid, and the superior rectal artery (the continuation of the inferior mesenteric artery) (**Figure 1.18**).

26.4 Longitudinal folds of simple columnar epithelium line the upper two-thirds. The lower one-third is lined by stratified squamous epithelium, blending with the skin. The dentate line divides these areas.

26.5 The foregut runs from the mouth to the duodenum, as far as the entry of the bile duct (D2). The midgut ends two-thirds of the way along the transverse colon. The hindgut ends two-thirds of the way along the anal canal at the dentate line.

26.6 The paracolic gutters are peritoneal recesses on the posterior abdominal wall, lying lateral respectively to the ascending and descending colon. Their significance is that substances such as bile or pus can travel along their length and settle at sites remote from their origin. The left paracolic gutter is limited superiorly by the phrenicocolic ligament, and inferiorly by the attachment of the lateral limb of the sigmoid mesocolon at the pelvic brim. The right paracolic gutter is superiorly continuous with the hepatorenal pouch (Morrison's pouch), and inferiorly with the pelvis. The right paracolic gutter is continuous with the lesser sac.

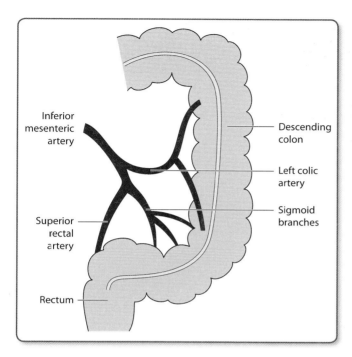

Figure 1.18 Branches of the inferior mesenteric artery.

26.7 The hepatorenal pouch (Morrison's pouch) is the most dependent part of the abdomen and is a common site for accumulation of fluid/pus/blood.

26.8 Rectal adenocarcinoma spreads via the following routes:
- local spread: direct invasion of other structures in the pelvis
- lymph node spread: regional and then distal
- blood-borne distal spread: to the liver, lungs, and bone
- peritoneal spread to other abdominal organs.

Station 27

27.1 A Inferior vena cava. Enters the diaphragm at T8, accompanied by the right phrenic nerve.

27.2 B Oesophageal hiatus

27.3 C Aorta. Traverses the diaphragm at T12, accompanied by the thoracic duct and azygous/hemiazygous veins.

27.4 D Sternum

  E Vertebral body

  F Spinal cord

27.5a The vagi accompany the oesophagus through the diaphragm at T10.

27.5b T8 or T9.

27.5c T10.

Table 1.8 summarises the structures traversing the diaphragm.

Table 1.8 Structures traversing the diaphragm		
Vertebral level	**Main structure transmitted**	**Additional structures transmitted**
T8	Inferior vena cava opening	Right phrenic nerve
T10	Oesophageal opening	Vagi, branches of the left gastric vessels
		Lymphatics
		Thoracic duct
T12	Aortic opening	Azygos, and hemiazygos veins
T12 (crura)	Splanchnic nerves	

27.6 The splanchnic nerve traverses the crura of the diaphragm, and the sympathetic chain passes behind the diaphragm deep to the medial arcuate ligament.

27.7 The phrenic nerves (C3– C5; mnemonic: 'C3, 4, 5 keeps the diaphragm alive'). These contain motor, sensory, and sympathetic nerve fibers. There is sometimes an accessory phrenic nerve (often a branch of the nerve to the subclavius).

27.8 The phrenic nerves originate at the C3–C5 vertebral levels. They run vertically downwards over the anterior scalene muscles deep to the prevertebral layer of deep cervical fascia. They enter the thorax by passing over the subclavian arteries. The right phrenic nerve passes along the right side of the brachiocephalic artery, posterior to the subclavian vein, and then crosses anterior to the root of the right lung, over the pericardium of the right atrium, and then leaves the thorax by passing through the caval opening in the diaphragm. The left phrenic nerve travels lateral to the left subclavian artery and passes in front of the root of the left lung and over the pericardium of the left ventricle to pierce the muscular diaphragm to supply the peritoneum on its under surface.

27.9 The central tendon is formed by the septum transversum. The peripheral rim comes from the body wall. There are also contributions from the oesophageal mesentery and the pleuroperitoneal membranes.

27.10 The most common acquired hernias are termed 'sliding' and 'rolling'. Sliding hernias consist of the projection of the upper part of the stomach through the diaphragm in to the chest when the patient lies or bends. It predisposes to gastroesophageal reflux due to incompetence of the lower oesophageal sphincter. A rolling hernia describes the fundus of the stomach rolling up through the diaphragm in front of the oesophagus. Patients with this condition do not experience reflux.

27.11 Herniation may occur posteriorly through the foramen of Bochdalek. This is the most common form of congenital diaphragmatic hernia and is due to developmental failure of the posterolateral diaphragmatic foramina. It most commonly occurs on the left side. A hernia through the foramen of Morgagni is located anteromedially, between the costal and sternal origins of the diaphragm. Other forms of congenital hernia include a deficiency of the central tendon, or a large oesophageal hiatus.

Station 28

28.1 T12–L3

28.2 A Minor calyx of the left kidney

B Major calyx of the left kidney

C Left renal pelvis

28.3 D The right ureter. The three narrowest parts of the ureter are (i) the pelviureteric junction, (ii) where the ureter crosses the pelvic brim and (iii) the vesicoureteric junction.

28.4 Like most long tubes the ureter has a segmental blood supply from vessels that it passes close to: the aorta, the renal artery, the testicular/ovarian artery, the internal iliac artery and the inferior vesical vessels.

28.5 The renal vein is anterior to the renal artery, which is anterior to the renal pelvis.

28.6 Yes, this is often cut during open aortic aneurysm repair (remember that the left renal vein reaches across the aorta to reach the inferior vena cava). This is possible due to sufficient collateral drainage via the adrenal and inferior phrenic veins.

28.7 Pancreas, kidneys, ureters, adrenals, aorta, para-aortic lymph nodes, lumbar sympathetic chain ascending/descending colon, the duodenum beyond the first few centimetres, inferior vena cava, rectum. The spleen is *not retroperitoneal*, a common incorrect answer given in the exam!

28.8 The distal part of the pronephros develops in to the mesonephric duct. A diverticulum of the lower end of the mesonephric duct develops in to the metanephric duct. Tissue overlying the end of this duct develops in to the kidneys (metanephros), whilst the duct itself develops in to the collecting tubules, calyces, pelvis, and ureter.

28.9 The inferior mesenteric artery.

Station 29

29.1 A The rectum

B The pubic symphysis

C The bladder

29.2a D The uterus

29.2b See **Figure 1.19**.

> **Fundus:** lies above the entrance of the fallopian tubes.
>
> **Body:** the part that lies below the fallopian tubes.
>
> **Cervix:** projects in to the vagina.
>
> **Cavity:** hollow space within the uterus.
>
> **Internal os:** communication in to the uterus.
>
> **External os:** communication in to the vagina.

29.2c The uterine artery (internal iliac artery), and the ovarian artery (abdominal aorta).

29.2d The most common position is anteverted, where the long axis of the uterus is bent forwards. The uterus is also usually anteflexed (bent forward at the level of the internal os). It follows that the uterus can also be retroverted and retroflexed.

29.3a E The cavity of the vagina.

29.3b The relations of the vagina are important to know for the purposes of vaginal examination. Anteriorly lies the bladder, urethra, and symphysis pubis. Posteriorly lies the Pouch of Douglas (in which fluid and bowel may be felt) and the rectum. Laterally are the levator ani muscles, pelvic fascia and the ureters. At the apex of the vagina is the cervix.

29.3c the vagina is supplied by the vaginal, uterine, internal pudendal, and middle rectal arteries (all branches of the internal iliac artery). It is drained by the vaginal vein (internal iliac vein).

29.3d the vagina and vaginal cervix are lined by stratified squamous epithelium. The uterine cervix is lined by tall columnar cells (which secrete the cervical mucus plug). The uterus is lined by cuboidal ciliated cells forming tubular glands.

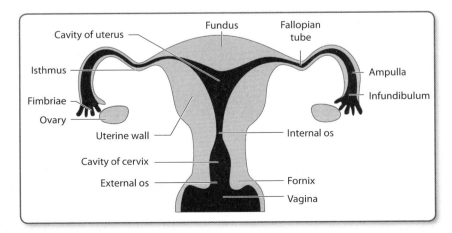

Figure 1.19 The uterus.

29.4 See **Figure 1.19**. The infundibulum is the most lateral part and opens in to the peritoneal cavity via the ostium. This joins the wide ampulla, becoming the narrow isthmus before piercing the uterine wall.

29.5 These are two glands located in the labium magus. They secrete mucus to provide vaginal lubrication. They can become obstructed, forming Bartholin's cysts, which are prone to infection.

29.6 The broad ligaments are folds of peritoneum that connect the lateral sides of the uterus to the pelvic sidewalls. The fallopian tubes lie in the free edge of the broad ligaments and open into the cornu of the uterus. The ligaments also carry the ovary (attached by the mesovarium to the posterior aspect of the uterus), the round ligament, the ovarian ligament, the uterine vessels and their branches, lymphatics and nerves.

29.7 The round ligaments maintain anteversion of the uterus during pregnancy. They are attached to the uterine horns (where the uterus and the fallopian tubes meet) and travel in the anterior layer of the broad ligament to leave the pelvis via the internal inguinal ring. They then pass through the inguinal canal to attach to the labium majora.

29.8 The *cardinal (or cervical) ligaments* pass laterally from the cervix and upper vagina to the sidewalls of the pelvis. The *uterosacral ligaments* pass backwards from the posterolateral cervix and from the lateral vaginal fornices to attach to the periosteum in front of the sacroiliac joints and the lateral part of the sacrum. The *pubocervical fascia* extends from the cardinal ligament to the pubis, either side of the bladder (acting as a sling).

Station 30

30.1 A Right psoas major muscle

    B Right external iliac artery

    C Left iliacus muscle

    D Left ureter

    E Superior hypogastric plexus

    F Left internal iliac artery

    G Left external iliac vein

    H Left common femoral artery

30.2 The anterior vertex is the pubic symphysis and the two other vertices are the ischiopubic rami of the pelvic bone. Its contents in males are the penis and scrotum. In females, the triangle contains the external genitalia, the urethra, and the vagina (**Figure 1.11**).

30.3 The bladder is supplied by the superior and inferior vesical arteries (internal iliac artery). It drains to the vesical venous plexus (iliac vein).

30.4 The bladder is innervated by sympathetic and parasympathetic fibres. The sympathetic fibres originate at L1–2. These fibres inhibit contraction of the detrusor and stimulate tonic contraction of the internal urethral sphincter. The parasympathetic preganglionic fibres originate at S2–4 as the pelvic splanchnic nerves, and synapse with postganglionic neurones in the bladder wall. Most of the afferent impulses (initiated by stretch) travel through these fibres. The parasympathetic fibres stimulate contraction of the detrusor and inhibit the internal urethral sphincter. In the continent individual there are fibres originating in the cerebral cortex that inhibit the micturition reflex until it is required.

30.5 A mnemonic for the layers of scrotum is: **S**ome **D**amn **E**nglishman **C**alled **I**t **T**estes: **S**kin, **D**artos, **E**xternal spermatic fascia, **C**remaster, **I**nternal spermatic fascia, **T**unica vaginalis, **T**estis.

30.6 The lymph drainage of the testis and epididymis is via the spermatic cord and ends at the para-aortic lymph nodes at L1. The scrotum, in contrast, drains to the superficial inguinal lymph nodes.

30.7 The testicular arteries both branch off from the aorta at L2, they then travel in the inguinal canal to reach the testes. Note that it is the left testicular vein not artery that drains in to the left renal vein, whereas the right joins the inferior vena cava.

30.8 The male urethra is approximately 20 cm long. The prostatic urethra is the area surrounded by prostate. It is about 3 cm and has a central elevated area called the urethral crest, with a depressed area either side termed the prostatic sinuses (into which prostatic ducts empty). The crest has a short tract – the verumontanum – into which opens the prostatic utricle. The ejaculatory ducts open either side of the utricle. The membranous urethra is about 2 cm and traverses the external sphincter urethrae and perineal membrane. The spongy urethra is the area within the corpus spongiosum of the penis.

30.9 Ejaculation is a sympathetic process, whereas erection is parasympathetic. A useful mnemonic is **P**oint = **P**arasympathetic, **S**hoot = **S**ympathetic.

30.10 Transitional cell epithelium.

Station 31

31.1 **A** Piriformis

   B Coccygeus and sacrospinous ligament

   C Obturator internus

   D Internal pudendal artery

   E Left common iliac

   F L5 vertebral body

   G Obturator nerve

   H Anterior trunk of internal iliac

   I External iliac artery

31.2 The piriformis (A) originates from the anterior surface of the lateral mass of the sacrum. Its tendon traverses the greater sciatic foramen to insert in to the upper border of the greater trochanter. It is innervated by the nerve to the piriformis (L5–S2) and is an external rotator of the hip.

31.3 The obturator internus (C) originates from the inner surface of the anterolateral wall of the pelvis and the obturator membrane. It inserts in to the greater trochanter. The muscle is innervated by the nerve to obturator internus (sacral plexus), and is a lateral rotator of the femur.

31.4 L1–L4.

31.5 All of the branches of the lumbar plexus arise from the lateral border of the psoas (iliohypogastric nerve, ilioinguinal nerve, lateral cutaneous nerve of the thigh, femoral nerve) except for the genitofemoral nerve (anterior aspect), and obturator nerve (medial border).

31.6 L2–L4.

31.7 L4–S4.

31.8 The lumbar sympathetic chain is a continuation of the thoracic chain as it passes under the medial arcuate ligament of the diaphragm and travels on the lumbar vertebral bodies. On the left, it runs posterolateral to the aorta, on the right underneath the inferior vena cava. They converge on the coccyx at a structure known as the ganglion impar.

31.9 Lumbar sympathectomy is performed for patients with non-reconstructible arterial disease or vasospastic conditions of the lower limbs. It involves excision of a variable number of the L1–L2 ganglia to denervate the sympathetic supply to the leg and hence increase its blood supply.

31.10 The vagus nerve is the main parasympathetic nerve of the abdominal organs. It supplies the gastrointestinal tract as far as the proximal transverse colon. There is also parasympathetic supply from S2–S4 in the form of the pelvic splanchnic nerves. These supply the distal transverse colon as well as the rectum, internal anal sphincter, bladder wall, internal vesicle sphincter, penis and clitoris.

Station 32

32.1 The image displays a barium meal.

32.2 **A** Lesser curve

   B Pylorus

   C Antrum

   D Fundus

   F Greater curve

   G Body

32.3 E Stomach rugae. These are longitudinal folds in the mucous membrane of the stomach that flatten out when the stomach distends.

32.4 All of the arteries that supply the stomach are derived from the coeliac axis (**Figure 1.12**). The left gastric is the only direct branch of the axis, and passes upwards and to the left to reach the oesophagus (which it also supplies) before descending along the lesser curvature. The right gastric arises from the common hepatic artery and runs up the lesser curvature. The short gastric arises from the splenic artery at the hilum of the spleen and travels in the gastrosplenic ligament to supply the upper greater curvature. The left gastroepiploic also originates from the splenic artery and travels in the greater omentum to supply the greater curvature. The right gastroepiploic is a branch of the gastroduodenal artery (which in turn comes off the hepatic artery). It supplies the inferior greater curvature.

32.5 Sympathetic fibres arise from the coeliac plexus. They carry afferent pain fibres, cause reduction in secretory and motor function, and cause constriction of the pylorus. The parasympathetic fibres arise from the vagus nerves. Parasympathetic fibres are secretomotor to the stomach and cause relaxation of the pylorus. The left vagus nerve forms the anterior vagal trunk and enters the abdomen on the anterior surface of the oesophagus. It gives off branches to the anterior stomach wall, the liver, and the pylorus of the stomach. The posterior vagal trunk enters the abdomen on the posterior surface of the oesophagus and supplies the posterior wall of the stomach. The posterior trunk also gives off branches to the coeliac and superior mesenteric plexuses to supply the pancreas and the colon as far as the splenic flexure.

32.6 Highly selective vagotomy is division of those branches of the anterior and posterior vagus nerves that supply the acid-secreting body of the stomach. The nerve of Latarjet is preserved, maintaining function of the pyloric antrum.

32.7 The anterior relations of the stomach are: the anterior abdominal wall, the left costal margin, the left pleura and lung, the diaphragm, and the left lobe of the liver. The posterior relations are: the lesser sac, the spleen and splenic artery, the pancreas, the left suprarenal gland, the left kidney, and transverse colon and mesocolon.

32.8 The junction of pylorus of the stomach from the duodenum is marked by an external constriction and the constant vein of Mayo.

32.9 The cardiac sphincter is a physiological rather than anatomical sphincter. Tonic constriction of the circular layer of smooth muscle at this level prevents gastric contents from regurgitating upwards. It relaxes ahead of peristaltic waves caused by the swallowing of food. There are mucosal folds at the junction which act as valves, and the right crus of the diaphragm also exerts external pressure.

32.10 The lymph drainage follows the arterial supply. The superior two-thirds of the stomach drain along the left and right gastric vessels. The right greater curvature of the stomach drains along the right gastroepiploic arteries to the subpyloric nodes. The left part of the greater curve drains alongside the short gastric and splenic vessels to the suprapancreatic nodes. All lymph eventually passes to the coeliac nodes.

Station 33

33.1 See **Figure 1.20** demonstrating the vessels within the splenic hilum.

    A Portal vein origin (confluence of the splenic and superior mesenteric veins)

    B Splenic vein

    C Spleen

    D Origin of the coeliac axis

    E Splenic artery

    Note how the density of the splenic artery mimics that of the aorta in an arterial phase scan. This knowledge helps you identify that the vessel here labeled 'E' is an artery and not a vein.

33.2 The Epstein–Barr virus causes glandular fever and is associated with splenomegaly.

33.3 The diaphragm ensures that the spleen enlarges downwards, but the left colic flexure and phrenicocolic ligament direct the spleen medially. The notched anterior border of the spleen is palpable as it projects below the costal margin.

33.4 Posteriorly: the diaphragm (behind which is the pleura, left lung and 9–11th ribs).

    Anteriorly: the stomach, the tail of the pancreas.

    Inferiorly: the splenic flexure of colon.

    Medially: the left kidney.

33.5 The spleen is intraperitoneal (and hence mobile).

33.6 Splenorenal (or lienorenal), gastrosplenic, splenocolic, and splenophrenic ligaments (or we also accept: 'all of them').

33.7 The splenic artery originates from the coeliac axis (see **Figure 1.12**). It runs a tortuous course along the upper border of the pancreas giving off multiple

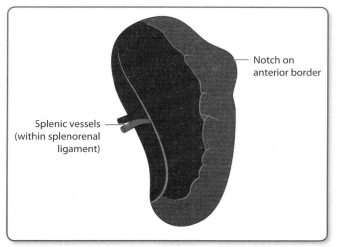

Figure 1.20 The spleen.

Notch on anterior border

Splenic vessels (within splenorenal ligament)

branches to the pancreas (the largest of which is the arteria pancreatica magna), the short gastric artery, the left gastroepiploic artery, and the posterior gastric artery.

33.8 In the foetus the spleen has haematopoietic properties up until the 5th month of gestation. In the adult it has immune functions (via humoral and cell-mediated pathways) and filters red blood cells.

33.9 The spleen develops as multiple thickenings of mesenchyme in the dorsal mesentery. In most people these masses fuse, although approximately 10% of people have more than one spleen.

33.10 The medulla of the adrenal gland receives preganglionic sympathetic fibres from the greater splanchnic nerve. It can be considered a specialised sympathetic ganglion, except that it releases its adrenergic secretions directly into the bloodstream. The cortex is regulated by hormones from the pituitary and hypothalamus, well as the renin–angiotensin system.

33.11 The adrenal glands have an outer yellow cortex, and a dark brown inner medulla. The medulla secretes adrenaline and noradrenaline in response to sympathetic stimulation. The cortex produces corticosteroid hormones and is further divided in to a zona glomerulosa (producing mineralocorticoids), zona fasciculata (producing cortisol), and zona reticularis (producing androgens).

Station 34

34.1 A Common hepatic artery

B Common hepatic duct

C Portal vein

D Inferior vena cava

E Tail of the pancreas

34.2 The liver has a connective tissue layer, Glisson's capsule, which covers its surface and invests its blood vessels. Bleeding from the liver can be contained within this capsule, although this may rupture and blood can leak in to the peritoneal cavity.

34.3 The gross liver can be divided into left and right segments by the attachments of the falciform ligament, ligamentum teres, and ligamentum venosum. However, it is functionally divided by a plane that passes through the gallbladder and the inferior vena cava fossae. These functional lobes have separate blood supply and biliary drainage, and can thus be resected separately. In the Couinaud or 'French' system, these functional lobes are divided into a total of eight sub-segments.

34.4 The liver receives parasympathetic and sympathetic supply from the coeliac plexus. The anterior vagal trunk also gives off a branch to the liver.

34.5 The falciform ligament is a two-layered fold of peritoneum that contains the ligamentum teres (the remnant of the umbilical vein, see **Figure 1.16**). It attaches the umbilicus to the anterior surface of the liver before splitting in to two layers on its posterior surface. The right layer forms the upper coronary ligament and the left the upper triangular ligament.

34.6 The ligamentum venosum is the remnant of the foetal ductus venosus, which shunts blood from the umbilical vein to the inferior vena cava. It adheres to the left branch of the portal vein and travels in a fissure on the visceral surface of the liver to attach superiorly to the inferior vena cava.

34.7 The bile duct lies anterior and to the right, the hepatic artery lies anterior and to the left, and the portal vein lies posteriorly.

Station 35

35.1 A Wing of the ileum

    B Iliopectineal line (with the ischial spine behind it)

    D Ala of sacrum

    E Coccyx

    F Superior pubic ramus

35.2 C Obturator foramen. The obturator nerve and vessels pass through this space.

35.3 The sacroiliac joint is a synovial plane joint.

35.4 The sacrococcygeal joint is a secondary cartilaginous joint.

35.5 The pelvic inlet (or brim) is bounded anteriorly by the symphysis pubis, laterally by the iliopectineal lines, and posteriorly by the sacral promontory.

35.6 The false pelvis is a space within the abdomen bounded posteriorly by the lumbar vertebrae, laterally by the iliac fossae and iliacus muscles, inferiorly by the pelvic inlet, and anteriorly by the anterior abdominal wall.

35.7 The pudendal (Alcock's) canal is a fascial space in the lateral wall of the ischioanal fossa containing the pudendal nerve and internal pudendal vessels.

35.8 Medial is the ischioanal fossa, and laterally are the obturator internus and ischial tuberosity.

35.9 The superior hypogastric plexus is a continuation of the aortic plexus with contributions from the third and fourth lumbar sympathetic ganglia. It lies on the promontory of the sacrum and may be damaged during operations in the pelvis, e.g. open aortic aneurysm repair. Injury results in erectile dysfunction in males and bladder dysfunction in females.

35.10 The pudendal nerve is a branch of the sacral plexus. It leaves the pelvis via the greater sciatic foramen, and enters the perineum through the lesser sciatic foramen. Its branches are:

- inferior rectal nerve: supplies the external anal sphincter, the mucous membrane of the lower half of the anal canal, and the perianal skin.
- dorsal nerve of the penis/clitoris

- perineal nerve: has a superficial branch that supplies the skin of the posterior scrotum/labia majora, and a deep branch supplying the muscles of the urogenital triangle.

Station 36

36.1 See **Figure 1.21**.

    A Corpora cavernosa of the penis

    B Corporum spongiosum of the penis

    C Right testis

    D Epididymis

36.2 The seminiferous tubules are located in the lobules of the testis. Each testis has 200–300 lobules and each lobule contains one to three coiled tubules. The tubules drain in to a plexus termed the rete testis, and thence in to efferent ductules. This pierces the tunica albuginea at the upper testis and passes into the head of the epididymis. The efferent ductules coalesce upon a single much coiled tube, which forms the body and tail of the epididymis. This is a 6 metre long tube that allows for storage and maturation of spermatozoa. The tube continues from the tail as the vas deferens, which travels through the inguinal canal in the spermatic cord. It emerges from the deep inguinal ring and then travels downwards and backwards on the lateral wall of the pelvis (intersecting the ureter at the ischial spine), before running medially and downwards on the posterior bladder. The final part of the vas forms an ampulla before combining with the duct of the seminal vesicle to form the ejaculatory duct. The two ejaculatory ducts pierce the posterior surface of the prostate to open in to the prostatic urethra either side of the prostatic utricle.

36.3 The testis and epididymis are supplied by the testicular arteries, which come off the aorta at L2 and pass through the inguinal canal. The venous drainage is the testicular veins, via the pampiniform plexus. The right vein drains in to the inferior vena cava, and the left to the left renal vein.

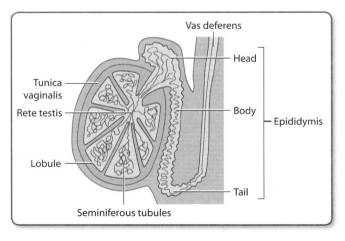

Figure 1.21 The testis.

36.4 The Sertoli cells form the epithelium of the seminiferous tubules. Their function is to nurture developing sperm cells through spermatogenesis. The cell is activated by follicle-stimulating hormone (FSH) and in turn secretes a number of hormones and proteins. Leydig cells are interstitial cells that produce androgens in response to luteinizing hormone (LH).

36.5 The testes develop on the posterior abdominal wall and descend during the latter stages of pregnancy, explaining the distant origin of their vascular and nervous supply. If descent is incomplete they may be found at any point along this path: the abdomen, the inguinal canal, superficial ring, or high in the scrotum.

36.6 A varicocele is a dilatation of the pampiniform plexus. The majority of varicoceles occur on the left side and this is probably due to the testicular vein on the left side entering the left renal vein rather than the inferior vena cava.

36.7 A hydrocele is fluid within the tunica vaginalis, and may be associated with a patent processus vaginalis. The processus vaginalis is an embryological outpouching of peritoneum in to the scrotum, and surrounds the front and sides of the testis. The processus normally closes soon after birth. A persistent patent processus vaginalis allows for fluid and peritoneal contents to travel in to the scrotum. Persistency is more common on the right side. Hydroceles can also be caused by inflammation of the testis without communication to the peritoneal cavity.

36.8 Both the testis and epididymis have appendages. The former is derived from the paramesonephric (Müllerian) ducts, and the latter from the mesonephric tubules. The testicular appendage is called the hydatid of Morgagni, and is present in most individuals. As these appendages exist on stalked bodies, they may both undergo torsion. This, in itself, is not a problem, but the clinical presentation may mimic torsion of the testes. Clinically a 'blue dot' is visible through the scrotal skin.

36.9 Fournier's gangrene is a necrotising infection of the perineum and associated structures. The condition is associated with diabetes and immunosuppression, and a mixture of both aerobic and anaerobic organisms is usually responsible. It can be rapidly spreading and requires urgent admission, antibiotics and debridement.

Station 37

37.1 A Bladder

B Pubic symphysis

C Penis

D Prostate

E Rectum

37.2 BPH stands for benign prostatic hyperplasia (not hypertrophy). Hyperplasia is the abnormal but benign proliferation of cells of the same type. It is often a response to a specific external stimulus. Hypertrophy, in contrast, is a benign increase in the size of the cells.

37.3 The transition zone is affected in benign prostatic hyperplasia, compressing the surrounding peripheral zone. The zones of the prostate are outlined in **Table 1.9**.

37.4 Prostate carcinoma usually occurs in the peripheral zone.

37.5 The prostate is supplied by prostatic branches of the inferior vesical arteries (both ultimately originating from the internal iliac artery).

37.6 Cancer can spread via the prostatic venous drainage. The veins of the prostate form a venous plexus in front of the vertebral bodies, outside of the prostatic capsule, before draining in to the internal iliac veins. There are connections between the prostatic venous plexus and the vertebral veins. The veins in the plexus do not have valves, and therefore during periods of raised abdominal pressure (e.g. coughing or straining) the direction of flow may be directed in to the vertebrals, allowing seeding to the vertebral bodies.

37.7 The seminal colliculus or verumontanum is an elevation of the posterior wall of the prostatic urethra in the middle of the urethral crest. At its margins open the prostatic utricle and the ejaculatory and prostatic ducts. During transurethral resection of the prostate the surgeon works above this level to avoid damage to the urethral sphincter.

37.8 The prostatic utricle is a blind ending pouch on the posterior wall of the prostatic urethra at the apex of the urethral crest, on the seminal colliculus (verumontanum). It is derived from the paramesonephric (Müllerian) duct, which in the female becomes the fallopian tubes, uterus and upper vagina.

37.9 The body of the penis comprises two dorsal corpora cavernosa and a ventral corpus spongiosum. The corpus spongiosum expands distally to form the glans penis. The penis is enclosed in Buck's fascia and has a foreskin that is connected to the glans penis by the frenulum. The urethra travels within the corpus spongiosum.

37.10 The arterial supply is the internal pudendal artery (internal iliac). The corpus spongiosum is supplied by the artery of the bulb, the corpora cavernosa are

Table 1.9 The zones of the prostate		
Central	Wedge shaped region that surrounds the ejaculatory ducts (extends from bladder base to the veru)	< 5% of prostatic cancer
Peripheral	Posterolateral part of the prostate, surrounding the central zone	70% of prostatic cancer
Transition	Surrounds the prostatic urethra proximal to the veru	20% of prostatic cancer Benign prostatic hyperplasia arises here
Anterior fibromuscular zone (or stroma)	Anterior region composed of fibrous and muscular tissue	Not affected by cancer

supplied by the deep arteries of the penis, and the sheath of the corpora cavernosa are supplied by the dorsal artery of the penis. The veins of the penis drain to the internal pudendal vein.

Station 38

38.1 A Right ureter

B Bladder

C Uterus

D Rectum

E Levator ani

38.2 The ovary is supplied by the ovarian artery, which branches from the abdominal aorta at L1. The corresponding veins drain in to the inferior vena cava on the right, and the left renal vein on the left. This is identical to the blood supply of the testicles.

38.3 The lymph drainage follows the arterial supply into paraaortic nodes at the L1 level.

38.4 The neurovascular and lymphatic structures travel via the suspensory ligament (also known as the infundibulopelvic ligament) of the ovary and thence through the mesovarium, to enter the hilum of the ovary.

38.5 The ovary is attached to the following ligaments:
- the mesovarium: attaches the ovary to the broad ligament of the uterus
- the round ligament of the ovary: connects the ovary to the lateral margin of the uterus.
- the suspensory ligament of the ovary: connects the mesovarium to the lateral wall of the pelvis.

38.6 The ovary (and testis) is surrounded by the tunica albuginea.

38.7 Ca125.

Station 39

39.1 A Left ureter

B Psoas major

C Superior hypogastric plexus

D Left hypogastric nerve

39.2 The lumbar plexus is formed in the psoas muscle from the anterior rami of L1–L4.

39.3 The genitofemoral nerve (L1, L2) supplies the cremaster muscle of the scrotum and scrotal skin (genital branch) and the skin of the anterior thigh (femoral branch) (**Table 1.10**).

Table 1.10 The nerves of the lumbar plexus

Nerve	Motor supply	Sensory supply
Iliohypogastric (T12–L1)	External oblique Internal oblique Transversus abdominis	Lower abdominal wall Buttock
Ilioinguinal (L1)	External oblique Internal oblique Transversus abdominis	Upper medial thigh Root of penis and scrotum Mons pubis Labia majora
Genitofemoral (L1–L2)	Cremaster muscle	Anterior thigh
Lateral cutaneous nerve of the thigh (L2–L3)	None	Anterior and lateral thigh
Obturator (L2–L4)	Obturator externus Gracilis, adductor brevis Adductor longus Pectineus Adductor magnus (adductor part)	Medial thigh
Femoral (L2–L4)	Iliacus, sartorius Pectineus Quadriceps femoris	Anterior thigh Medial leg and foot (saphenous branch)
Muscular branches	Psoas Quadratus lumborum Iliacus	None

39.4　The ilioinguinal nerve supplies the external oblique, the internal oblique, transversus abdominis, the skin of the upper medial thigh, the base of the penis and scrotum, the mons pubis and the labia majora.

39.5　The cremasteric reflex can be elicited by lightly stroking the medial thigh. The afferent limb of the reflex is the femoral branch of the genitofemoral nerve. This causes contraction of the cremaster via the efferent limb, which is the genital branch of the genitofemoral nerve. The function of the cremasteric reflex is to raise the testis for warmth and protection. It may be absent in testicular torsion.

39.6　The sympathetic trunk enters the abdomen behind the medial arcuate ligament.

Chapter 2

Limbs and spine

Syllabus topics

The following topics are listed within the Intercollegiate MRCS Examination syllabus for limbs and spine anatomy. Tick them off as you revise these topics to ensure you have covered the syllabus.

Upper limb

- ❑ Pectoral girdle
- ❑ Breast
- ❑ Axilla
- ❑ Brachial plexus
- ❑ Scapular region
- ❑ Cubital fossa
- ❑ Muscles of the arm and forearm
- ❑ Carpal tunnel
- ❑ Shoulder joint
- ❑ Elbow joint
- ❑ Radio-ulnar joints
- ❑ Wrist joint
- ❑ Hand joints
- ❑ Thumb movements
- ❑ Arteries and pulses (surface and imaging anatomy)
- ❑ Nerves: axillary, radial, musculocutaneous, ulnar and median
- ❑ Arteriography
- ❑ Venography
- ❑ Dermatomes & tendon reflexes
- ❑ Superficial veins and lymphatics

Lower limb

- ❑ Gluteal region
- ❑ Thigh, front, medial side, back
- ❑ Femoral triangle
- ❑ Femoral sheath and canal
- ❑ Femoral hernia
- ❑ Adductor canal
- ❑ Popliteal fossa
- ❑ Leg, compartments
- ❑ Hip joint
- ❑ Knee joint
- ❑ Ankle joint
- ❑ Foot, arches
- ❑ Foot joints

Spine

- ❑ Vertebral column
- ❑ Vertebral canal

Station 1

A 31-year-old lactating woman presents with a hard, painful, erythematous lump in the right breast. A diagnosis of breast abscess is made and arrangements are made for a percutaneous drainage to be performed.

This photograph demonstrates the anterior aspect of the female chest:

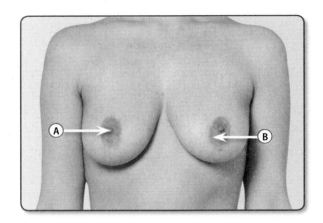

1.1 In which dermatome is the region indicated by A located?

1.2 Other than lactiferous ducts, what other secretory glands are found in area B?

1.3 What embryological structures does the breast develop from?

1.4 Where is milk produced? What does it travel through to leave the breast?

1.5 How does the structure of the breast alter during pregnancy?

1.6 Why does skin dimpling occur with malignant infiltration of the breast?

1.7 What is meant by the terms *simple* and *radical* mastectomy?

1.8 Define the boundaries of the quadrangular space and name the structures that traverse it.

1.9 Define the boundaries of the triangular space and name the structures that traverse it.

Station 2

A 32-year-old woman presents to the breast clinic with a mobile, painless lump in the upper, outer quadrant of the left breast. A mammogram is undertaken.

On the following page the projection labelled (a) is lateral-oblique and the projection labelled (b) is cranio-caudal.

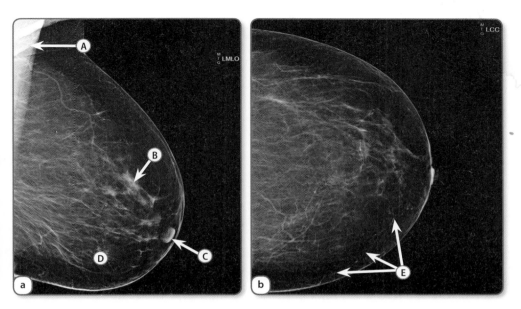

2.1 Describe the surface anatomy of the adult female breast in relation to the thoracic skeleton.

2.2 Identify the structures labelled A to E.

2.3 What is the blood supply to the breast?

2.4 What is the lymphatic drainage of the breast? Classify the groups of lymph nodes within the axilla.

2.5 What is the surgical relevance of the lymphatic drainage of the breast?

2.6 What are the boundaries of the axilla?

2.7 What structures are contained within the axilla?

2.8 In which quadrant of the breast are malignancies most commonly found?

Station 3

A 19-year-old workman accidentally drops and breaks a plate of glass while fitting a window. A shard of glass is impaled in his right forearm.

Images (a) and (b) on the following page show the anterior aspect of the right arm.

3.1 In which dermatomes are the points labelled A, B and C located?

3.2 Which cutaneous nerves supply regions labelled A, B, C?

3.3 Name the prominent muscle that accounts for the bulge at D that originates from the lateral supracondylar ridge of the humerus and inserts onto the radial styloid process? What is its motor innervation?

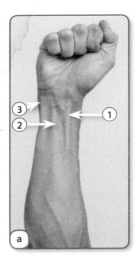

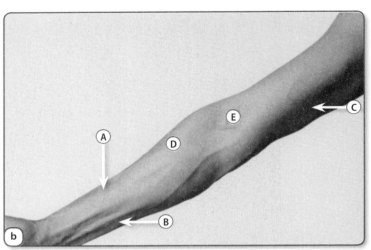

3.4 Which vein is commonly cannulated at position E?

3.5 Which muscles cause supination of the forearm?

3.6 Classify the compartments of the forearm.

3.7 List the muscles that belong to the superficial group in the flexor compartment of the forearm.

3.8 Identify the tendons labelled 1, 2 and 3.

Station 4

A 76-year-old woman presents to the outpatients clinic with a cold, pale left hand. She has absent arterial pulses and monophasic Doppler signals in the left brachial and radial arteries. You request an angiogram.

The image on the following page is a normal arteriogram of the left upper limb.

4.1 Identify the arteries labelled A to D.

4.2 What is the origin of the artery labelled A?

4.3 Is the artery labelled A medial or lateral to its corresponding vein?

4.4 Name the branches of the artery labelled A.

4.5 Name the branches of the artery labelled D.

4.6 Describe the blood supply to the structure labelled E.

4.7 What are the branches of the artery labelled C?

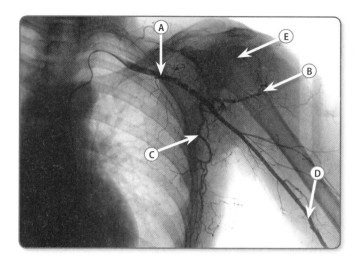

Station 5

A 22-year-old woman falls off her horse and extends her hand to break her fall. She feels a sudden and severe pain in the shoulder region. On clinical examination of the patient in the emergency department, there is an obvious deformity in the clavicular region and bony fragments can be palpated.

This is the clavicle viewed from below (demonstrating normal anatomy):

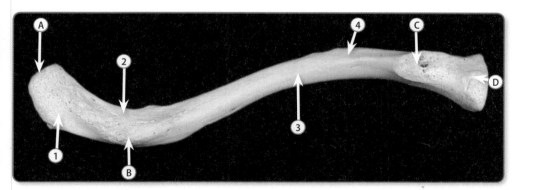

5.1 To which side of the body does this bone belong?

5.2 What are the functions of the clavicle?

5.3 With which bone does the medial end of the clavicle articulate?

5.4 Identify the parts labelled A to D.

5.5 Which muscles attach to the areas labelled 1 to 4?

5.6 Which part of the bone is most likely to fracture when the clavicle is subjected to an indirect stress of sufficient force?

5.7 What structures are at risk in clavicular fractures at this point?

5.8 What type of joint is the sternoclavicular joint?

5.9 Which ligaments stabilise the sternoclavicular joint?

5.10 What muscle separates the clavicle from the subclavian vessels and brachial plexus?

5.11 What is the normal range for passive shoulder flexion and extension?

5.12 What is the normal range for passive elbow flexion and extension?

Station 6

A 50-year-old patient requires cannulation of the cubital vein. The colleague who carried it out calls you soon after. He is concerned that he may have inadvertently cannulated an artery instead of a vein.

This is a dissection of the left cubital fossa:

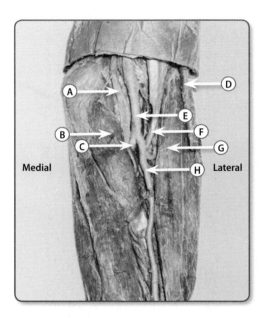

6.1 Identify the structures labelled A to H.

6.2 What are the origin, insertion, action and innervation of muscle G?

6.3 What are the boundaries of the cubital fossa?

6.4 What layer protects the brachial artery when blood is drawn from the median cubital vein?

6.5 What is the annular ligament?

6.6 What are the humeral attachments of the common flexor and extensor tendons of the forearm?

6.7 What is the function of the anconeus muscle?

6.8 Is the ulnar nerve medial or lateral to the ulnar artery at the wrist?

6.9 At the wrist which tendon lies lateral (radial) to the median nerve?

Station 7

A 69-year-old man with multiple myeloma is discovered to have a pathological fracture of the shaft of humerus. It is decided that he is to undergo internal fixation of the fracture.

This image shows the anterior aspect of the normal humerus:

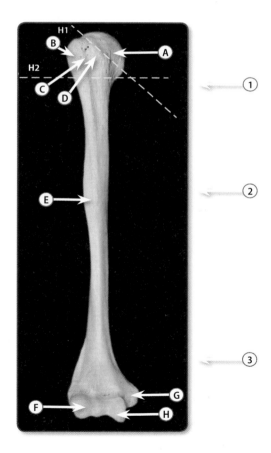

7.1 To which side of the body does this bone belong?

7.2 Which of the two lines (H1 or H2) denotes the surgical neck of the humerus?

7.3 Identify the parts labelled A–H.

7.4 What tendons attach to the region labelled B?

7.5 What tendons attach to the region labelled D?

7.6 What group of tendons attach to the region labelled G?

7.7 What are the origins and what is the insertion of the triceps brachii muscle?

7.8 Which nerves are particularly vulnerable in fractures at levels indicated by 1, 2 and 3?

7.9 In a subject with an anterior shoulder dislocation what is the most laterally situated palpable bony prominence in the shoulder region?

7.10 Describe the muscles involved in abducting the arm above your head.

7.11 What bony structures are commonly fractured in association with elbow dislocation?

Station 8

A 63-year-old female patient on haemodialysis presents with pain and generalised swelling of the left arm, following the creation of an arteriovenous (brachiocephalic) fistula. Obstruction of the deep veins impeding venous return is suspected. As the resident in charge of the patient you wish to refresh your knowledge of upper limb vascular anatomy

The following image is a contrast study of a normal left upper limb:

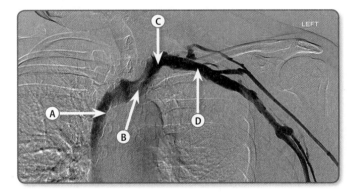

8.1 What is the name of the investigation above?

8.2 Identify the structures labelled A to D.

8.3 Where does the structure labelled D originate?

8.4 What are the tributaries of the structure labelled D?

8.5 Which other structure (not demonstrated on this investigation) joins structure C to form the structure labelled B?

8.6 In the axilla what runs more superficially: the axillary artery or the axillary vein?

8.7 Describe the courses of the basilic and cephalic veins.

8.8 Describe the deep veins that drain the hand.

Station 9

A 55-year-old man falls over whilst intoxicated and presents to the emergency department with a severely painful right shoulder that he is unable to move. He is seen to be supporting the painful limb with the other hand. A diagnosis of shoulder dislocation is made on clinical examination.

A plain anteroposterior radiograph of the right shoulder is taken after reduction of the dislocation:

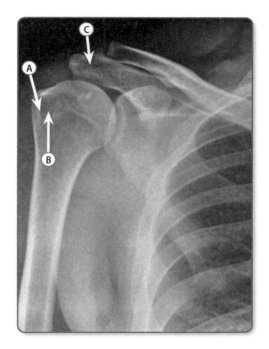

9.1 What type of joint is the shoulder joint?

9.2 Identify the part labelled A. What muscles/tendons insert here?

9.3 Which muscles/tendons attach to the part labelled B?

9.4 What is the name given to the part labelled C?

9.5 What structures stabilise the shoulder joint?

9.6 What is the most common type of shoulder dislocation, and what structures may be damaged during such an injury?

9.7 Name the two bursae surrounding this joint.

9.8 Define the terms Bankart's lesion and Hill–Sachs' lesion.

9.9 Classify the compartments of the arm.

9.10 What major nerves, arteries and muscles run in the posterior compartment of the arm?

Station 10

A 30-year-old postman falls off his bike and lands on his right hand. One week after the injury he is still experiencing pain in the wrist and he attends the emergency department.

This is the dorsum of the right hand:

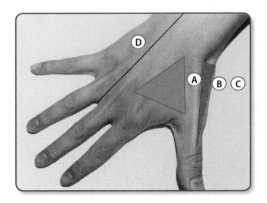

10.1 What is the name given to the orange shaded region?

10.2 What is the most likely structure to have been injured if a patient complains of pain on palpation within this region?

10.3 What other structure is contained within this anatomical space?

10.4 Name the tendons labelled A, B and C that form the boundaries of this space?

10.5 Which peripheral nerve is responsible for sensation within the green shaded area on the back of the hand?

10.6 Describe the course of the radial nerve.

10.7 Which muscles does the radial nerve innervate?

10.8 What is the result of radial nerve damage:

    10.8a Within the axilla?

    10.8b At the level of the mid humerus?

    10.8c At the wrist?

10.9 In which dermatome is the region of skin labelled D?

10.10 Which nerve innervates the skin over the region D?

Station 11

A 29-year-old woman falls onto her left shoulder whilst ice-skating. On clinical examination there is bruising and tenderness over the upper, outer aspect of the shoulder region.

Image (a) demonstrates the surface anatomical features of the left shoulder in a normal subject:

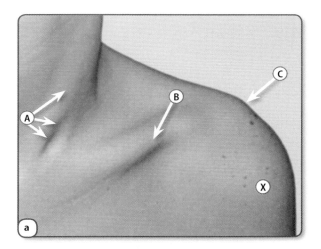

11.1 Identify the muscle indicated by the arrows labelled A.

11.2 What are the attachments and action of this muscle?

11.3 What bony structure is palpable at point B?

11.4 Regarding the joint at point C:

    11.4a What is its name?

    11.4b What type of joint is this?

    11.4c Which ligaments help stabilise this joint?

11.5 Which nerve provides cutaneous innervation to the area labelled X? How is it commonly damaged?

11.6 Name the muscles innervated by this nerve.

11.7 Which cord of the brachial plexus does this nerve originate from?

This is an axial prosection of the left shoulder region and upper thorax at the level of the humeral head, viewed from above:

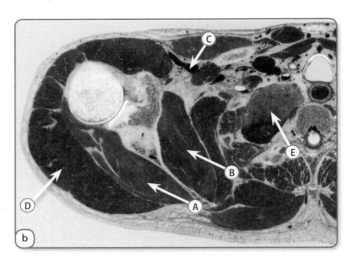

11.8 Identify the structures labelled A, B, C and E.

11.9 Which muscles form the rotator cuff of the shoulder joint?

11.10 What is the motor innervation of these muscles?

11.11 Identify the muscle labelled D. What is the action of this muscle?

Station 12

A 78-year-old woman falls down a flight of stairs. She is taken to the emergency department complaining of a swollen painful right wrist. A plain radiograph confirms a fracture of the distal radius.

This is the anterior aspect of the right radius:

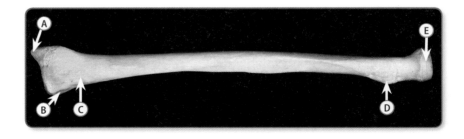

12.1 Identify the parts labelled A, D and E.

12.2 What articulates with the point labelled B?

12.3 What muscle attaches at the region labelled C?

12.4 What is the innervation and action of this muscle?

12.5 What is the origin, insertion and innervation of the supinator muscle?

12.6 What attaches at the part labelled D?

12.7 What structure encircles the part labelled E?

12.8 Describe Galeazzi fracture.

12.9 Describe Monteggia fracture.

Station 13

A 39-year-old presents to the emergency department with a painful swelling to the right elbow. You suspect bursitis.

This is the lateral aspect of the right ulna:

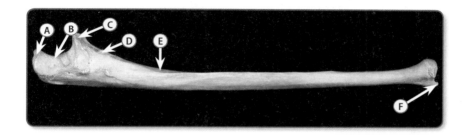

13.1 Identify the parts labelled A, B, C, D and F.

13.2 Which end of the ulna is conventionally termed the head?

13.3 Where is the coronoid process and what does it articulate with?

13.4 What muscle attaches at the region labelled E?

13.5 What is the innervation and action of the abductor pollicis longus?

13.6 The interosseous membrane joins the radius and ulna. What is the name for this type of joint?

13.7 Which muscles contribute to:

    13.7a elbow flexion?

    13.7b elbow extension?

13.8 What is a bursa? What causes bursitis?

Station 14

A 34-year old builder falls from a height of 12 feet on to the pavement. Along with bilateral rib fractures he is discovered to have a fracture of the scapula neck.

The image on the following page is the dorsal aspect of the scapula (demonstrating normal anatomy).

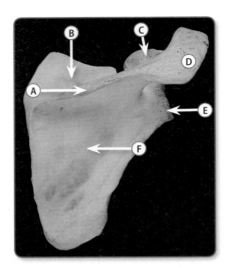

14.1 To which side of the body does this bone belong?

14.2 Identify the parts labelled A to F.

14.3 What muscles attach to the parts labelled B, F and A?

14.4 At what vertebral level is the inferior angle of the scapula?

14.5 At what vertebral level is the most medial part of the spine?

14.6 Name three muscles that attach to the part labelled C.

14.7 Which muscle/tendon originates from the supraglenoid tubercle?

14.8 Which muscle/tendon originates from the infraglenoid tubercle?

14.9 Which muscles are responsible for flexion and extension of the shoulder?

14.10 Which muscles are responsible for internal and external rotation of the shoulder?

Station 15

A 25-year-old man punches a window whilst drunk and suffers lacerations to the forearm. He presents to the emergency department and you are called to assess him. On clinical examination he has weakness of the thumb.

Images (a) and (b) on the following page display movement of the thumb in two different planes.

15.1 What movement of the thumb is being demonstrated in (a)?

15.2 Which muscles are responsible for this action and what is their innervation?

15.3 Which movements of the thumb are being demonstrated by the red and blue arrows in (b)?

15.4 Which muscles are responsible for these actions and what are their innervations?

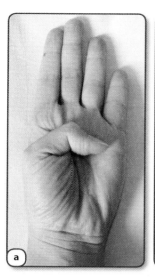
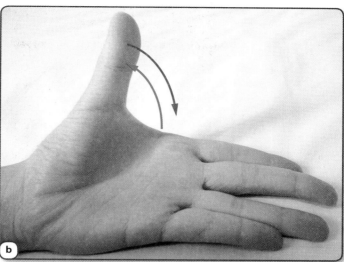

a

b

15.5 Which two other movements of the thumb have not been demonstrated?

15.6 How would you classify the joints of the body?

15.7 What type of joint allows the thumb to perform all the movements described?

Image (c) demonstrates a patient trying to straighten his thumb flat against his index finger but being unable to do so.

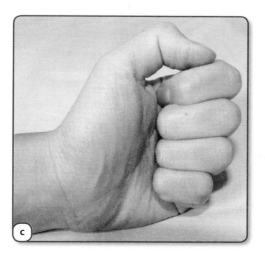

c

15.8 What is this clinical sign called?

15.9 What nerve has been injured. Give three causes of this sign.

15.10 What other actions would you expect this patient to find difficult?

15.11 Describe the course of the ulnar nerve within the upper limb.

15.12 What do you understand by the term 'ulnar paradox'?

Station 16

A 67-year-old man is working in his garage with a circular saw when he accidently slices into the distal interphalangeal joint of the index finger. You review him in the hand clinic the following day.

This is the left palm (demonstrating normal anatomy):

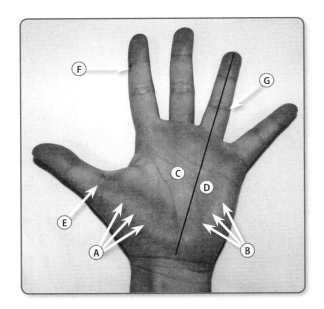

16.1 Which muscles comprise the thenar eminence, indicated by the arrows labelled A?

16.2 Which muscles comprise the hypothenar eminence, indicated by the arrows labelled B?

16.3 Which peripheral nerve supplies sensation to the area labelled C?

16.4 Which peripheral nerve supplies sensation to the area labelled D?

16.5 What is the name of the joint labelled E? Which muscle is responsible for flexion of this joint?

16.6 What are the names of the joints labelled F and G? Which muscles flex these joints?

16.7 What are the actions of the lumbricals?

16.8 What are the interossei muscles and what is their action?

16.9 Which is encountered closer to the skin: the digital nerve or digital artery?

Station 17

A 27-year-old male snowboarder attends your clinic after falling on the slopes whilst on holiday the previous week. He remembers falling onto his outstretched right hand and is complaining of pain between his thumb and index finger.

The radiographs below are in a series known as 'scaphoid views'. They all demonstrate normal anatomy:

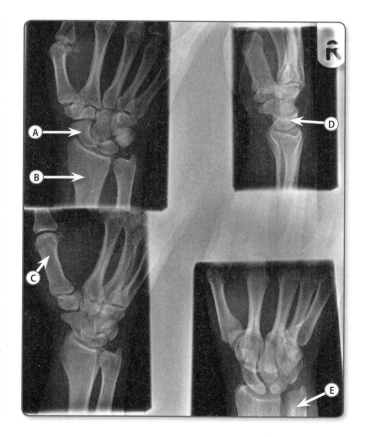

17.1 Identify the structures labelled A to E.

17.2 Given the clinical scenario and the fact that an initial plain film did not reveal a fracture, does this exclude the diagnosis of scaphoid injury.

17.3 Describe the blood supply to the scaphoid bone.

17.4 What may be the clinical consequences of missing a scaphoid fracture?

17.5 Which part of the scaphoid bone is most prone to this complication?

17.6 Name three other bones within the upper or lower limbs that may also be at risk of this complication.

17.7 In the absence of trauma, what medical conditions or risk factors should be asked about in the history when contemplating this diagnosis?

Station 18

A 32-year-old male gardener presents with an acute onset of pain and swelling in his left little finger. The pain started 1 week previously, shortly after he pricked the tip of his finger, and there is now erythema and tenderness tracking along the finger into the palm.

Image (a) displays the left palm and (b) the dorsal aspect of left thumb:

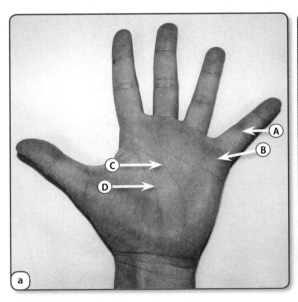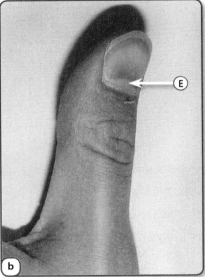

18.1 What types of joints are A and B? Which ligaments protect these joints?

18.2 What are the names of the arterial arches that would be found beneath points labelled C and D?

18.3 What is the medial boundary of the thenar space?

18.4 What is the lateral boundary of the mid-palmer space?

18.5 Why are infections of the little finger and thumb more likely to spread into the palm than infections in the other fingers?

18.6 What are the cardinal signs of infectious digital flexor tenosynovitis?

18.7 Define the term 'paronychia'.

18.8 What is the name of the light area on the proximal nail labelled E?

18.9 Define the term 'felon'. What may be the consequences of neglecting a felon?

Station 19

A 54-year-old female secretary presents to the orthopaedic clinic with numbness and tingling in the left thumb and index finger, along with weakness of the thumb.

This is an axial MRI of the carpal tunnel of the left wrist (demonstrating normal anatomy):

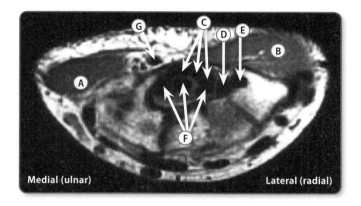

19.1 Identify the muscles labelled A and B.

19.2 What are the names given to the tendons labelled C, D, E and F?

19.3 What are the contents of the carpal tunnel?

19.4 To which carpal bones does the flexor retinaculum (transverse carpal ligament) attach?

19.5 Name the structures at risk during carpal tunnel release.

19.6 What is the structure labelled G in the MRI image?

19.7 Is this structure ever involved in carpal tunnel syndrome?

19.8 What is the innervation of the muscles whose tendons reside within the carpal tunnel?

19.9 Describe Tinel's test.

19.10 Where is Guyon's canal and what runs through it?

Station 20 (Specialty)

A 37-year-old male office worker attends the orthopaedic clinic complaining of elbow pain, from which he has suffered for the previous 2 months. He complains that the pain is inhibiting his tennis playing.

Image (a) is an anteroposterior radiograph of the left elbow joint (demonstrating normal anatomy):

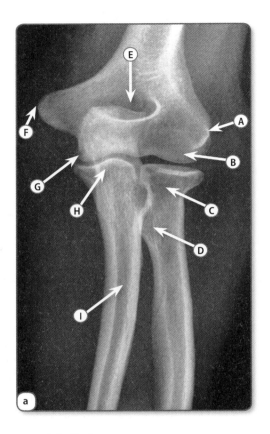

20.1 Identify the structures labelled A to I.

20.2 What tendon attaches to the structure labelled D?

20.3 What are the origins of this muscle?

20.4 What muscle attaches to structure labelled H?

20.5 What is the action of this muscle?

20.6 Describe the deformity associated with:

    20.6a Colles' fracture.

    20.6b Smith's fracture.

Image (b) on the following page is an axial view of a prosection through the right elbow viewed from above.

20.7 Identify the structures labelled A to E.

20.8 What would be the clinical consequences of damage to the ulnar nerve?

20.9 Describe the course of the median nerve.

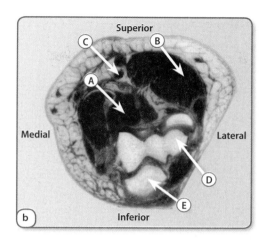

20.10 What would be the result of an injury to the median nerve at:

20.10a the elbow?

20.10b the wrist?

20.11 What is the origin and what are the names of the branches of the brachial artery?

Station 21

A 16-year-old boy catches a cricket ball at close range and suffers severe pain in the right metacarpophalangeal joint of his middle finger. A plain film shows a fracture of the metacarpal head of this finger. You are called to the emergency department to assess the patient.

The image below is the volar aspect of an articulated right hand (demonstrating normal anatomy):

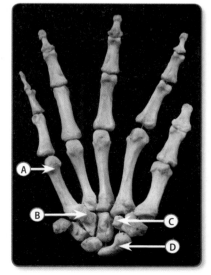

21.1 Identify the bones labelled A to D.

21.2 What type of bone is the pisiform bone?

21.3 Which structures attach to the pisiform bone?

21.4 Which carpal bones articulate with the radius?

21.5 Define Bennett's fracture.

21.6 Where do the tendons of flexor digitorum profundus and flexor digitorum superficialis insert?

21.7 Where does flexor pollicis longus originate and insert?

21.8 What is 'mallet finger'? How is this treated?

21.9 What is 'trigger finger'? How is this treated?

21.10 What is the function of the cruciform and annular pulleys of the hand?

Station 22

A 22-year-old man is attacked by a dog and suffers lacerations to the dorsum of his left hand. On exploration of his wound in theatre he is found to have several damaged tendons. Your registrar is assisting you in theatre whilst you perform the tendon repairs.

This is a dissection of the dorsal aspect of the left hand (demonstrating normal anatomy):

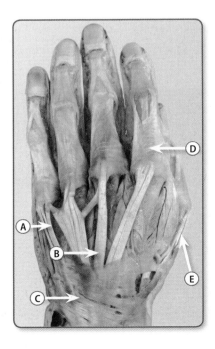

22.1 Identify the structures labelled A to E.

22.2 Which nerves supply the muscles attached to the tendons labelled B?

22.3 Where is the origin and insertion of the extensor digitorum communis muscle?

22.4 Why is it difficult to fully extend the ring finger alone at the metacarpophalangeal joint?

22.5 What is the origin and insertion of the extensor carpi ulnaris muscle?

22.6 What is the origin and insertion of the extensor carpi radialis longus muscle?

22.7 What is the structure labelled C attached to?

22.8 What is 'de Quervain's tenosynovitis'?

22.9 What is 'Volkmann's contracture' of the hand?

Station 23

A 32-year-old man spins out of control on a wet road whilst on a motorbike and collides with the roadside barriers. The emergency personnel note, as they extract him, that he is bleeding from a deep laceration to the left hand. You are asked to assess him.

This is a dissection of the palmer aspect of the left hand (demonstrating normal anatomy):

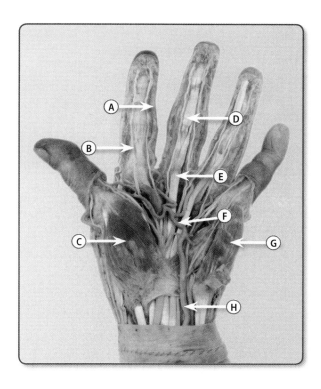

23.1 Identify the structures labelled A to H.

23.2 What is the origin of the anterior and posterior interosseous nerves?

23.3 Which muscles do they innervate?

23.4 What are the origins of the anterior and posterior interosseous arteries?

23.5 Which forearm flexor is commonly used as a graft for tendon transfers?

23.6 What is the name of the terminal branches of the radial and ulnar arteries?

23.7 Describe Allen's test.

Station 24

A 20-year-old man is involved in an accident whilst riding his motorbike and lands on his right shoulder. In hospital it is noted that his arm is internally rotated with the forearm pronated. On performing a neurological examination of the limbs you note numbness of the lateral aspect of the arm and forearm.

This is a dissection of the right brachial plexus (demonstrating normal anatomy):

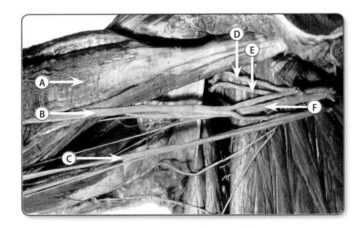

24.1 Identify the muscle labelled A, and the nerves labelled B to F.

24.2 Which muscles does the nerve labelled D supply?

24.3 What are the root values for the radial, median, musculocutaneous and axillary nerves?

24.4 What are the branches of the posterior cord of the brachial plexus?

24.5 Where do the roots, trunks, divisions and cords of the brachial plexus lie?

24.6 What would be the clinical consequences of an upper trunk brachial plexus lesion?

24.7 What would be the clinical consequences of a lower brachial plexus lesion?

24.8 Which muscle does the long thoracic nerve supply and how would you test for a deficit of this nerve?

24.9 Which branch of the brachial plexus gives a contribution to the accessory phrenic nerve (when it is present)?

24.10 List the branches of the brachial plexus that come off at the level of the trunks?

24.11 The cords of the brachial plexus are named after their relationship to which structure?

Station 25

A 23-year-old man presents to the orthopaedic clinic with pain and swelling of the lower right thigh. On palpation you feel a hard mass just above the right knee.

This is an axial dissection through the right thigh, viewed from above at the level of the distal femur:

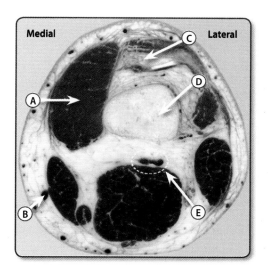

25.1 Identify the structures labelled A to E.

25.2 What are the origin, insertion, and action of the quadratus femoris muscle?

25.3 What are the origin, insertion, and action of the semitendinosus muscle?

25.4 What is the innervation of the adductor magnus muscle?

25.5 Why is hip pain sometimes referred to the knee joint?

25.6 What are the roots of the obturator nerve?

25.7 What area of skin, and group of muscles does the obturator nerve innervate?

Station 26

A 32-year-old professional male rugby player presents to the orthopaedic clinic with a limp and left hip pain.

This photograph illustrates a man undergoing a hip examination. The patient is being asked to resist a force indicated by arrow A.

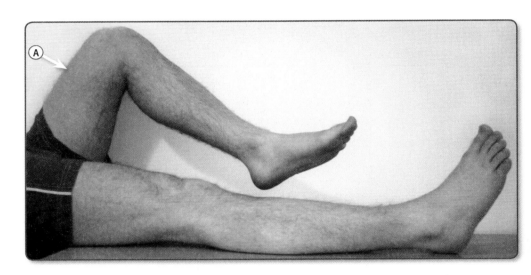

26.1 What action is being tested by pressing on area A in the image above?

26.2 Which dermatome does the arrow point to?

26.3 What muscles and nerve roots are involved in resisting the force of the arrow?

26.4 What is the normal range of motion for flexion and extension of the hip?

26.5 What is the normal range of motion for internal and external rotation of the hip?

26.6 What is the normal range of motion for flexion and extension of the knee?

26.7 What is the normal range of motion for internal rotation of the knee?

26.8 How do you measure 'real' and 'apparent' leg length? What do these terms mean?

26.9 How do you perform McMurray's test, and what does it test for?

26.10 How do you perform Lachman's test, and what does it test for?

Station 27 (Generic)

A 62-year-old man presents to the orthopaedic clinic with right hip pain. On examination he has a positive Trendelenburg test and restricted hip movements.

This is a prosection of the right gluteal region (demonstrating normal anatomy):

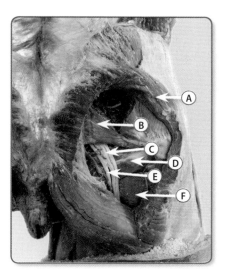

27.1 Identify the structures labelled A to F.

27.2 What is the clinical significance of Trendelenburg's test, and which muscles are involved?

27.3 What are the innervation and blood supply of the structure labelled A?

27.4 Regarding structure C:

    27.4a What are its root values?

    27.4b What are its main branches?

27.5 Regarding structure B:

    27.5a What are its origin, insertion, and function?

    27.5b What vessels leave the greater sciatic foramen below B?

    27.5c What nerves leave the greater sciatic foramen below B?

27.6 What is the 'fascia lata'?

27.7 What is the 'iliotibial tract', which muscles insert into it, and what is its function?

27.8 What is the surface landmark for safe intramuscular injection into the buttocks?

Station 28

A 54-year-old woman presents to the emergency department with a severe painful lump in the right groin region. When you examine her you find that the lump is below and lateral to the pubic tubercle and there is a positive cough reflex.

This is a dissection of the right femoral region (demonstrating normal anatomy):

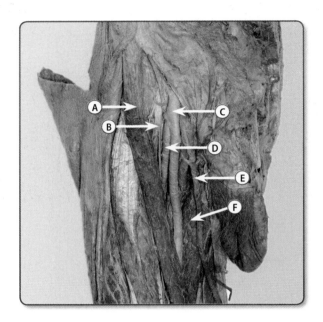

28.1 Using anatomical principles, give a differential for a lump in the groin.

28.2 Identify the structures labelled A to F.

28.3 What is the origin and course of structure C?

28.4 Through which opening does a femoral hernia pass, and what are the boundaries of this opening?

28.5 What are the normal contents of this opening, and what is its physiological significance?

28.6 What are the boundaries of the femoral triangle?

28.7 What is the 'femoral sheath'?

28.8 What are the boundaries of the adductor canal ('Hunter's canal')?

28.9 Tingling or numbness of the lateral thigh is a common condition. Which nerve is responsible for this and what is this condition called?

Station 29

A 45-year-old female cleaner presents to the orthopaedic clinic with a painful swelling just below her right knee, which has been present and worsening for 6 months. You assess her and request some radiographs.

Images (a) and (b) on the following page are anteroposterior and lateral radiographs of the right knee.

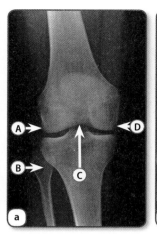
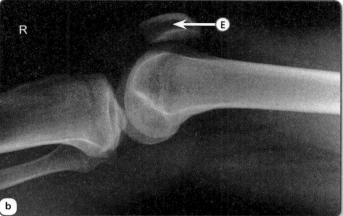

29.1 Identify the bony landmarks labelled A to D.

29.2 Regarding the bone labelled E:

　　29.2a What is it? What type of bone is it?

　　29.2b Comment on its position.

　　29.2c What is the function of this bone?

　　29.2d Which direction does it most commonly dislocate?

29.3 Which joints connect the tibia and fibula and what type of joints are these?

29.4 Which four muscles comprise the quadriceps femoris?

29.5 Define the terms 'housemaid's knee', and 'clergyman's knee'.

29.6 Where can the common peroneal nerve be palpated?

29.7 What are the clinical consequences of injury to the common peroneal nerve?

29.8 After section of the sciatic nerve, some flexion of the knee is still possible. Which muscles allow this?

Station 30

An 82-year-old woman falls at home. In the emergency department she complains of severe pain in the hip and on examination the leg is seen to be shortened and externally rotated. There is a deep laceration down the posterior aspect of the thigh.

Image (a) on the following page is a medial view of the upper end of the femur.

30.1 To which side of the body does this bone belong?

30.2 Identify the bony landmarks labelled A, B, C, D.

30.3 Which arteries supply the head of the femur?

30.4 How does this differ in the young child?

30.5 Why do some fractures of the femoral neck result in avascular necrosis?

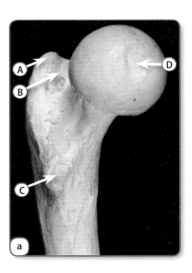

Image (b) is a prosection of the muscles of the posterior right thigh:

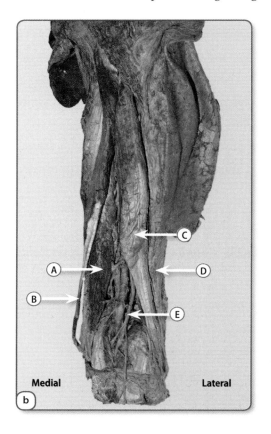

30.6 Identify the structures labelled A to E.

30.7 What is the blood supply to the gracilis muscle?

30.8 What is the innervation of the gracilis muscle?

30.9 What is the origin and insertion of the gracilis muscle?

30.10 Which other muscles contribute to hip adduction?

Station 31

A 34-year-old male jockey presents to the surgical outpatients clinic with a lump in the right popliteal region. On examination, the lump is approximately 2 × 2 cm, non-tender and pulsatile.

This is a dissection of the right popliteal fossa:

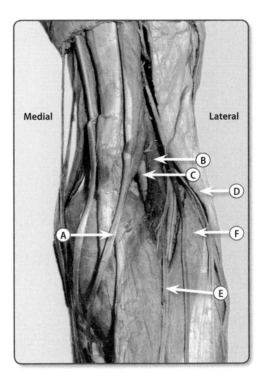

31.1 Using anatomical principles give a differential for a lump in the popliteal region.

31.2 Identify the structures labelled A to F.

31.3 What is the definition of an aneurysm?

31.4 What are the boundaries of the popliteal fossa?

31.5 What is the deepest structure in the popliteal fossa?

31.6 What are the branches of the popliteal artery?

31.7 In which compartment does the tibial nerve run in the lower leg?

31.8 What would be the consequences of a high section of the tibial nerve?

31.9 In which compartment does the deep peroneal nerve run?

31.10 What would be the consequences of section of the superficial peroneal nerve?

31.11 What is the function of the popliteus muscle?

Station 32

Whilst intoxicated, a 55-year-old man falls off his bicycle and suffers a fracture to the mid-tibia. Six hours after open reduction and internal fixation he complains of severe pain in the calf. On examination you find evidence of compartment syndrome and the patient is brought back to theatre immediately for fasciotomies.

This prosection demonstrates the left leg from its anterolateral aspect (demonstrating normal anatomy):

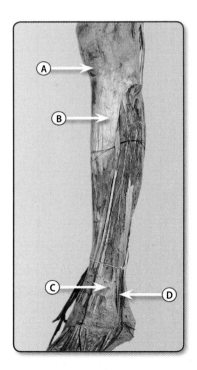

32.1 What bony prominence is palpable at the part labelled A?

32.2 Identify the structures labelled B to D.

32.3 What are the symptoms and signs of anterior compartment of the leg syndrome?

32.4 Classify the fascial compartments of the lower leg and give their principal blood supply.

32.5 In which compartment is the extensor digitorum longus muscle?

32.6 In which compartment does the tibial nerve run?

Station 33

A 72-year-old man with a history of atrial fibrillation presents to the emergency department with an acutely painful right leg. He undergoes urgent investigation to determine the blood supply to his lower limbs.

This is a contrast study of the right lower limb (demonstrating normal anatomy):

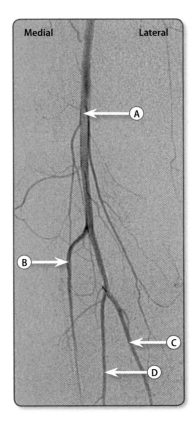

33.1 What is the name of the above investigation?

33.2 Identify the vessels labelled A to D.

33.3 What are the signs and symptoms of an acutely ischaemic limb?

33.4 In which compartment does the vessel labelled D run?

33.5 What are the terminal branches of the vessel labelled C?

33.6 What is the origin of the dorsalis pedis artery?

33.7 What does the sural nerve supply, and what is its origin?

33.8 Between which structures at the medial malleolus does the vessel labelled C run?

Station 34

A 32-year-old male motorcyclist spins off his bike on a motorway. On arrival in the emergency department he is complaining of severe pain in the right hip and a pelvic radiograph confirms dislocation. After assessment you reduce the hip.

A post-reduction radiograph of the right hip is taken:

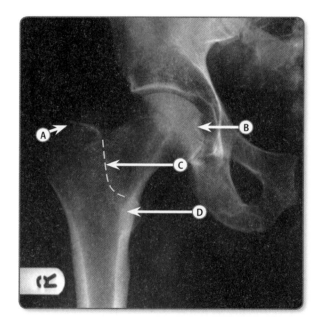

34.1 Identify the structures labelled A, B, C, D.

34.2 What structure attaches to the part labelled B?

34.3 What muscles insert into the part labelled D?

34.4 In which direction does the head of the femur dislocate most commonly?

34.5 Which nerve is at particular risk during the above dislocation?

34.6 How would one clinically assess for damage to this structure?

34.7 Which strong ligaments prevent dislocation of the hip?

34.8 Where is the glenoid capsule attached to the neck of the femur?

Station 35

A 28-year-old woman presents to the orthopaedic clinic 1 week after her knee gave way during the middle of a football match. She has been suffering from pain and swelling since then.

This is a posterior view of the right knee ligaments (demonstrating normal anatomy):

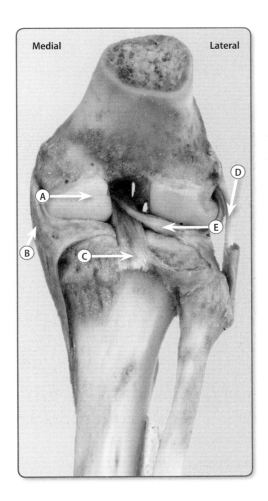

35.1 Identify the structures labelled A to E.

35.2 Which muscles flex and extend the knee?

35.3 What are the common nerve roots for these actions?

35.4 Which ligaments protect the knee?

35.5 What are the attachments of these ligaments?

35.6 What is the function of the menisci of the knee?

35.7 What are the usual actions that cause meniscal tears of the knee?

35.8 What tissue type are the menisci composed of?

Station 36

A 71-year-old woman undergoes elective total hip replacement. She suffers post-operative bleeding and requires emergency evacuation and washout. Five days after this second operation you observe her mobilising on the ward and note that she is suffering from foot drop.

This is a photograph of the buttocks and posterior thigh region:

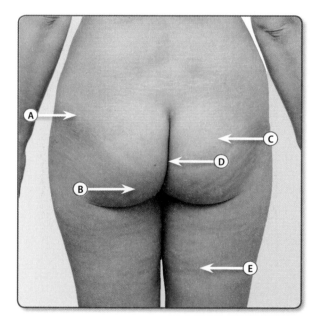

36.1 What bony prominences are palpable at A and B?

36.2 What bulky muscles are palpable at C and E?

36.3 What is the anatomical term for the skin crease at point D?

36.4 What are the surface markings of the sciatic nerve?

36.5 What does Hilton's law state?

36.6 Which muscles comprise the hamstring group?

36.7 What is the origin and insertion of the semimembranosus muscle?

36.8 What is the innervation of the semimembranosus muscle?

Station 37

A 36-year-old man falls off his motorbike whilst travelling at high speed. He complains of severe pain in the pelvis and pelvic radiography reveals fractured pubic rami and bilateral dislocation of the sacroiliac joints.

This is a normal hemipelvis viewed from its lateral surface:

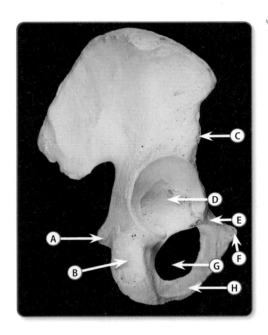

37.1 To which side of the body does this bone belong?

37.2 Identify the parts labelled A to H.

37.3 What attaches to it the part labelled A?

37.4 Which muscles attach to the part labelled B?

37.5 Which muscles attach to the part labelled C?

37.6 What bones comprise the pelvis?

37.7 What type of joint is the symphysis pubis?

37.8 List 3 ways the male differs from the female pelvis.

37.9 What is the origin and insertion of the obturator internus muscle?

37.10 What are the boundaries of the greater sciatic foramen?

37.11 What are the boundaries of the lesser sciatic foramen?

37.12 Over what part of the pelvis does the common iliac artery bifurcate?

37.13 What are the branches of the external iliac artery?

37.14 What are the posterior branches of the internal iliac artery?

Station 38

A 65-year-old diabetic man presents to the vascular clinic with claudication of the right calf. On examination, you detect monophasic signals in the limb and want to investigate further. You discuss the patient with your consultant, who quizzes you on the arterial supply of the lower limb.

This is a digital subtraction angiogram of the lower limbs:

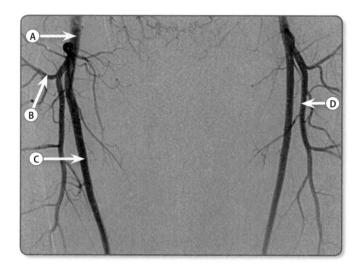

38.1 Identify the arteries labelled A, B, C and D.

38.2 What are the branches of the common femoral artery?

38.3 What are the surface landmarks for palpation of the dorsalis pedis and the posterior tibial arteries?

38.4 By which route can blood reach the foot in complete obstruction of the superficial femoral artery?

38.5 What are the contents of the adductor canal?

38.6 Where does the superficial femoral artery become the popliteal artery?

38.7 Where would you position a Doppler probe to detect the peroneal artery?

Station 39 (Generic)

A 62-year-old man presents to the vascular clinic with varicosities of the right medial ankle. Six months previously he suffered a deep vein thrombosis of this leg.

These images display the medial (a) and posterior (b) aspect of the right leg:

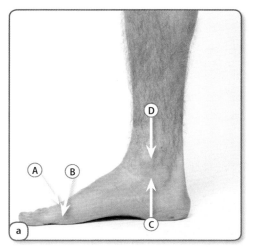
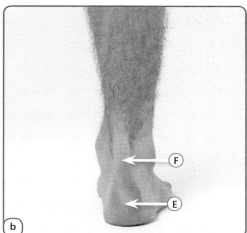

39.1 What tendons run at the points labelled A (with the big toe in extension) and F?

39.2 What bony prominences can be palpated at the points labelled B, C, D, E and F?

39.3 What superficial vein is present in front of the point labelled D?

    39.3a Describe the course of this vein.

    39.3b What nerve accompanies this vein in the lower leg?

    39.3c What tributaries does this vein recieve just before it terminates?

39.4 What superficial vein runs up the posterior midline of the lower leg?

    39.4a Describe the course of this vein.

    39.4b What nerve accompanies this vein in the lower leg?

39.5 Describe the deep venous return of the leg.

39.6 Why might stripping the superficial venous system not be the optimal solution for this patient?

Station 40

A 29-year-old woman sustains a stab wound to the right anterior thigh during a fight. You attend the trauma call and are asked to conduct the secondary survey.

The image on the following page shows the anterior aspect of the thighs. The wounds are indicated by the points labelled A, C and E.

40.1 In which dermatomes are the points B and D located?

40.2 Which cutaneous nerves innervate the points labelled B and D?

40.3 What bulky muscle would a knife probably first encounter at the point labelled C?

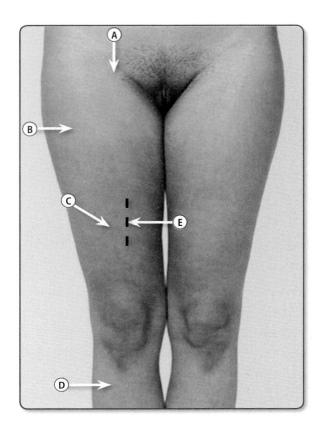

40.4 The wound at point E is opened up by the linear incision shown. What important vessels and nerves would be encountered here?

40.5 What would be the clinical consequences of section of the major nerves encountered at point E?

40.6 Which common nerve roots control flexion and extension of the hip?

40.7 Which muscles cause flexion and extension of the hip?

40.8 What are the origin, insertion and function of the tensor fasciae latae?

Station 41

A 35-year-old woman has been experiencing inferior heel pain and has been diagnosed with plantar fasciitis by her general practitioner. The condition has been refractory to medical treatment, however, and she has been referred to the orthopaedic clinic.

These images display the plantar (a) and dorsal (b) surfaces of the right foot:

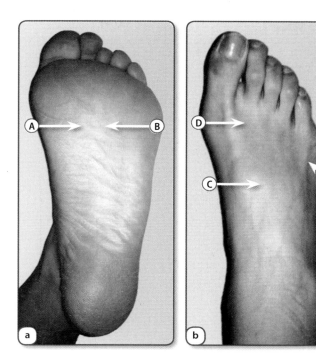

41.1 Which cutaneous nerves supply the points A to E?

41.2 Which dermatomes do the points A to E reside in?

41.3 What are the attachments of the plantar fascia?

41.4 Define the 'sustentaculum'. The tendon of which muscle attaches to it?

41.5 Name the three arches of the foot.

41.6 Where is the insertion of the peroneus longus?

41.7 Where is the insertion of the peroneus brevis?

41.8 Where is the insertion of the peroneus tertius?

41.9 What is the function of the peroneus tertius?

Station 42

A 23-year-old woman trips whilst playing hockey and suffers severe pain and swelling in her left ankle. She presents to the emergency department with a suspected fracture and you are asked to assess her.

The radiographs below show the anteroposterior (a) and lateral (b) radiographs of a normal left ankle joint:

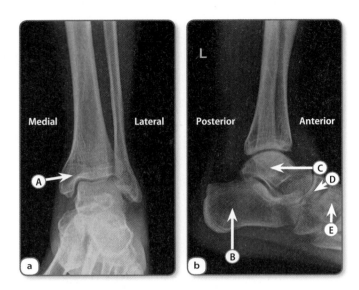

42.1 Identify the bony structures labelled A to E.

42.2 What type of joint is the ankle joint?

42.3 What bones comprise this joint?

42.4 Which nerves supply this joint?

42.5 What are the attachments of the deltoid ligament?

42.6 Which tendons pass behind the lateral malleolus?

42.7 What is the syndesmosis of the ankle?

42.8 What classification system is used for distal fibular fractures?

Station 43

A 24-year-old female dancer trips and stubs her foot whilst performing in a musical play. The foot becomes very painful and swollen over its medial aspect. You assess her in the emergency department and suspect that she has suffered a fracture.

The image on the following page is a radiograph of the bones of the normal left foot.

43.1 Identify the bones labelled A to E.

43.2 Where does the tibialis anterior muscle insert?

43.3 Where does the tibialis posterior muscle insert?

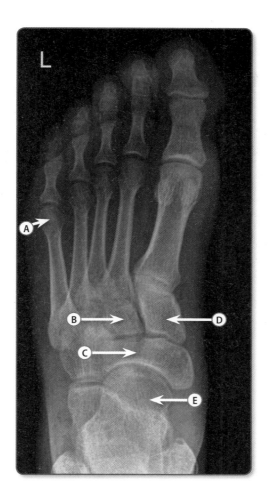

43.4 What muscles cause inversion and eversion of the foot?

43.5 At which bony articulation does inversion/eversion occur?

43.6 What muscles dorsiflex and plantarflex the foot?

43.7 What muscles flex and extend the big toe?

Station 44

A 34-year-old male builder falls from a height onto his back and is taken to the emergency department complaining of severe back pain. A computed tomography scan of his spine reveals multiple fractures in the thoracic and cervical regions and he is taken to theatre for operative fixation.

Image (a) is a vertebra viewed from above:

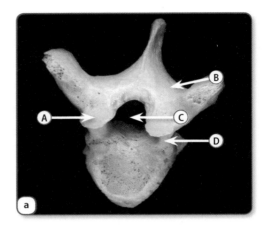

44.1 What segment of the vertebral column is this vertebra from?

44.2 Identify the parts labelled B, C and D.

44.3 What is the part labelled A?

    44.3a What does it articulate with?

    44.3b What type of joint is this?

Image (b) is the same vertebra viewed from the side:

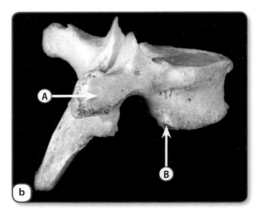

44.4 Identify the part labelled A. What does it articulate with?

44.5 Identify the part labelled B. What does it articulate with?

44.6 Describe the structure and function of the intervertebral discs.

44.7 What layers from skin downwards does a needle pass through during a lumbar puncture to enter the subarachnoid space?

44.8 At what vertebral level does the pia mater end?

44.9 What are the surface landmarks for the correct level to insert a needle during lumbar puncture?

Image (c) is a vertebra from another part of the vertebral column, viewed from above:

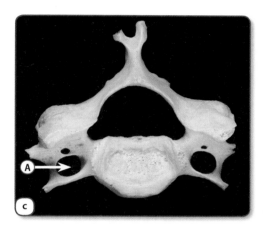

44.10 Which part of the vertebral column is this vertebra from?

44.11 What is the name of the foramen labelled A and what runs in here?

Station 45

A 44-year-old woman presents to the orthopaedic clinic with back pain, which has progressively worsened over the last 6 months. You perform an examination of her back to identify the problem.

The photograph on the next page illustrates some aspects of the surface anatomy of the back.

45.1 What muscle mass is palpable at the point labelled A, attaching to the inferior angle of the scapula?

45.2 What is the action of this muscle?

45.3 What muscle mass is palpable at the points labelled B?

45.4 What parts does this muscle have, what is its innervation, and what action does it exert?

45.5 What muscle mass is palpable at the points labelled C?

45.6 What are its action, origin and insertion?

45.7 In which dermatome is the point labelled D located?

45.8 What bony landmark is palpable at the point labelled E?

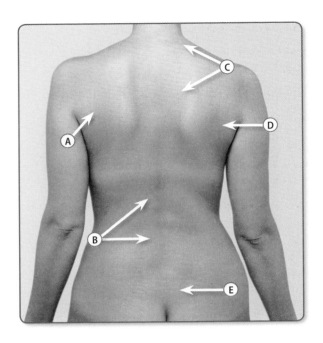

Station 46

A 61-year-old man with prostate cancer presents to the emergency department with severe acute back pain that came on 24 hours ago. He is having trouble walking and confesses to incontinency of urine. You assess him and organise urgent imaging of the spine.

This is a sagittal T2-weighted MRI of a normal spine:

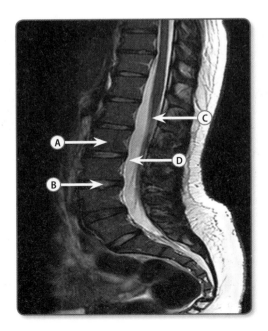

46.1 Identify the structures labelled A to D.

46.2 At what vertebral level does the spinal cord terminate?

46.3 What are the contents of the vertebral canal below this level?

46.4 What is the arterial supply of the spinal cord?

46.5 What is the function of the anterior and lateral spinothalamic tracts?

46.6 What is the function of the posterior columns?

46.7 Do the L3 spinal nerves leave the spinal canal above or below their respective vertebral pedicles?

Station 47

A 46-year-old male porter attends the surgical outpatients clinic complaining of lumbar back pain associated with a sharp shooting pain down his left leg, and some numbness over his big toe and the front of his shin. He has been off work due to the pain for the last month and complains that the lifting he does at work makes the pain worse.

The image below is an axial MRI of a normal lumbar spine at the L5 vertebral level (demonstrating normal anatomy):

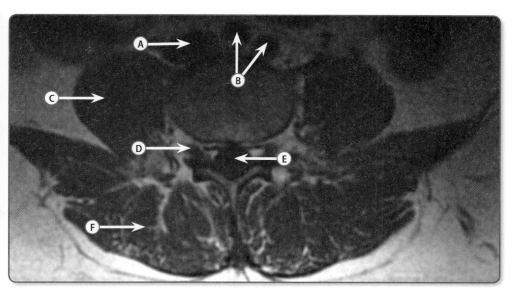

47.1 Identify the structures labelled A to E.

47.2 Given the clinical scenario what is your working diagnosis?

47.3 At what vertebral level do you think the pathology is?

47.4 What is the arterial supply to the intervertebral discs of the lumbar spine?

47.5 What is the venous drainage of the lumbar spine?

Station 48

A 54-year-old male builder attends the emergency department with backache. He has had the pain for the last 6 months but it is a bit worse this afternoon and he wanted to get it 'checked out'. He does not describe any neurological symptoms, but cannot get comfortable despite taking the maximum doses of the painkillers his general practitioner has prescribed him.

The image below is a sagittal MRI of a normal lumbar spine:

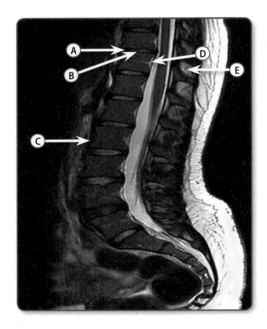

48.1 Identify the parts of the intervertebral disc labelled A and B.

48.2 What type of tissue is the structure labelled A composed of?

48.3 What is the function of the part labelled B within the intervertebral disc?

48.4 Identify the spinal ligaments labelled C, D and E.

48.5 What other unlabelled spinal ligaments provide stability to the vertebral column?

48.6 Where do the spinal ligaments labelled C and D attach?

48.7 Which muscles are responsible for flexion and extension of the lumbar spine?

Station 49

A 19-year-old male medical student is brought into the emergency department after sustaining an injury to his neck during a rugby match. He is complaining of severe neck pain and this was immobilised on scene. He does not report any neurological symptoms.

This is a lateral radiograph of a normal cervical spine:

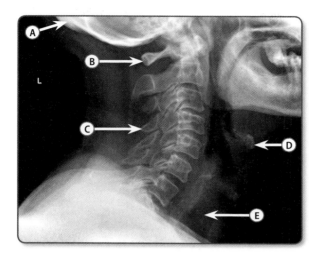

49.1 Identify the structures labelled A to E.

49.2 How does one clinically 'clear' the neck of cervical fracture?

49.3 Which types of cervical fractures are classified as unstable?

49.4 What features of the first cervical vertebra make it different to the cervical vertebrae C3–C7?

49.5 Does an absence of the posterior arch (or lamina) of the first cervical vertebrae cause instability of the cervical vertebral column?

49.6 What features of the second cervical vertebrae (C2) make it different to vertebrae C3–C7?

49.7 Which ligaments confer stability to the atlantoaxial joint?

49.8 How many intervertebral discs are there between the C1 to C7 vertebral bodies?

Answers

Station 1

1.1 T4

1.2 Montgomery's glands (or areolar glands) are sebaceous glands that lubricate the areola and nipple. They are seen as 4–28 tubercles on the areolar surface.

1.3 The breasts develop from a thickening of the ectoderm called the milk ridge (or mammary ridge), which extends from the axilla to the inguinal region. In humans the ridge persists only in the pectoral region. The area thickens and sends off 15–20 cords that grow into underlying mesenchyme. The mesenchyme proliferates and becomes raised to form the nipple.

1.4 Milk is produced in alveoli lined with milk-secreting cuboidal cells. The alveoli form lobules, and groups of lobules form lobes. The average breast has about 15–20 lobes that drain in to lactiferous ducts, which in turn drain in to the lactiferous sinus before departing the body through the nipple.

1.5 A number of changes occur during pregnancy. The secretory alveoli expand and further alveoli bud off. There is an increase in length and branching of the duct system. The vascularity of the connective tissue increases in order to supply the greater demands of the glands. The nipple increases in size and darkens, and the areolar area expands. Growth slows in the latter stages of pregnancy but the breasts continue to increase in size because of alveoli filling with colostrum.

1.6 The lobes of the breast are separated by fibrous septa, the suspensory ligaments of the breast (Cooper's ligaments), which are connected to the subcutaneous tissue. If a malignancy infiltrates the septa then they contract, causing the skin to be drawn inwards.

1.7 During a *simple* mastectomy the entire breast contents are removed but the axillary contents are left untouched. *Radical* mastectomy involves removal of the entire breast along with the axillary lymph nodes. In a classical radical mastectomy the pectoralis major and minor muscles are also removed. In a *modified radical* mastectomy, the pectoral muscles are left intact.

1.8 The 'quadrangular space' is an anatomical space within the axilla (**Figure 2.1**). Its borders are:
- superiorly – subscapularis and teres minor
- inferiorly – teres major
- medially – long head of triceps
- laterally – surgical neck of humerus.

This space transmits the axillary nerve and the posterior circumflex humeral artery and veins.

1.9 The 'triangular space' lies adjacent (medial) to the quadrangular space (**Figure 2.1**). It transmits the circumflex scapular artery. Its borders are:

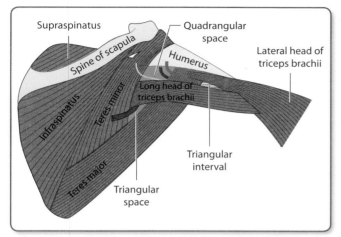

Figure 2.1 The right scapular and axillary regions viewed from behind, showing the triangular space (containing the circumflex scapular artery), triangular interval and quadrangular space (containing the axillary nerve and posterior circumflex humeral vessels).

- superiorly – subscapularis and teres minor
- laterally – long head of triceps
- inferiorly – scapula and teres major.

Note: the 'triangular space' is distinct from the 'triangular interval'. The latter is an area that lies inferolateral to the quadrangular space, with teres major as their shared borders. It transmits the radial nerve and profunda brachii vessels. The boundaries of the triangular interval are:

- superiorly – teres major
- laterally – humerus and lateral head of triceps
- medially – long head of triceps.

Station 2

2.1 The breast extends from the 2nd–6th ribs, from the lateral sternal edge to the midaxillary line. The floor is the pectoralis major muscle, with contributions from the serratus anterior, external oblique muscles and superior rectus sheath.

2.2 A Pectoralis major

   B Fibroglandular tissue

   C Nipple

   D Adipose tissue (breast volume is due to the amount of interposed fatty tissue)

   E Cooper's ligaments (fibrous bands that pass from the chest wall to skin)

2.3 The blood supply to the breast is from perforating branches of the internal thoracic, lateral thoracic and thoracoacromial arteries.

2.4 Most (75%) of the lymph from the breast drains into ipsilateral axillary lymph nodes. Lymph from the nipple and areola drains first into the subareolar plexus before draining into the axillary lymph nodes. The axillary lymph nodes are arranged in five groups (**Table 2.1** and **Figure 2.2**), the position of which is variable.

Table 2.1 The axillary lymph nodes		
Group	**Situated**	**Drains**
Anterior (pectoral)	Medial axillary wall along the lateral thoracic artery	The major part of the lymph drainage from the breast
Posterior	Medial axillary wall behind the anterior group with the subscapular artery	Axillary tail and posterior upper trunk
Lateral	Medial side of axillary vein	Upper limb
Central	The fatty tissue that fills the axilla	The upper three groups of nodes
Apical	The axillary apex	All of the above. Drains into the supraclavicular nodes and to the thoracic duct or right lymphatic trunk.

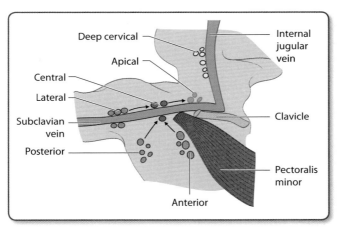

Figure 2.2 The axillary lymph nodes.

Within the deeper aspects of the breast the lymphatics follow the perforating branches of the internal thoracic artery. They travel next with the intercostal arteries and drain into the para-aortic lymph nodes. In this way, cancer may spread from the breast into the thorax. Lymphatic connection across the midline means breast cancer can spread to the contralateral breast.

2.5 Cancer of the breast spreads via the lymphatics. Occasionally the first sign of breast cancer is an isolated enlarged axillary lymph node. The pattern of lymph node involvement is important for staging. Axillary lymph nodes are classified as being at one of three levels depending on their relationship to the pectoralis minor (note, the axillary artery is also divided into three parts according to its relation to the pectoralis minor muscle).

Level 1 – nodes lie distal to the lower border of pectoralis minor

Level 2 – nodes lie deep to the pectoralis minor muscle

Level 3 – nodes lie medial to the upper border of pectoralis minor.

2.6 The axilla is pyramid-shaped with its base comprising deep fascia and overlying skin and its truncated apex formed by the interval between the clavicle, scapula, and first rib. The boundaries of the axilla are:

- medial wall: lateral aspects of ribs 1–4, intervening intercostal spaces, with overlying digitations of serratus anterior
- lateral wall: humerus (specifically the bicipital groove)
- anteriorly: pectoralis major, pectoralis minor and clavipectoral fascia
- posteriorly: scapula, subscapularis, teres major, latissimus dorsi.

2.7 Contents of the axilla:

- axillary artery and its branches
- axillary vein: this vessel lies anteromedial to the axillary artery throughout the axilla
- axillary lymph nodes
- branches of the brachial plexus: the cords enter the axilla from above and surround the second part of the axillary artery. The cords are named after their relationship to the axillary artery (medial, lateral and posterior).
- long and short heads of the biceps brachii and coracobrachialis

2.8 The upper, outer quadrant.

Station 3

3.1 A C6 (**Figure 2.6**)

   B C8

   C T1/T2

3.2 A lateral cutaneous nerve of the forearm

   B medial cutaneous nerve of the forearm

   C medial cutaneous nerve of the arm

3.3 The brachioradialis. Its origin is the upper part of the lateral supracondylar ridge of the humerus, and it inserts onto the styloid process of the radius. Being a posterior compartment muscle it is innervated by the radial nerve.

3.4 E Median cubital vein

3.5 Muscles responsible for supination and pronation at the elbow:

- supination: biceps, supinator
- pronation: pronator teres, pronator quadratus.

3.6 The forearm compartments are divided into: anterior superficial, anterior deep, and posterior superficial and posterior deep.

3.7 The muscles and innervation of the compartments of the forearm are outlined in **Table 2.2**.

Table 2.2 Compartments of the forearm, their muscles, and their innervation

Compartment	Muscles	Innervation
Anterior superficial	Flexor carpi radialis Palmaris longus Pronator teres	Median nerve, except for the flexor carpi ulnaris (ulnar nerve) and ulnar half of flexor digitorum profundus (ulnar nerve)
	Flexor digitorum superficialis Flexor carpi ulnaris	Flexor pollicis longus and pronator quadratus innervated by the anterior interosseous branch of the median nerve
Anterior deep	Flexor digitorum profundus Flexor pollicis longus Pronator quadratus	
Posterior superficial	Brachioradialis Extensor carpi radialis longus Extensor carpi radialis brevis Extensor carpi ulnaris Extensor digitorum Extensor digiti minimi Anconeus	Radial nerve and its derivatives, the deep branch of the radial nerve and the posterior interosseous nerve
Posterior deep	Abductor pollicis longus Extensor pollicis brevis Extensor pollicis longus Extensor indicis Supinator	

3.8 **1** Flexor carpi radialis tendon

2 Flexor digitorum superficialis (this individual lacks a palmaris longus).

3 Flexor carpi ulnaris tendon

Station 4

4.1 **A** Axillary artery

B Circumflex humeral arteries

C Subscapular artery

D Brachial artery

4.2 The axillary artery (A) commences at the lateral border of the first rib (as the continuation of the subclavian artery), and ends at the inferior border of teres major to become the brachial artery.

4.3 The axillary artery is lateral to the axillary vein.

4.4 The axillary artery can be divided into three parts based upon its relationship to pectoralis minor: the first part is medial; the second part is deep; and the third part is distal. The branches of the axillary artery are:

- from the first part: superior thoracic artery
- from the second part: thoracoacromial artery, lateral thoracic artery
- from the third part: subscapular artery, anterior circumflex humeral artery, posterior circumflex humeral artery.

4.5 Branches of D (the brachial artery): ulnar, radial, profunda brachii, superior ulnar collateral, inferior ulnar collateral.

4.6 E Humeral head. The blood supply is from the arcuate artery, a branch of the anterior humeral circumflex artery. It enters the bone between the greater and lesser tubercles. There is also a less important supply from the posterior circumflex humeral artery to an area on the posteroinferior aspect of the head.

4.7 The circumflex scapular artery and the thoracodorsal artery.

Station 5

5.1 Right clavicle. The clavicle is the most frequently fractured long bone in the body. Taken out of its articulations with the manubrium and acromion it can be difficult to orientate, so it is worth familiarizing yourself with a real specimen if possible. The medial two-thirds are circular in cross-section and the lateral one-third is flat. The medial end articulates with the manubrium at the sternoclavicular joint. This synovial joint has an articular disc and allows movement in anteroposterior and vertical planes (allowing a minor degree of rotation). At the lateral end it articulates with the acromion of the scapula at the acromioclavicular joint.

5.2 It functions (i) as an attachment for muscles and (ii) as a strut that transmits forces from the upper limb to the axial frame.

5.3 The sternum (manubrium sterni).

5.4 See **Figure 2.3**.

    A Acromial end and articular surface

    B Conoid tubercle

    C Costoclavicular impression

    D Sternal articular

5.5 See **Figure 2.3**.

    1 Trapezius

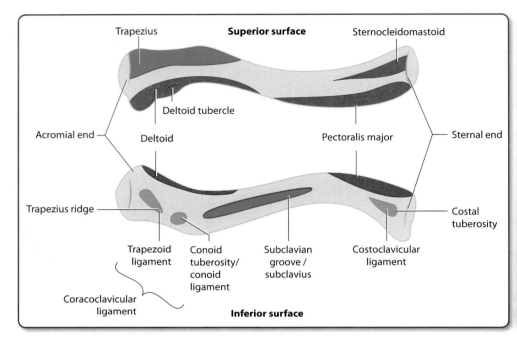

Figure 2.3 The clavicle and its muscular attachments. Red, origin; blue, insertion; green, ligament.

   2 Deltoid

   3 Subclavius

   4 Pectoralis major

5.6 The junction of the middle and outer third as this is the narrowest and weakest part of the bone.

5.7 Clavicular fractures may result in damage to the subclavian vessels and trunks of the brachial plexus, although these neurovascular injuries are quite rare.

5.8 The sternoclavicular joint is an atypical synovial joint.

5.9 The sternoclavicular ligaments anteriorly and posteriorly, and the costoclavicular ligament inferolaterally.

5.10 The subclavius muscle.

5.11 Approximate normal values for shoulder range of movement are given in **Table 2.3**.

5.12 Approximate normal values for elbow range of movement are given in **Table 2.4**.

Station 6

6.1 A Left median nerve

   B Left pronator teres muscle

Table 2.3 Normal values for shoulder range of movement (from the anatomical position)

Flexion	120°
Extension	30°
Abduction	165°
Adduction	55°
External rotation	70°
Internal rotation	105°

Table 2.4 Normal values for elbow range of movement (from the anatomical position)

Flexion	145°
Extension	0-5°
Supination	90°
Pronation	90°

C Left ulnar artery

D Left cephalic vein

E Left brachial artery

F Left biceps tendon

G Left brachioradialis muscle

H Left radial artery

6.2 Brachioradialis (G) originates from the lateral supracondylar ridge of the humerus, and inserts onto the base of the styloid process of the radius. It is a flexor of the semi-pronated elbow and is innervated by the radial nerve (being a posterior compartment muscle).

6.3 Boundaries of the cubital fossa:
- lateral: brachioradialis
- medial: pronator teres
- proximal: a line running from the medial to lateral epicondyles of the humerus
- roof: deep fascia
- floor: brachialis.

6.4 The bicipital aponeurosis lies between the median cubital vein and the brachial artery.

6.5 The annular ligament wraps around the radial head and neck and is attached to the margins of the radial notch of the ulna. It allows rotation of the radius about a virtually fixed ulna.

6.6 Common flexor origin: anterior aspect of medial epicondyle.

Common extensor origin: anterior aspect of lateral epicondyle.

6.7 The anconeus is a small muscle that originates from the lateral epicondyle and inserts onto the olecranon process of the ulna. It aids in extension of the elbow and stabilises the joint.

6.8 The ulnar nerve is medial to the ulnar artery.

6.9 The flexor carpi radialis tendon is lateral to the median nerve.

Station 7

7.1 Right humerus.

7.2 H2 is the surgical, and H1 is the anatomical neck of the humerus.

7.3 See **Figure 2.4**.

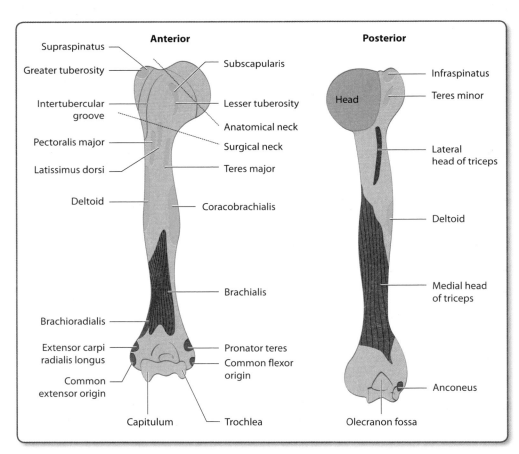

Figure 2.4 The humerus and its muscular and ligamentous attachments. Red, origin; blue, insertion.

   A Head of humerus

   B Greater tubercle

   C Intertubercular sulcus

   D Lesser tubercle

   E Shaft of humerus

   F Capitulum

   G Medial epicondyle

   H Trochlea

7.4 B Supraspinatus, infraspinatus, teres minor.

7.5 G Subscapularis.

7.6 H This is the common flexor origin of the forearm.

7.7 Origin: long head – infraglenoid tubercle of scapula. Medial and lateral head – dorsal surface of humerus (the medial head is more distal than the lateral head). Insertion: olecranon process of the ulna.

7.8 1 Axillary nerve

   2 Radial nerve

   3 Median nerve

7.9 The acromion process.

7.10 The supraspinatus initiates abduction of the arm to about 15°, the deltoid then abducts to 90°. Movement from 90 to 180° is achieved through rotation of the scapula by the trapezius and serratus anterior.

7.11 Fractures of the radial head and neck, medial epicondyle and coronoid process.

Station 8

8.1 This is a digital subtraction venogram of the left upper limb.

8.2 See **Figure 2.5**.

   A Superior vena cava

   B Left brachiocephalic vein (or left innominate vein)

   C Left subclavian vein

   D Left axillary vein

8.3 D (the axillary vein) originates at the inferior border of the teres major where it receives its superficial tributaries (the basilic and cephalic veins). It is a continuation

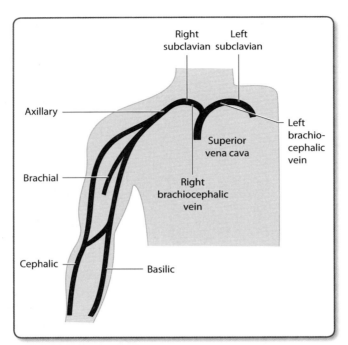

Figure 2.5 Superficial veins of the upper limb.

of the brachial vein (a deep vein). It terminates at the lateral border of the first rib where it continues as the subclavian vein.

8.4 Tributaries of D (axillary vein) include the brachial, cephalic and basilic veins and various other unnamed tributaries in the axilla.

8.5 The internal jugular vein joins the subclavian to form B, the brachiocephalic (or innominate) vein bilaterally, which then drain into the superior vena cava.

8.6 The axillary vein is superficial to the axillary artery.

8.7 The superficial veins begin as a network over the dorsum of the hand. The cephalic vein has a constant position behind the radial styloid and runs up the lateral border of the forearm. In the upper arm it lies lateral to the biceps and perforates the clavipectoral fascia to run deep, and drains in to the axillary vein.

The basilic vein runs up the medial border of the forearm and lies medial to the biceps brachii in the upper arm. It pierces the deep fascia halfway between the elbow and the axilla. The median cubital vein joins the basilic and cephalic veins to each other slightly distal to the elbow.

8.8 The deep veins of the hand and forearm resemble the arteries, with superficial and deep palmer arches draining in to ulnar and radial veins before merging to form the brachial vein.

Station 9

9.1 The shoulder joint is a ball and socket joint consisting of the head of the humerus articulating with the glenoid fossa of the scapula. It is deepened by the cartilaginous glenoid labrum. It is a synovial joint and hence has a capsule lined by synovial membrane, extending down to the diaphysis of the humerus.

9.2 A Greater tubercle of humerus. This is the insertion point of the supraspinatus, infraspinatus, and teres minor muscles.

9.3 B Intertubercular sulcus (or bicipital groove). Attachments: Teres major, latissimus dorsi, and pectoralis major.

9.4 C Acromion process.

9.5 The glenoid cavity of the shoulder is shallow compared to the hip socket. This allows it a greater degree of freedom but also makes it at higher risk of dislocation. The rotator cuff group of muscles are the main stabilisers of the shoulder. These consist of the supraspinatus, infraspinatus, teres minor (all of which insert in to the greater tuberosity of the humerus), and the subscapularis (which inserts in to the lesser tuberosity). The shoulder is also stabilised to a lesser extent by other surrounding muscles such as the deltoid, latissimus dorsi, and pectoralis major. The long head of the biceps brachii, running through the joint capsule, also contributes to joint stability.

9.6 The most common type of dislocation is anterior (more specifically, anteroinferior) in approximately 95% of cases. Commonly damaged structures include: nerves of the brachial plexus (especially the axillary and the radial nerves), the axillary artery, and the humeral head.

9.7 Subacromial, subscapular bursae.

9.8 A Bankart's lesion is the avulsion of the anteroinferior glenoid labrum at its attachment to the glenohumeral ligament complex. The joint capsule and inferior glenohumeral ligaments are damaged.

A Hill–Sachs lesion is an indentation fracture in the posterolateral region of the humeral head, caused when the humeral head impacts against the anterior glenoid rim during dislocation.

9.9 The arm is divided by an intermuscular septum in to anterior and posterior compartments.

The contents of the compartments of the upper arm are given in **Table 2.5**.

Table 2.5 Compartments of the upper arm		
	Posterior compartment	**Anterior compartment**
Muscles	Triceps brachii Anconeus	Biceps brachii Coracobrachialis Brachialis
Arteries	Profunda brachii Ulnar collateral	Brachial
Nerves	Ulnar Radial	Ulnar Median Musculocutaneous

Station 10

10.1 The anatomical snuff box.

10.2 Scaphoid bone. The clinical recognition of scaphoid fracture is important, as fractures do not always appear on radiographs in the acute stage. Untreated fractures may lead to avascular necrosis of the proximal segment due to the retrograde vascular supply of this part.

10.3 Contents of the anatomical snuffbox: radial artery (the cephalic vein and radial nerve overlie this space).

10.4 **A** Medial border of snuff box: extensor pollicis longus.

B & C Lateral border of snuff box: abductor pollicis longus and extensor pollicis brevis.

Note: to remember this imagine that extensor pollicis is on either side of the snuff box, however 'brevis' is too 'little' to be on the outer edge all on its own and so is accompanied by abductor pollicis longus.

The floor is the scaphoid and trapezium. The proximal border is the styloid process of the radius.

10.5 Superficial branch of the radial nerve (this actually innervates a wider space, but the area that is shown is without overlap from other nerves).

10.6 The radial nerve originates from the posterior cord of the brachial plexus (C5–T1). It leaves the axilla and traverses the triangular space of the arm. It then descends in the extensor compartment behind the medial head of triceps brachii (supplying the extensors of the upper arm) before occupying the radial groove on the posterior surface of the humerus. The nerve pierces the lateral intermuscular septum to emerge in the anterolateral aspect of the forearm between the brachioradialis (superficial) and brachialis (deep). At this level it divides into its *superficial* and *deep* branches.

The *deep* branch is known as the *posterior interosseous nerve* after it passes between the two heads of the supinator muscle and is responsible for the motor innervation of all forearm extensors. At the mid forearm the nerve passes close to the anterior interosseous artery and passes deep to extensor digitorum in the extensor retinaculum, ending at the back of the wrist to supply the wrist joint. The *superficial* branch is sensory. It passes down the forearm lateral to the radial artery eventually passing over the anatomical snuffbox to innervate the dorsal first web space.

10.7 The muscles that the radial nerve innervates are given in **Table 2.6**.

10.8 The consequences of radial nerve damage are given in **Table 2.7**.

10.9 **D** C8 dermatome (**Figure 2.6**).

10.10 Dorsal cutaneous branch of the ulnar nerve.

Table 2.6 Muscles innervated by the radial nerve

Muscular branches within the upper arm	Triceps brachii (lateral and medial heads)	Extends the elbow joint
	Anconeus	Assists triceps in elbow extension
	Brachioradialis	Flexes the elbow joint
	Extensor carpi radialis longus	Extends the wrist joint
Deep branches	Extensor carpi radialis brevis	Extends the wrist joint
		Abducts the thumb
	Supinator	Supinates the forearm
Posterior interosseus nerve (a continuation of the deep branches)	Extensor digitorum	Extends proximal phalanges and wrist
	Extensor digiti minimi	Extends the little finger
	Extensor carpi ulnaris	Extends wrist (with an ulnar deviation)
	Extensor pollicis longus	Extends interphalangeal joint of the thumb
	Extensor pollicis brevis	Extends and abducts the thumb
	Extensor indicis	Extends the index finger, wrist and midcarpal joints
	Abductor pollicis longus	Abducts the thumb

Table 2.7 Consequences of radial nerve damage

Type of nerve damage	Causes	Motor	Sensory
Radial nerve within the axilla	Compression injuries such as ill-fitted crutches and 'Saturday night palsy' (falling asleep with an arm hung over the back of a chair)	Loss of the elbow extensors (including triceps reflex), wrist drop due to loss of wrist extensors, weakness of extensors of fingers. Note that with loss of wrist extension it becomes very difficult to grip objects and hence flexion of the fingers is also impaired	Loss of sensation over the back of the arm/forearm (posterior cutaneous nerve of arm), lower lateral part of arm (inferior lateral cutaneous nerve of arm) and a patch of skin over the dorsal first web space
Radial nerve at level of humerus	Fractures of humerus	Same as above, but with preservation of elbow extensors	Loss of sensation over the lateral forearm and a patch of skin over the dorsal first web space

Contd...

Table 2.7 cont.

Type of nerve damage	Causes	Motor	Sensory
Posterior interosseus nerve in forearm	Fractures/dislocations of radial head	Same as above, except that wrist extension is preserved due to the extensor carpi radialis longus	None (due to preservation of superficial radial nerve)
Posterior interosseus nerve at wrist	Traumatic laceration	None	None (due to preservation of superficial radial nerve)
Superficial radial nerve	Traumatic laceration	None	Patch of skin over the dorsal first web space

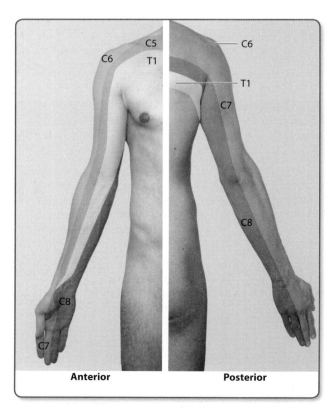

Figure 2.6 Upper limb dermatomes.

Station 11

11.1 A Sternocleidomastoid

11.2 Working by itself each sternocleidomastoid muscle flexes the neck and simultaneously rotates the neck to the other side. Working together, the two sternocleidomastoids are powerful flexors of the neck. The sternocleidomastoid has two heads: a tendinous sternal head (arising from the anterosuperior surface of the manubrium sterni) and a clavicular head (arising from the medial third of the upper surface of the clavicle). It inserts into the lateral surface of the mastoid process and the superior nuchal line just medial to the mastoid process. The muscle is innervated by the spinal accessory nerve.

11.3 The clavicle.

11.4a The acromioclavicular (AC) joint.

11.4b Atypical synovial joint. A joint capsule provides a tough fibrous layer. This is lined on the inside with synovial membrane (that secretes synovial fluid). The joint surfaces are covered in fibrocartilage and not articular hyaline cartilage, as are most synovial joints. The AC joint has an intraarticular disc of fibrocartilage.

11.4c Two ligaments stabilize the joint predominantly: the acromioclavicular ligament, and the coracoclavicular ligament. The acromioclavicular ligament is important for horizontal stability. The coracoclavicular ligament comprises two parts: the conoid and trapezoid ligaments which together help maintain vertical stability.

11.5 The axillary nerve (C5 and C6, via the upper lateral cutaneous nerve of the arm) supplies this area of skin, known as the 'regimental badge'. This nerve can be damaged during anteroinferior dislocation of the humerus, and so its presence should be tested before reducing these injuries. It can also be damaged during fractures of the surgical neck of the humerus, or after prolonged heavy compression with a crutch.

11.6 The axillary nerve innervates deltoid and teres minor.

11.7 Posterior cord.

11.8 A Infraspinatus

B Subscapularis

C Axillary artery (with the accompanying subclavian vein just superficial.

Note: how the thinner walled vein is easily compressed and does not maintain its circular cross-sectional structure unlike the thicker walled artery).

D Deltoid muscle

E Lung

11.9 The rotator cuff muscles of the shoulder can be remembered by the mnemonic **SITS**: **S**upraspinatus, **I**nfraspinatus, **T**eres minor, and **S**ubscapularis (**Figure 2.7**).

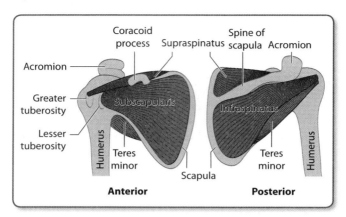

Figure 2.7 The rotator cuff muscles.

11.10 **Table 2.8** illustrates the actions, and other important features of the rotator cuff.

11.11 **D** Deltoid muscle. Due to its macroscopic structure comprising anterior, posterior, and lateral fibres, it assists in the actions mainly of shoulder abduction but also plays a smaller part in shoulder flexion and extension.

Table 2.8 The rotator cuff muscles

Muscle	Origin	Insertion	Innervation	Action
Supraspinatus	Supraspinous fossa of the scapula	Greater tubercle of humerus	Suprascapular nerve	Initiates abduction Internal rotation
Infraspinatus	Infraspinous fossa of the scapula	Greater tubercle of humerus	Suprascapular nerve	External rotation
Teres minor	Dorsum of lateral border of the scapula	Greater tubercle of humerus	Axillary nerve	External rotation
Subscapularis	Subscapular fossa on the anterior surface of the scapula	Lesser tubercle of humerus	Upper and lower subscapular nerves	Internal rotation Adduction

Station 12

12.1 **A** Styloid process

   D Bicipital (or radial) tuberosity

   E Radial head

12.2 The ulna.

12.3 The pronator quadratus.

12.4 This is a pronator of the forearm and is innervated by the anterior interosseous nerve. It originates from the anteromedial aspect of the distal ulnar shaft, and inserts onto the anterolateral aspect of the distal part of the shaft of the radius and the interosseous membrane.

12.5 Supinator has two heads: one arises from the lateral epicondyle of the humerus and the annular ligament, and the other arises from the ulna. It inserts onto the neck and shaft of the radius. The muscle is a supinator of the forearm when the elbow is extended, and is innervated by the posterior interosseous nerve.

12.6 The biceps tendon.

12.7 The annular ligament.

12.8 Galeazzi's fracture is a fracture of the proximal third of the radius with dislocation of the distal radioulnar joint.

12.9 Monteggia's fracture is a fracture of the shaft of the ulna with anterior dislocation of the radial head (with rupture of the annular ligament). It is often caused by a direct blow to the back of the upper forearm.

Station 13

13.1 **A** Olecranon

    B Trochlear notch

    C Coronoid process

    D Tuberosity

    F Styloid process

13.2 The head is at the distal end of the ulna, unlike the radius where it is proximal.

13.3 The triangular coronoid process is on the anterior surface of the ulnar below the olecranon process (C). On its lateral surface it has a radial notch for articulation with the radius.

13.4 **E** Flexor digitorum profundus.

13.5 The abductor pollicis longus arises from the upper posterior ulna, the posterior shaft of the radius, and the interosseous membrane. The muscle inserts into the base of the first metacarpal bone. It is an abductor and extensor of the thumb and is innervated by the deep branch of the radial nerve.

13.6 A syndesmosis joint (a slightly movable articulation where the bony surfaces are united by an interosseous ligament).

13.7a Elbow flexion: biceps brachii, brachialis, brachioradialis, forearm flexors.

13.7b Elbow extension: triceps, anconeus.

13.8 A bursa is a fibrous sac lined by synovial membrane filled with a film of viscous fluid. They occur close to joints and reduce friction between tendons and other structures. A synovial sheath is a tubular bursa surrounding a tendon. Bursitis is inflammation of a bursa. It can be caused by repetitive movement or by inflammatory conditions such as rheumatoid arthritis.

Station 14

14.1 This is the right scapula. This bone can be difficult to side, but remember that the glenoid fossa faces outwards, the coracoid process forwards and the spine faces backwards.

14.2 A Spine

   B Supraspinous fossa

   C Coracoid process

   D Acromion process

   E Margin of the glenoid cavity

   F Infraspinous fossa

14.3 B Supraspinatus

   F Infraspinatus

   A Trapezius, deltoid

   Table 2.9 and **Figure 2.8** lists the muscular attachments of the scapula.

Table 2.9 Muscular attachments of the scapula	
Dorsal (posterior) aspect	Supraspinatus attaches superior to the dorsal spine
	Infraspinatus attaches inferior to the spine
Lateral border (superior to inferior)	The long head of triceps
	Teres minor
	Teres major
	Latissimus dorsi (from the tip of the angle of the scapula)
Medial border	Rhomboid major
	Rhomboid minor
	Levator scapula
Costal (internal/anterior) surface	Subscapularis occupies the majority of the surface
	Serratus anterior is attached along the medial and inferior borders
Spine	Trapezius is attached along the superior aspect of the spine
	Deltoid is attached along the inferior aspect of the spine

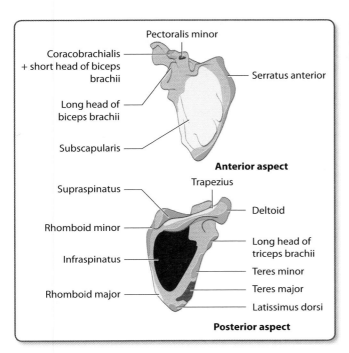

Figure 2.8 Muscular attachments of the scapula.

14.4 T7

14.5 T3

14.6 Attachments to C (coracoid process): pectoralis minor, coracobrachialis and short head of biceps brachii muscle.

14.7 The long head of biceps brachii muscle originates from the supraglenoid tubercle.

14.8 The long head of the triceps brachii muscle originates from infraglenoid tubercle.

14.9 Muscles responsible for movements at the shoulder are given in **Table 2.10**.

Table 2.10 Muscles causing movements of the shoulder	
Adduction	Pectoralis major, latissimus dorsi, teres major, triceps, subscapularis
Abduction	Deltoid, supraspinatus
Flexion	Pectoralis major, anterior fibres of the deltoid, coracobrachialis, biceps brachii
Extension	Latissimus dorsi, posterior fibres of the deltoid, triceps and teres major
Medial (internal) rotation	Subscapularis, pectoralis major, anterior fibres of deltoid, latissimus dorsi, teres major
Lateral (external) rotation	Infraspinatus, teres minor, posterior fibres of the deltoid

14.10 See **Table 2.10**.

Station 15

15.1 Flexion of the thumb

15.2 Flexor pollicis longus and brevis, median nerve.

15.3 Red arrow: adduction.
Blue arrow: abduction.

15.4 **Table 2.11** lists the movements of the thumb, the muscles involved, and their innervation.

Table 2.11 Movements of the thumb		
Movement	**Muscles involved**	**Innervation**
Flexion	Flexor pollicis longus	Median nerve
	Flexor pollicis brevis	
Extension	Extensor pollicis longus	Radial nerve
	Extensor pollicis brevis	
	Abductor pollicis longus	
Abduction	Abductor pollicis brevis	Median nerve
Adduction	Adductor pollicis	Ulnar nerve
Opposition	Opponens pollicis	Median nerve

15.5 The other actions include opposition and extension.

15.6 The main classification of joints is outlined in **Table 2.12**.

15.7 The carpometacarpal joint of the thumb is a saddle joint.

15.8 Froment's sign. A piece of paper is placed between the thumb and index finger and the patient is asked to hold it there whilst the examiner pulls it out. Patients with ulnar nerve damage have impaired adductor pollicis, but cheat by using their flexor pollicis longus to hold the paper in place (median nerve).

15.9 Ulnar nerve injury. Traumatic laceration, fracture of the humerus, cubital tunnel syndrome.

15.10 Commonly tested are abduction and adduction of the fingers. There may be weakness of any of the muscles supplied by the ulnar nerve. These are outlined in **Table 2.13**.

15.11 The ulnar nerve is the continuation of the medial cord of the brachial plexus (C8–T1). It descends in the arm behind the brachial artery, angling backwards and

Table 2.12 Classification of joints

Type of joint	Structures	Examples
Fibrous (immoveable)	Held together by a ligament	Radioulnar Talofibular joint
Cartilaginous (slightly moveable)	The articulating surfaces of the bones are cartilaginous. • *Primary* cartilaginous joints (known as 'synchondroses') are joined by hyaline cartilage, which may ossify with age. • *Secondary* cartilaginous joints (known as 'symphyses') have a compressible pad of fibrocartilage between the hyaline covered bone endings.	Primary: the first sternocostal joint Secondary: pubic symphysis
Synovial (freely moveable)	A synovial capsule surrounds the joint with an inner synovial membrane that secretes synovial fluid. Hyaline cartilage is at the articulating ends of the bones. There are six subtypes of synovial joints classified by the shape of the joint.	Ball and socket: glenohumeral joint Saddle: carpometacarpal joint of the thumb Condyloid: metacarpophalangeal joints Hinge: elbow joint Pivot: atlantoaxial joint Gliding: intercarpal joints

passing through the intermuscular septum behind the medial epicondyle of the humerus and anterior to the olecranon. Within the upper arm it does not give off any branches. In the forearm the nerve passes between the two heads of the flexor carpi ulnaris on the surface of the flexor digitorum profundus. It emerges at the wrist medial to the ulnar artery (lateral to the flexor carpi ulnaris) and crosses the wrist above the flexor retinaculum (transverse carpal ligament).

The branches of the ulnar nerve comprise:

- muscular branches supplying flexor carpi ulnaris and medial half of flexor digitorum profundus
- palmar cutaneous branch supplying skin over the medial part of the palm
- dorsal cutaneous branch supplying skin to medial one and a half digits dorsally
- superficial branch supplying only the palmaris brevis muscle
- a deep branch supplying the adductor pollicis, hypothenar, interossei and ulnar lumbricals.

Table 2.13 Muscles supplied by the ulnar nerve

Muscle type	Muscles	Movement
Muscular branches within the upper arm	Flexor carpi ulnaris	Flexes and adducts wrist
	Flexor digitorum profundus (medial part)	Flexes the fingers and wrist
Deep branch within the hand	Adductor pollicis	Adducts the metacarpal of the thumb (deep branch of ulnar nerve)
	Abductor digiti minimi	Abducts the little finger
	Flexor digiti minimi	Flexes and abducts the little finger
	Opponens digiti minimi	Opposes little finger with thumb
	Three palmar interossei	Deep branch of ulnar nerve, adduct the fingers and thumb. In addition, they flex the metacarpophalangeal joint and extend the interphalangeal joints.
	Four dorsal interossei	Deep branch of ulnar branch, abduct the index, middle and ring fingers at metacarpophalangeal joint. Flex a straight finger.
	Lumbricals (third and fourth)	Flexes the metacarpophalangeal joint and extends the interphalangeal joints simultaneously
Superficial branch within hand	Palmaris brevis	Deepens the hollow in the palm of the hand (superficial branch)

15.12 With ulna nerve lesions, 'clawing' may occur due to denervation of the medial two lumbricals of the hand. The lumbricals normally flex the metacarpophalangeal joints and so their denervation causes these joints to become extended by the newly unopposed action of the forearm extensors. The 'claw' is completed by slight flexion of the interphalangeal joints occurs due to the pull of the flexor digitorum profundus (ulnar nerve for these fingers). However, in higher lesions the profundus is also paralysed and so the fingers look less like a claw.

Station 16

16.1 The thenar eminence is formed from three muscles: flexor pollicis brevis, abductor pollicis brevis and opponens pollicis. Adductor pollicis is not part of the thenar eminence and the remaining muscles that act on the thumb (flexor pollicis longus, adductor pollicis, and abductor pollicis longus) are located within the forearm.

16.2 Hypothenar muscles: flexor digiti minimi brevis, abductor digiti minimi, and opponens digiti mini. Note that the names of the hypothenar muscles complement the thenar muscles.

16.3 C Median nerve (C5–T1)

16.4 D Ulnar nerve (C8–T1)

16.5 E Metacarpophalangeal joint of the thumb. Flexion is achieved with flexor pollicis longus and flexor pollicis brevis.

16.6 F Distal interphalangeal joint of the index finger. Flexion is achieved with flexor digitorum profundus.

G Proximal interphalangeal joint of the ring finger. Flexion is achieved with flexor digitorum superficialis and flexor digitorum profundus.

16.7 The lumbrical muscles flex the metacarpophalangeal joints whilst extending the interphalangeal joints. Other muscles acting on the fingers include the flexor digitorum superficialis, flexor digitorum profundus, and interossei. The flexor digitorum superficialis inserts into the middle phalanx and flexes the proximal interphalangeal joints primarily, but also the metacarpophalangeal and wrist joints to a lesser extent. The flexor digitorum profundus tendons insert into the distal phalanx and cause distal interphalangeal joint flexion, but also flexion of the proximal, metacarpophalangeal and wrist joints to a lesser extent.

16.8 The *dorsal interossei* are bipennate muscles that have two heads originating from adjacent metacarpals. They insert into the bases of the proximal phalanx and extensor expansions of their corresponding digits. Their primary function is to flex the metacarpophalangeal joints and extend the interphalangeal joints (like the lumbricals). Their secondary function is to abduct the fingers away from the axis of the middle finger.

The *palmer interossei* are unipennate muscles that originate from the sides of the metacarpals and insert in to the base of the proximal phalanx of the same digit. Their function is to adduct the fingers towards the middle finger.

A mnemonic for the actions of the interossei is: **DAB** (short for **Dorsal AB**ducts) and **PAD** (short for **Palmar AD**ducts).

16.9 The digital nerve.

Station 17

17.1 A Scaphoid bone

B Radius bone

C First metacarpal bone

D Lunate bone (It looks very 'lunar')

E Ulnar bone

17.2 No. It is quite common for a scaphoid fracture to be unnoticeable on an initial plain film of the carpal bones and a repeat film taken 7–10 days after the initial injury is recommended to ensure that any developing necrosis of the bone is not missed.

17.3 The blood supply to the scaphoid bone is from the radial artery via two routes. The main supply is via dorsal branches of the radial artery that enter the scaphoid on its dorsal surface at approximately the 'waist' of the bone. These vessels supply the waist and proximal pole of the scaphoid bone in a retrograde fashion. The remainder of the blood supply is via palmar branches of the radial artery that supply the distal aspect of the bone. These branches enter the scaphoid at its distal pole (**Figure 2.9**).

17.4 It is important to detect an injury to the scaphoid early as the blood supply to the bone may be impaired. Should this occur, there is a high likelihood of avascular necrosis.

17.5 The proximal pole of the scaphoid is most at risk of avascular necrosis due to its lack of collateral blood supply. A fracture at the distal pole and waist of the scaphoid poses less of a risk of avascular necrosis compared to one more proximal that disrupts the major arterial supply to the bone (**Figure 2.10**).

17.6 Bones which are commonly affected by avascular necrosis are listed in **Table 2.14**.

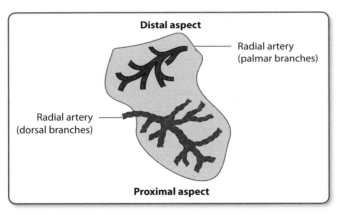

Figure 2.9 Vascular arterial supply to the scaphoid bone.

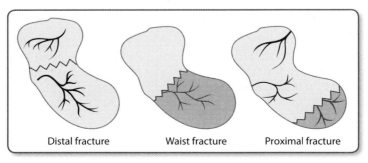

Figure 2.10 Demonstration of how various fractures of the scaphoid bone result in the likelihood of avascular necrosis (area at risk shaded in pink).

Table 2.14 Common sites for avascular necrosis

Bone affected	Eponymous name of fracture	Comments
Scaphoid	None	The proximal pole of the scaphoid is at risk of avascular necrosis due to its lack of collateral blood supply
Lunate	Kienböck's disease	Rare Affects the dominant hand of the patient in over two-thirds of cases
Head of the second or third metatarsal bones	Freiberg's infarction	Seen in young female runners Pain is usually felt in the forefoot and may resolve spontaneously
Talus	Diaz disease	Can lead to total loss of the ankle joint with destruction and deformity in severe cases.
Navicular	Kohler's disease	Frequently self-limiting and unilateral More common in males
Femoral head	Perthes' disease (in children), Chandler's disease (if cause is idiopathic in adults)	Presents with hip pain The treatment is to avoid remove force on this joint until the condition has resolved

17.7 Other medical conditions to ask about include sickle cell disease, previous radiotherapy, corticosteroid usage, and autoimmune conditions such as rheumatoid arthritis and systemic lupus erythematosus.

Station 18

18.1 A The proximal interphalangeal joint is a synovial hinge joint. It has a palmar ligament (known as the volar plate), and two collateral ligaments.

B The metacarpophalangeal joint is a synovial condyloid joint. It is protected by palmer and collateral ligaments. The deep transverse metacarpal ligament unites the palmer ligaments of the 2nd–5th joints.

18.2 C Superficial palmar arch

D Deep palmar arch

18.3 The thenar space is a potential compartment in the hand in to which infection can spread (**Figure 2.11**). The boundaries of the thenar space are:
- medially: the intermediate palmer septum (which connects the deep surface of the lateral part of the palmar aponeurosis to the front of the third metacarpal bone)
- laterally: lateral palmar septum
- anteriorly: the lateral part of palmar aponeurosis
- posteriorly: adductor pollicis
- distally: proximal transverse crease of palm
- proximally: distal margin of flexor retinaculum (transverse carpal ligament).

18.4 The boundaries of the mid-palmar space (**Figure 2.11**):
- medially: medial palmar septum
- laterally: intermediate palmar septum (the lateral border of the mid-palmar space is the medial border of the thenar space)
- anteriorly: medial part of palmar aponeurosis, and flexor tendons to medial three fingers
- posteriorly: fascia covering the medial three metacarpal bones and interosseous muscles
- distally: distal transverse crease of palm
- proximally: distal margin of flexor retinaculum (transverse carpal ligament).

18.5 The flexor tendons of the digits travel within fibrous flexor sheaths. The distal limit of the sheaths is the insertion of the profundus tendon at the base of the distal phalanx. The proximal limit of the sheaths of the 2nd–4th digits is the metacarpal heads, but the sheaths of the little finger and thumb extend past the wrist. This continuation of the sheath for the thumb is termed the radial bursa and that for the little finger the ulnar bursa. Infections of the thumb and little finger can therefore readily spread into the palm.

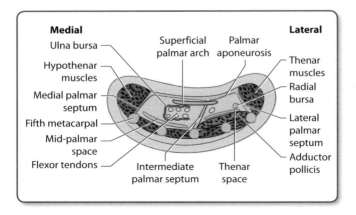

Figure 2.11 Spaces of the hand, axial view from below.

18.6 Kanavel described four cardinal signs of infectious flexor tenosynovitis:
- fusiform digital swelling
- semi-flexed digital posture
- pain on passive extension
- tenderness along the flexor tendon sheath.

18.7 Paronychia is infection of the soft tissues folds surrounding the proximal nail. The lateral nail fold is termed the paronychial fold, and the infection usually starts here. It may extend to the proximal fold, the eponychium, and even to the contralateral paronychial fold ('horseshoe infection'). *Staphylococcus aureus* is the typical organism and the treatment is antibiotics and drainage.

18.8 E Lunula. This is a crescent shaped area that is the visible part of the germinal matrix of the nail.

18.9 Felon is infection of the distal volar pulp space of the digits. This space is composed of fat broken up between multiple fibrous septa connecting the subcutaneous layer to the bone. If one of these compartments becomes infected and oedematous then there is little room for expansion and the pressure increases. Not only is this extremely painful but it can compromise the blood supply and cause necrosis of the tip of the distal phalanx. Other complications include proximal spread of infection, flexor tenosynovitis, osteomyelitis, septic arthritis of the distal interphalangeal joint, and paronychia.

Station 19

19.1 See **Figure 2.12**.

   A Hypothenar muscles

   B Thenar muscles

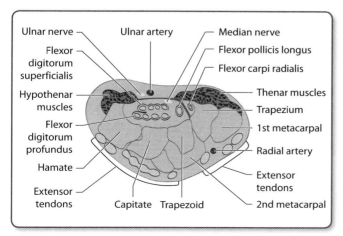

Figure 2.12 The carpal tunnel, axial view from below.

Note

The MRI in this station can be confusing to the unfamiliar candidate because of its orientation. The best method to determine the orientation of the scan is to remember that the flexor carpi radialis, whilst within the carpal tunnel, does not lie within the same fascial compartment as the other ten structures. Once you identify this structure you know that the side where this tendon lies is therefore radial (lateral).

19.2 **C** Flexor digitorum superficialis muscle tendons

D Flexor pollicis longus muscle tendon

E Flexor carpi radialis muscle tendon

F Flexor digitorum profundus muscle tendon

19.3 The contents of the carpal tunnel are:
- the four tendons of the flexor digitorum profundus
- the four tendons of the flexor digitorum superficialis
- median nerve (this is in the most superficial structure)
- the tendon of the flexor pollicis longus.

19.4 The flexor retinaculum (transverse carpal ligament) is a strong fibrous sheath that attaches to the tubercle of the scaphoid and the pisiform bone laterally and the hook of hamate and tubercle of the trapezium medially.

19.5 Structures at risk during a carpal tunnel release include:
- palmar cutaneous branch of the median nerve giving sensation to the thenar eminence
- recurrent branch of median nerve, which is the motor branch to the thenar muscles
- ulnar nerve
- median nerve
- flexor tendons within the wrist.

19.6 **G** Ulnar artery (the ulnar nerve is smaller in diameter and lies medial to the artery)

19.7 No. The ulnar artery lies outside of the carpal tunnel and is not affected by the carpal tunnel syndrome.

19.8 All the muscles are supplied by the median nerve and its branches except for the medial half of flexor digitorum profundus (ulnar nerve).

19.9 Tinel's test consists of tapping over the median nerve, causing tingling in the thumb/index and middle finger, indicating some degree of carpal tunnel compression. In Phalen's test, the subject holds their wrist in exaggerated flexion, increasing the pressure in the carpal tunnel. This, again, may reproduce the symptoms of carpal tunnel syndrome in sufferers.

19.10 Guyon's canal is a fibro-osseous tunnel that begins at the proximal extent of flexor retinaculum (transverse carpal ligament) and ends at the aponeurotic arch of the hypothenar muscles. Its walls are the pisiform, the hook of the hamate, the volar carpal ligament, and pisohamate ligament. It contains the ulnar artery and the ulnar nerve.

Station 20

20.1 A Lateral epicondyle of the humerus

B Capitulum

C Radial head

D Radial tuberosity

E Olecranon fossa

F Medial epicondyle of the humerus

G Trochlea notch of ulna

H Coronoid process of ulna

I Ulnar shaft

20.2 The biceps brachii tendon attaches to D (radial tuberosity).

20.3 The biceps brachii muscle has two heads: the long head originates from the supraglenoid tubercle of the scapula; the short head originates from the coracoid process of the scapula. The biceps brachii inserts on to the posterior border of radial tuberosity, and the bicipital aponeurosis to deep fascia and the border of the subcutaneous ulna.

20.4 The brachialis muscle attaches to H (coronoid process of ulna).

20.5 The brachialis muscle aids in flexion of the forearm. However, it does not participate in supination unlike the biceps brachii muscle.

20.6a Colles' fracture is a transverse fracture of the radius about 2.5 cm proximal to the wrist joint. The distal fragment is displaced posteriorly and angulated, giving a 'dinner fork' like appearance.

20.6b Smith's fracture is a fracture of the distal radius where the distal fragment is displaced anteriorly.

20.7 A Brachialis muscle

B Brachioradialis muscle

C Ulnar artery

D Lateral epicondyle of the humerus

E Olecronon of the ulna

20.8 **Table 2.15** describes the results of damage to the ulnar nerve at various levels.

Table 2.15 Consequences of ulnar nerve section

Type of damage	Causes	Motor	Sensory
Ulnar nerve at wrist	Traumatic laceration, fractures.	Weakness of intrinsic muscles of hands (tested by abduction and adduction of fingers), clawing of the hand (except less clawing in second and third digits compared to 'Klumpke's palsy' due to intact supply of the lumbricals).	If the division is above the palmar and dorsal cutaneous branches (5 cm above the wrist) then there is loss of sensation to the medial 1.5 fingers on the volar and dorsal surfaces, and the corresponding palm.
Ulnar nerve at elbow	Fractures (especially medial epicondyle) or dislocations of elbow, cubital tunnel syndrome	Similar weaknesses of intrinsic muscles of hand. There is less clawing of the fourth and fifth fingers, as the flexor digitorum profundus to those fingers is paralysed (the 'ulnar paradox'). There is a radial deviation of the wrist due to paralysis of flexor carpi ulnaris	Loss of sensation to the medial 1.5 fingers on the volar and dorsal surfaces, and the corresponding palm.

20.9 The median nerve is a continuation of the medial cord of the brachial plexus (C5–T1). During its descent within the arm it remains in the flexor compartment accompanied by the brachial artery, deep to biceps brachii. In the cubital fossa the median nerve lies medial to the brachial artery. It continues into the forearm by passing deep to pronator teres and flexor digitorum superficialis origin, here it gives off the anterior interosseous branch. At the wrist the nerve emerges on the lateral side of the superficialis tendons and gives off another branch, the palmar cutaneous branch, before travelling with the flexor digitorum superficialis tendons through the carpal tunnel under the flexor retinaculum (transverse carpal ligament).

The median nerve supplies the palmar aspect of the thumb and lateral 2.5 fingers. **Table 2.16** lists muscles supplied by the median nerve.

20.10 Median nerve damage (A) can occur at several levels (**Table 2.17**).

20.11 The brachial artery is the continuation of the axillary artery at the distal border of the teres major muscle. Branches of the brachial artery are: profunda brachii, superior ulnar collateral, inferior ulnar collateral, nutrient branches to the humerus, and the two terminal branches – the radial artery and ulnar artery (**Figure 2.13**).

Table 2.16 Muscles supplied by the median nerve

Nerve	Muscles	Movements
Anterior interosseous nerve	Flexor pollicis longus	Flexes terminal phalanx of thumb
	Flexor digitorum profundus (lateral half)	Flexes distal interphalangeal joints of the fingers and wrist
	Pronator quadratus	Pronates forearm
Muscular branches	Pronator teres	Pronates forearm, flexes wrist
	Flexor carpi radialis	Flexes wrist
	Flexor digitorum superficialis	Flexes proximal interphalangeal joints of the fingers
	Palmaris longus	Flexes the wrist
	First two lumbricals	Flexes the metacarpophalangeal joints whilst extending the interphalangeal joints
	Abductor pollicis brevis	Abducts the thumb
	Opponens pollicis	Opposes thumb
	Flexor pollicis brevis	Flexes proximal phalanx of thumb

Table 2.17 Consequences of median nerve damage

Location of damage	Causes	Motor	Sensory
Wrist	Traumatic laceration Carpal tunnel syndrome	Weakness of the lateral two Lumbricals, Opponens pollicis, Abductor pollicis brevis, and Flexor pollicis brevis muscles (LOAF muscles). This is tested by abducting the thumb with the dorsum of the hand flat on the table	If the lesion is above the palmer cutaneous branch in the forearm then there is loss of sensation to the volar surface of skin below and including the radial 3.5 digits. If the lesion is below this level, then the sensation to the palm (but not the digits) is preserved
Supracondylar level	Supracondylar fractures of the humerus, rarely elbow dislocation.	As well as above consequences: loss of forearm pronation, weak wrist flexion (as it now solely depends on flexor carpi ulnaris and medial half of flexor digitorum profundus, supplied by the ulnar nerve)	Loss of volar cutaneous sensation below and including the radial 3.5 digits

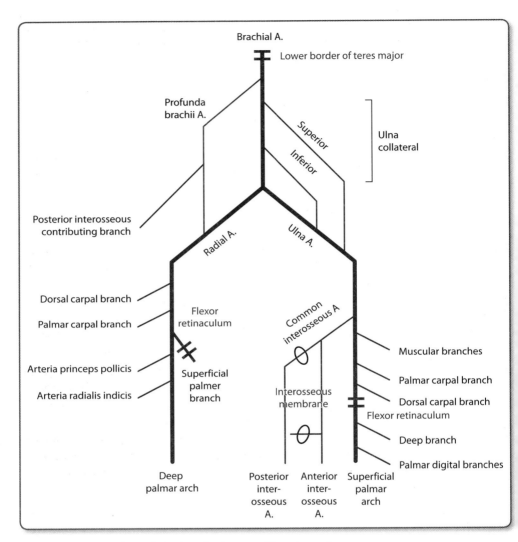

Figure 2.13 Branches of the brachial artery. (A. = Artery).

Station 21

21.1 A Metacarpal head of the little finger

  B Hook of the hamate

  C Trapezoid

  D Scaphoid

21.2 It is a sesamoid bone, meaning that it is embedded within a tendon (that of flexor carpi ulnaris).

21.3 The flexor retinaculum (transverse carpal ligament), the flexor carpi ulnaris and the abductor digiti minimi (to complete the list: pisometacarpal ligament, pisohamate ligament, and volar carpal ligament).

21.4 The scaphoid, lunate, and triquetral bones.

21.5 Bennett's fracture is an intra-articular fracture dislocation of the base of the metacarpal of the thumb extending in to the first carpometacarpal (trapeziometacarpal) joint.

21.6 Flexor digitorum profundus: originates from the ulna, interosseous membrane, and fascia of the forearm and inserts in to the base of the distal phalanx of the medial four fingers.

Flexor digitorum superficialis: has humeroulnar and radial heads, and inserts into the middle phalanx of the medial four fingers.

21.7 The flexor pollicis longus muscle originates from the anterior surface of the radius and the interosseous membrane. It travels through the carpal tunnel and inserts in to the base of the distal phalanx of the thumb.

21.8 Mallet finger results from a hyperextension injury that avulses or ruptures the insertion of the extensor tendon in to the distal phalanx, resulting in flexion of the distal phalanx at rest due to pull from the flexor digitorum profundus. It is often treated in a finger splint for 6 weeks although occasionally surgery is required.

21.9 Trigger finger is catching of the finger during flexion or extension due to a disparity of size between the flexor tendon and the pulley system of the finger. The most common location is the A1 pulley. It can be treated with steroid injections, but surgical release of A1 pulley is a more definitive treatment.

21.10 The pulleys of the digits are thickenings of the flexor tendon sheath that keep the tendons tight to the bones. There are three cruciform pulleys and these prevent sheath collapse and expansion during digital motion. There are five annular ligaments that act to prevent bowstringing.

Station 22

22.1 A Extensor digiti minimi tendon

 B Extensor digitorum tendon of middle finger

 C Extensor retinaculum

 D Extensor expansion of index finger

 E Abductor pollicis longus tendon

22.2 The posterior interosseous branch of the radial nerve.

22.3 The extensor digitorum communis originates from the lateral epicondyle of the humerus. The tendons terminate in an aponeurotic extensor expansion over the proximal phalanges. They attach by a central slip in to the base of the middle phalanx, and two lateral slips in to the distal phalanx. The extensor expansion receives the attachments of the interossei and lumbricals.

22.4 There are attachments between the tendons of the extensor digitorum tendons of the little, ring, and middle fingers, making it difficult to fully extend each of these fingers alone.

22.5 The extensor carpi ulnaris originates from the lateral epicondyle of the humerus, and inserts in to the base of the 5th metacarpal.

22.6 The extensor carpi radialis longus originates from the lateral supracondylar ridge of the humerus, the lateral intermuscular septum, and the lateral epicondyle of the humerus. It inserts in to the dorsal surface of the base of the second metacarpal bone.

22.7 The extensor retinaculum (C) is attached laterally to the lateral margin of the radius, and medially to the triquetrum and pisiform.

22.8 de Quervain's tenosynovitis is inflammation of the sheath containing extensor pollicis brevis and abductor pollicis longus (both abductors of the thumb). It is commonly treated by steroid injection.

22.9 Volkmann's contracture is fibrosis and contraction of the long flexors and extensors of the forearm due to ischaemia and necrosis of the muscles. The wrist is usually flexed (as the forearm flexors are bulkier than the extensors), the metacarpophalangeal joints are extended (the long extensors insert into proximal phalanges), and the interphalangeal joints flexed.

Station 23

23.1 A Palmar digital artery of index finger

B Palmar digital nerve of index finger

C Abductor pollicis brevis

D Flexor digitorum profundus

E Flexor digitorum superficialis

F Superficial palmar arch

G Abductor digiti minimi

H Ulnar artery

23.2 The anterior interosseous nerve is a branch of the median nerve and the posterior interosseous nerve is a branch of the radial nerve.

23.3 The anterior interosseous nerve arises below the two heads of pronator teres and runs on the anterior surface of the interosseous membrane. It supplies the flexor pollicis longus, the pronator quadratus, and the radial half of flexor digitorum profundus.

The posterior interosseous nerve passes between the two heads of supinator in to the posterior compartment. This nerve supplies most of the extensors of the forearm.

23.4 Both the anterior and posterior interosseous arteries are branches of the ulnar artery.

23.5 The palmaris longus is a wrist flexor that is absent in about 13% of people. Its absence does not significantly weaken flexion and so is suitable for use as a tendon graft.

23.6 The radial artery ends as the deep palmar arch in the palm of the hand. This lies 1 cm proximal to the superficial palmar arch, which is the continuation of the ulnar artery.

The deep palmar arch gives off palmar metacarpal branches. The superficial palmar arch supplies the hypothenar eminence and gives off the digital arteries. There is an anastomosis between the deep and superficial arches and hence division of the radial or ulnar artery by itself is usually of little consequence.

23.7 Allen's test assesses the patency of the radial and ulnar arteries, and is useful before arterial cannulation or puncture. The radial artery is compressed at the wrist and the patient is asked to tightly clench their fist, which closes off the superficial and deep palmar arches. The patient then opens their hand. After a few seconds the hand should be fully perfused by blood from the ulnar artery via the palmar arches. These actions are repeated with compression of the ulnar artery to complete the test.

Station 24

24.1 A Biceps brachii (short head)

   B Median nerve

   C Ulnar nerve

   D Musculocutaneous nerve

   E Axillary nerve

   F Radial nerve

24.2 D Musculocutaneous nerve. It innervates the biceps brachii, brachialis, and coracobrachialis muscles (mnemonic: **BBC** – **B**iceps, **B**rachialis, and **C**oracobrachialis).

24.3 Radial: C5–T1

   Median: C5–T1

   Musculocutaneous: C5–C7

   Axillary: C5, C6

24.4 The branches of the posterior cord can be remembered using the acronym **STAR**: upper **S**ubscapular nerve, **T**horacodorsal nerve, **A**xillary nerve, and **R**adial nerve (note the thoracodorsal nerve is also known as the nerve to latissimus dorsi).

24.5 The *roots* (C5–T1) lie between the anterior and middle scalene muscles.

   The *trunks* (middle and lower) lie within the posterior triangle of the neck.

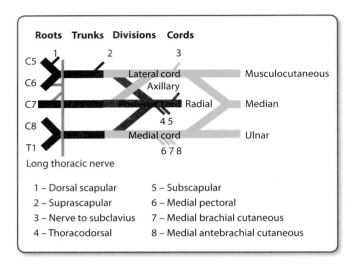

Figure 2.14 The brachial plexus.

The *divisions* (anterior and posterior) lie behind the clavicle.

The *cords* (lateral, posterior and medial) lie in the axilla.

Note: the brachial plexus can be difficult to memorise. Of the structures in **Figure 2.14**, the named nerves are the most important to remember; the less important nerves are numbered. Try also to take note of the roots and cords.

24.6 Upper brachial plexus injuries may occur due to shoulder dystocia. Injuries of this type are referred to as 'Erb–Duchenne' paralysis. The roots involved are C5 and C6 and hence muscles innervated by the axillary (deltoid and teres minor), suprascapular (supra- and infraspinatus), and musculocutaneous (biceps and brachialis) nerves are affected. The arm hangs limply, medially rotated and fully pronated – like giving a tip to the waiter behind your back ('waiter's tip palsy').

24.7 Lower brachial plexus injuries involve T1 roots, and can be caused by upward traction on the arm at birth. This injury is termed 'Klumpke's palsy'. T1 supplies the small muscles of the hand and so it takes on a 'clawed' appearance due to unopposed action of the long flexors and extensors (causing extension of the metacarpophalangeal joints and flexion of the interphalangeal joints).

24.8 The long thoracic nerve of Bell (C5–C7) supplies the serratus anterior muscle. Section of this nerve produces a 'winged scapula' appearance (prominent protrusion of the scapula). This appearance is exaggerated by pushing against resistance. There is weak anteversion and abduction of the arm above the head.

24.9 The nerve to the subclavius.

24.10 Suprascapular nerve (upper trunk). This supplies supraspinatus and infraspinatus.

24.11 The axillary artery (not anything 'brachial'!).

Station 25

25.1 **A** Vastus medialis muscle

    B Long (or great) saphenous vein

    C Patella

    D Distal femur

    E Popliteal vessels

25.2 Quadratus femoris arises from the lateral border of the ischial tuberosity. The muscle inserts in a vertical line that extends from the quadrate tubercle of the femur to the level of the lesser trochanter. It is an external rotator of the hip and is innervated by the nerve to the quadratus femoris (**Table 2.18**).

25.3 Semitendinosus arises from the upper posterior surface of the ischial tuberosity, and inserts in to the upper medial shaft of the tibia. It is a flexor and internal rotator of the knee, and an extensor of the hip. The muscle is innervated by the tibial part of the sciatic nerve.

25.4 Adductor magnus has two parts: *adductor* and *hamstring*. The *adductor* part arises from the ischiopubic ramus and inserts in to the lower gluteal line and linea aspera. This part is innervated by the posterior division of the obturator nerve. The *hamstring* portion arises from the posterior surface of the ischial tuberosity and inserts in to the adductor tubercle, and is innervated by the tibial portion of the sciatic nerve.

25.5 The same nerves that innervate the hip – the femoral, sciatic, and obturator nerves – also supply the knee. Hence, hip disease is an important differential to be considered in knee pain.

Table 2.18 Compartments of the thigh

Compartment	Muscles	Nerve supply	Blood supply
Anterior	Sartorius, iliacus, psoas. Pectineus, quadriceps femoris (rectus femoris, vastus lateralis, vastus medialis, vastus intermedius)	Femoral nerve (except psoas which is from the lumbar plexus)	Femoral artery
Medial	Gracilis, adductor longus, adductor brevis, adductor magnus (adductor), obturator externus	Obturator	Profunda femoris and obturator arteries
Posterior	Biceps femoris, semitendinosus, semimembranosus, adductor magnus (hamstring)	Sciatic nerve	Profunda femoris artery

Note: Adductor magnus has both adductor and hamstring portions, and different nerves innervate them.

25.6 The obturator nerve arises from the lumbar plexus from the anterior divisions of the anterior primary rami of L2–4. It emerges at the medial border of the psoas and splits in to anterior and posterior branches at the obturator groove before traversing the obturator foramen to supply the adductors of the thigh.

25.7 Sensory: the skin of the medial thigh.

Motor: adductor magnus (adductor part), adductor longus, adductor brevis, gracilis, pectineus, obturator externus.

Station 26

26.1 Hip flexion.

26.2 L2/L3

26.3 Iliacus and psoas major mainly. Other muscles that contribute are rectus femoris, sartorius, and pectineus. L2/L3.

26.4 Normal values for hip and knee ranges of movement are given in **Table 2.19**.

26.5 See **Table 2.19**.

26.6 See **Table 2.19**.

26.7 See **Table 2.19**.

26.8 'Real' leg length can be measured with the patient lying down with the pelvis square and legs positioned symmetrically in abduction. The measurement is from the medial malleolus to the anterior superior iliac spine. 'Apparent' leg length is measured with the legs parallel, from the medial malleolus to the xiphisternum (or other constant midline landmark). Real shortening is due to loss of bone length whereas apparent shortening is due to fixed deformity.

26.9 The McMurray circumduction test is performed to identify meniscal injury in the knee. With the patient supine, the knee is first flexed to 90° and the examiner's left hand is placed over the knee joint, with thumb laterally and index finger medially.

Table 2.19 Normal values for hip and knee range of movement* (from the anatomical position)		
	Hip	**Knee**
Flexion	120°	130°
Extension	30°	15°
Abduction	45°	*
Adduction	30°	*
External rotation	45°	*
Internal rotation	40°	10°
*These movements are not possible at the knee.		

The examiner's right hand applies an external rotation force to the foot while extending the knee and the left hand applies a valgus force to the knee. A torn medial meniscus may become trapped between the femoral and tibial condyles. The test is repeated with the knee being extended with internal rotation of the foot and varus stress. Pain, clicking, or crepitus indicates a positive test.

26.10 Lachman's test evaluates anterior cruciate ligament injury. The knee is flexed to 30° and the lower leg is grasped with one hand on the tibia and the other on the thigh. The leg is then pulled forward firmly. If the anterior cruciate ligament is deficient, there will be a greater forward translation of the joint than normal.

Station 27

27.1 A Gluteus maximus

B Piriformis

C Sciatic nerve

D Inferior gemellus

E Posterior femoral cutaneous nerve

F Quadratus femoris

27.2 Trendelenburg's test is ipsilateral sinking of the pelvis opposite the side of a pathological hip when standing on one leg ('sound side sags'). A normal (negative) test is indicated by a rise of the pelvis opposite the side on which the subject is standing. This is caused by contraction of the gluteus medius and minimus, and is necessary for normal gait. If there is weakness of either of these muscles, dislocation of the femoral head, or a defective femoral neck or angle then Trendelenburg's sign will be positive.

27.3 A Gluteus maximus. This is the largest muscle in the body. It originates from the outer surface of the ilium, sacrum, coccyx, and sacrotuberous ligament and inserts into the iliotibial tract and gluteal tuberosity of the femur. It is supplied by the inferior gluteal nerve (L5–S2) and the superior and inferior gluteal arteries (internal iliac artery). Its action is to extend and laterally rotate the hip, and it helps extend the knee (through the iliotibial tract).

27.4a C The sciatic nerve (the largest nerve in the body)

L4–S3.

27.4b The major branches of the sciatic nerve are: the tibial nerve, the common peroneal nerve, the nerve to quadratus femoris (also supplying the inferior gemellus and the hip joint), and the nerve to obturator internus (also supplying the superior gemellus).

27.5 B Piriformis muscle.

27.5a The piriformis originates from the front surface of the sacrum (**Figure 2.15**). It leaves the pelvis through the greater sciatic foramen, to insert on to the greater trochanter of the femur. It is supplied by branches of the sacral plexus and acts as a lateral rotator of the femur, and stabiliser of the hip.

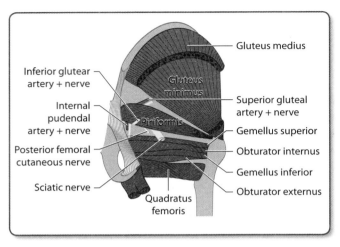

Figure 2.15
The gluteal region (gluteus maximus muscle removed but would overlie gluteus minimus).

27.5b Table 2.20 lists structures departing the greater sciatic foramen above and below the piriformis.

27.5c See **Table 2.20**.

27.6 The 'fascia lata' is the deep fascia of the thigh.

27.7 The iliotibial tract is a dense area of fascia lata over the lateral leg. It is attached superiorly to the tubercle of the iliac crest, and inferiorly to the lateral condyle of the tibia. It receives the tensor fasciae latae muscle and the insertion of the gluteus maximus. It has an important role in stabilising the hip and extending the knee when standing.

27.8 The upper outer quadrant of the buttock. The important structures (notably the sciatic nerve and its branches) run safely medial to this.

Table 2.20 Structures exiting the greater sciatic foramen

Location	Vessels	Nerves
Above piriformis	Superior gluteal vessels	Superior gluteal nerve
Below piriformis	Inferior gluteal vessels	Inferior gluteal nerve
	Internal pudendal vessels	Pudendal nerve
		Sciatic nerve
		Posterior femoral cutaneous nerve
		Nerve to obturator internus
		Nerve to quadratus femoris

Station 28

28.1 The differential for a lump in the groin is:

- soft tissue: sebaceous cyst, lipoma, sarcoma
- musculoskeletal: psoas abscess
- vessel: femoral artery aneurysm or pseudoaneurysm, saphena varix
- nerve: femoral neuroma
- enlarged lymph node
- femoral hernia.

28.2 Remember, the mnemonic for the order of the structures in the femoral triangle from lateral to medial is **NAVY: N**erve, **A**rtery, **V**ein, and **Y**-fronts!

A Sartorius

B Femoral nerve

C Common femoral artery

D Profundus femoris artery

E Long saphenous vein

F Adductor longus

28.3 The femoral artery (C) is the continuation of the external iliac artery as it passes under the inguinal ligament. It gives off the profunda femoris about 3.5 cm below the inguinal ligament to become the superficial femoral artery. The artery then travels in the adductor canal, lying first on adductor longus and then adductor magnus, underneath sartorius. It passes through the adductor hiatus in adductor magnus to become the popliteal artery.

28.4 Femoral hernias pass through the femoral canal. This is bounded anteriorly by the inguinal ligament, posteriorly by the pectineal ligament (overlying the superior pubic ramus), medially by the lacunar ligament (the pectineal part of the inguinal ligament), and laterally by the femoral vein.

28.5 Normally the canal contains fat and a lymph node (Cloquet's node). The space in the canal allows for expansion of the femoral vein, and allows a lymphatic pathway to the external iliac nodes.

28.6 The boundaries of the femoral triangle are (**Figure 2.16**):

- superiorly: the inguinal ligament
- medially: medial border of adductor longus
- laterally: the medial border of sartorius
- floor: iliacus, psoas, pectineus, and adductor longus muscles
- roof: fascia lata (pierced by the saphenous vein).

28.7 The femoral sheath is a protrusion of the fascial lining of the abdominal wall. It surrounds the femoral vessels and lymphatics for about 2.5 cm below the inguinal ligament.

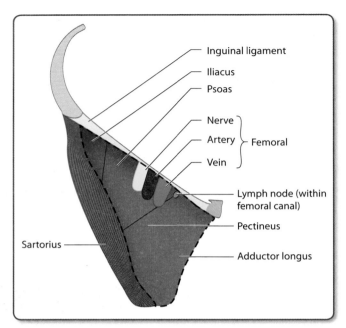

Figure 2.16 The right femoral triangle (triangle exists within dotted region).

Labels on figure:
- Inguinal ligament
- Iliacus
- Psoas
- Nerve ⎫
- Artery ⎬ Femoral
- Vein ⎭
- Lymph node (within femoral canal)
- Pectineus
- Sartorius
- Adductor longus

28.8 The adductor canal is bounded:
- anterolaterally – vastus medialis
- posteromedially – adductor longus and magnus
- anteromedially (i.e. the roof) – subsartorial fascia, on which lies sartorius.

28.9 The nerve involved is the lateral cutaneous nerve of the thigh, a branch of the lumbar plexus. The condition is termed meralgia paraesthetica.

Station 29

29.1 **A** Lateral femoral condyle

      B Head of the femur

      C Intercondylar fossa

      D Medial femoral condyle

29.2a **E** The patella. This is the largest sesamoid bone in the human body.

29.2b The patella is in its normal position with the knee in extension.

29.2c The patella protects the front of the knee. It may have a role in increasing the leverage that the tendon exerts on the femur during knee extension.

29.2d Laterally.

29.3 The tibia and fibula are connected at proximal and distal joints. The proximal tibiofibular joint is a synovial plane joint between the lateral condyle of the tibia and the head of the fibula. The distal tibiofibular joint is a fibrous joint between the fibular notch at the lower end of the tibia and the lower end of the fibula.

29.4 The rectus femoris, vastus medialis, vastus intermedius, and vastus lateralis.

29.5 'Housemaid's knee' – prepatellar bursitis, classically caused by prolonged kneeling forwards (as you would scrubbbing the floor).

'Clergyman's knee' – infrapatellar bursitis, classically caused by kneeling in the erect position (as you would praying).

29.6 The common peroneal nerve can be palpated as it winds around the neck of the fibula. Tight bandages and plaster casts can compress it.

29.7 **Table 2.21** outlines the result of damage to some of the major nerves of the lower limb.

29.8 The gracilis (obturator nerve), and the sartorius (femoral nerve).

Table 2.21 Consequences of section of major lower limb nerves

Nerve	Root values	Causes	Result of section	
			Motor	**Sensory**
Femoral	L2–L4	Operations on the hip, fractures of femur or pelvis, penetrating trauma of anterior thigh	Weakness of hip flexion and knee extension	Numbness of the anterior thigh and medial leg
Sciatic	L4–S3	Posterior dislocation of the hip, inadvertent intramuscular injection, penetrating trauma.	Paralysis of all muscles of leg except for adduction and flexion of hip and extension of knee	Numbness below the knee except area along medial malleolus and medial foot (saphenous nerve)
Tibial	Ventral divisions of L4–S3	Penetrating trauma of popliteal fossa	Paralysis of muscles of posterior compartment (plantarflexors) and sole of foot	Numbness along the back of the leg and sole of the foot
Common peroneal	Dorsal divisions of L4–S2	Penetrating trauma of popliteal fossa, tight bandages/casts, fracture of neck of fibula	Paralysis of muscles of anterior (dorsiflexors) and lateral (evertors) compartments	Numbness on anterolateral lower leg and upper surface of foot

Station 30

30.1 The left side (the lesser trochanter is prominent on the posterior surface of the femur, so this is the left side viewed from behind).

30.2 See **Figure 2.17**.

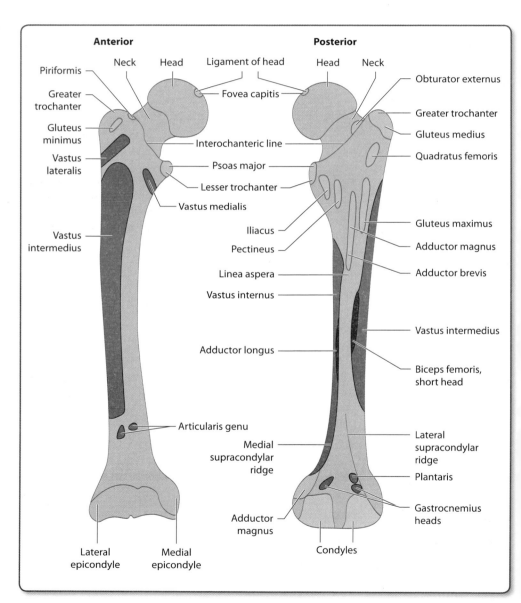

Figure 2.17 Muscular attachments of the femur.

A Greater trochanter

B Trochanteric fossa

C Lesser trochanter

D Fovea of head

30.3 There are three main blood sources to the head of the femur. The first is from vessels travelling up the diaphysis of the femur, the second is from reticular vessels piercing the capsule and travelling up the neck beneath the synovial membrane (from the medial femoral circumflex artery). The third, and least important in the adult, is from vessels in the ligamentum teres (derived from a branch of the obturator artery).

30.4 In the child the blood supply from arteries travelling in the ligamentum teres is much more important.

30.5 The most important factor is whether the fracture is intra- or extracapsular, as this determines whether the femur will receive enough blood to avoid avascular necrosis. Intracapsular fractures disrupt the reticular blood supply and the diaphyseal blood supply, and hence the only source of blood to the head is via the ligamentum teres. As this supply is poor in the adult it often results in necrosis of the head. Extracapsular fractures disrupt the diaphyseal blood supply but the retinacular supply is usually left intact, hence the risk of necrosis is lower. The degree of displacement of the femoral neck is an important factor in determining the patency of the retinacular vessels.

30.6 A Semimembranosus

B Semitendinosus

C Long head of biceps femoris

D Vastus lateralis

E Tibial nerve

30.7 The medial femoral circumflex artery. This muscle is commonly used as a pedicled or free flap based on this vessel.

30.8 The obturator nerve (anterior branch).

30.9 Gracilis originates from the outer surface of ischiopubic ramus. It inserts into the upper part of the shaft of the tibia on its medial surface.

30.10 Adductor longus, brevis and magnus, and pectineus.

Station 31

31.1 The differential for a popliteal lump includes:

- soft tissue: sebaceous cyst, lipoma, sarcoma
- vessel: short saphenous varicosity, popliteal aneurysm
- nerve: neuroma
- musculoskeletal: knee joint effusion, sarcoma, enlarged bursae, tumour of the femur or tibia
- enlarged lymph node

31.2 **A** Semitendinosus tendon

    B Popliteal vein

    C Popliteal artery

    D Biceps femoris muscle

    E Short saphenous vein

    F Lateral head of gastrocnemius

31.3 A localised widening of a portion of an artery, greater than 150% of its normal diameter. Aneurysms may be fusiform (expansion of the entire vessel circumstantially) or saccular (evagination of a segment of the circumference).

31.4 The boundaries of the popliteal fossa are listed below (**Figure 2.18**):
- superolateral: biceps femoris tendon
- superomedial: semimembranosus and semitendinosus
- inferomedial: medial head of gastrocnemius
- inferolateral: lateral head of gastrocnemius
- roof: deep fascia pierced by the short saphenous vein
- floor: popliteal surface of the femur, the posterior aspect of the knee joint, and the popliteus muscle.

31.5 The deepest structure is the popliteal artery. The space also contains the tibial nerve, the popliteal vein, the common peroneal nerve, sural and sural communicating nerves, lymph nodes and fat. The short saphenous vein and posterior femoral cutaneous nerves are in the fascia of its roof.

31.6 The branches of the popliteal artery are: the genicular arteries (the superior medial, superior lateral, middle, inferior medial and inferior lateral), the anterior tibial

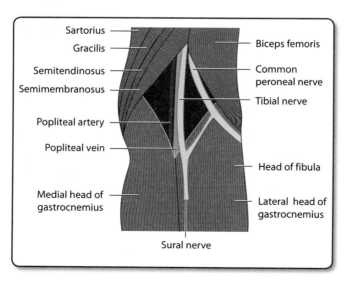

Figure 2.18 The right popliteal fossa.

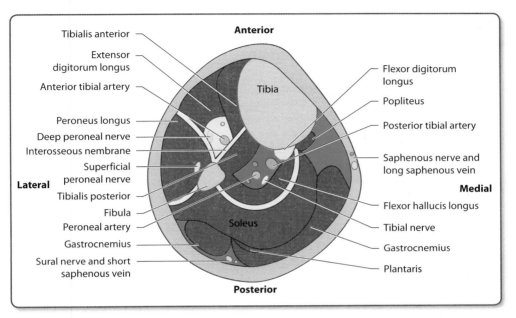

Figure 2.19 Axial section of the left lower leg, viewed from above, revealing the different compartments.

artery, and the tibial-peroneal trunk (which splits in to the posterior tibial artery and peroneal artery.

31.7 The deep posterior compartment (**Figure 2.19**).

31.8 Consequences of a high section of the tibial nerve:
- **sensory**: numbness of posterior surface of the leg, foot and 5th toe (via the sural nerve), the sole of the foot (via the medial and lateral plantar nerves).
- **motor**: loss of plantarflexion of the toes and inversion of the foot (**Table 2.21**).

31.9 The anterior compartment (**Figure 2.19**).

31.10 Consequences of section of the superficial peroneal nerve (**Table 2.21**):
- **sensory**: numbness of upper surface of the foot (apart from the first webspace, supplied by the deep peroneal nerve)
- **motor**: loss of eversion of the foot (paralysis of peroneus longus and brevis).

31.11 The popliteus muscle assists in the initial stages of flexion from full extension, as it internally rotates ('unscrewing' or 'unlocking') the joint. The muscle arises from the lateral condyle of the femur and is inserted in to the upper part of the posterior surface of the tibia.

Station 32

32.1 A Tibial prominence

32.2 B Fascia overlying tibialis anterior

   C Superior extensor retinaculum

   D Fibularis longus and brevis tendons

32.3 Compartment syndrome is caused by an increase in the compartment's pressure (or a reduction in its volume). This compromises capillary blood flow. Soft tissue oedema further raises the pressure, which then compromises first venous and lymphatic drainage and then arteriole perfusion causing ischaemia. It is commonly associated with soft tissue injury associated with fractures, and even open fractures can result in the syndrome. Pain out of proportion to clinical signs is suspicious of the condition. The leg is swollen and tender. Paraesthesia may be present. Active dorsiflexion, as well as stretching the muscles of the anterior compartment by passive plantarflexion increases the pain. As the pressure rises, dorsiflexion of the ankle and extension of the toes is lost, and sensation carried by the deep peroneal nerve (between the first and second webspace) is lost. Loss of pulses is a very late and worrying sign.

32.4 Compartments of the leg and blood supply (**Figure 2.19**):
   - anterior compartment (separated from the posterior by the interosseous membrane) – anterior tibial artery.
   - lateral compartment (separated from the anterior and posterior compartments respectively by the anterior and posterior fascial septa) – branches from the peroneal artery (which actually runs in the posterior compartment).
   - deep and superficial posterior compartments (divided by the deep transverse fascia) – posterior tibial artery.

Table 2.22 Compartments of the lower leg

Compartment	Muscles	Nerve supply	Blood supply
Anterior	Tibialis anterior Extensor digitorum longus Peroneus tertius Extensor hallucis longus Extensor digitorum brevis	Deep peroneal nerve	Anterior tibial artery
Lateral	Peroneus longus Peroneus brevis	Superficial peroneal nerve	Peroneal artery
Superficial posterior	Gastrocnemius Plantaris Soleus	Tibial nerve	Posterior tibial artery
Deep posterior	Popliteus Flexor digitorum longus Flexor hallucis longus Tibialis posterior	Tibial nerve	Posterior tibial artery

32.5 Extensor digitorum longus is in the anterior compartment of the leg. **Table 2.22** reviews the compartments of the lower leg.

32.6 The tibial nerve runs in the deep posterior compartment.

Station 33

33.1 This is a digital subtraction angiogram of the right lower limb.

33.2 See **Figure 2.16**.

   A Right popliteal artery

   B Right anterior tibial artery

   C Right posterior tibial artery

   D Right peroneal artery

33.3 The clinical features can be remembered using the '6 Ps': Pale, Pulselessness, Painful, Paralysed, Paraesthesia, Perishing cold.

33.4 Despite supplying the lateral compartment, the peroneal artery actually runs in the deep posterior compartment.

33.5 C (the posterior tibial artery) ends as the medial and lateral plantar arteries (**Figure 2.20**).

33.6 The dorsalis pedis is a continuation of the anterior tibial artery (**Figure 2.20**).

33.7 The sural nerve is the cutaneous branch of the tibial nerve. It is often joined by the sural communicating branch of the common peroneal nerve. It supplies the skin of the calf and back of the leg before accompanying the small saphenous vein behind the lateral malleolus to supply the skin along the lateral border of the foot and little toe.

33.8 The order of structures at the medial ankle from anterior to posterior can be remembered using the mnemonic 'Tom, Dick and Nervous Harry': Tibialis posterior, flexor Digitorum longus, Artery (posterior tibial), Nerve (tibial), flexor Hallucis longus.

Station 34

34.1 **A** Greater trochanter of the femur

   B Fovea capitis femoris

   C Intertrochanteric crest

   D Lesser trochanter of the femur

34.2 The ligament of the head of the femur (ligamentum teres) attaches to structure B (fovea capitis femoris). It contains the acetabular branch of the obturator artery, which is an important blood supply to the head in children but not so in later life.

34.3 The common tendon of the psoas and iliacus insert into structure D (lesser trochanter).

34.4 The femur is usually dislocated posteriorly. This is accompanied by fractures of the posterior acetabular lip if the hip is abducted at the time.

34.5 The sciatic nerve.

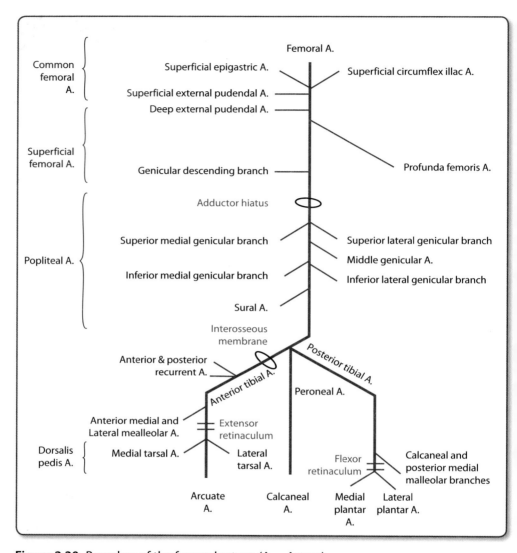

Figure 2.20 Branches of the femoral artery. (A. = Artery).

34.6 This would cause loss of all motor function of the leg besides adduction and flexion of the hip and extension of the knee. The patient would have foot drop. There would be loss of sensation of the lower leg and foot apart from the anteromedial thigh (femoral nerve) and a small strip down the medial side of the leg into the hallux (saphenous branch of femoral nerve) (**Table 2.21**).

34.7 **Table 2.23** lists the attachments of the ligaments of the hip.

Table 2.23 Ligaments of the hip

Ligament	Upper attachments	Lower attachment
Iliofemoral	Anterior inferior iliac spine	Upper and lower parts of the intertrochanteric line
Pubofemoral	Superior ramus of the pubis	Lower part of the intertrochanteric line
Ischiofemoral	Body of the ischium near the acetabular margin	Greater trochanter
Transverse acetabular	Acetabulum	Fovea capitis femoris

34.8 The capsule is attached on the anterior surface to the intertrochanteric line but on the posterior surface halfway up the femoral neck. Superiorly it is attached circumferentially around the glenoid labrum and transverse ligament.

Station 35

35.1 A Medial condyle of femur

   B Medial collateral ligament

   C Posterior cruciate ligament

   D Lateral collateral ligament

   E Lateral meniscus

35.2 The movements of the knee:
   - flexion: the hamstrings (semitendinosus, semimembranosus, and biceps femoris), gracilis, gastrocnemius, sartorius
   - extension: quadriceps femoris (rectus femoris, vastus lateralis, vastus medialis, vastus intermedius)
   - internal rotation: popliteus.

35.3 The nerve roots for flexion are L5 and S1. The nerve roots for extension are L3 and L4.

35.4 The knee has intracapsular and extracapsular ligaments. The intracapsular ligaments are the cruciates. The anterior cruciate ligament is attached to the anterior intercondylar area of the tibia and passes backwards and laterally to attach to the medial posterior surface of the lateral femoral condyle. The posterior cruciate ligament is attached to the posterior intercondylar area and passes forward and medially to be attached to the anterior lateral surface of the medial femoral condyle.

The medial and collateral ligaments are situated alongside the knee. The patellar ligament protects the anterior surface and is strengthened on each side of the patella by medial and lateral retinacula (from the vastus medialis and lateralis). The oblique popliteal ligament protects the posterior capsule and is derived from the semimembranosus.

Note: the main structures of the knee from anterior to posterior can be remembered by the mnemonic Treaves Is An Excellent Surgeon Especially In Piles: Transverse ligament, Internal meniscus, Anterior cruciate ligament, External meniscus, Spine, External meniscus, Internal meniscus, Posterior cruciate ligament.

35.5 *See answer to previous question.*

35.6 The menisci are C-shaped sheets composed of fibrocartilage, with the peripheral edges thickened and attached to the capsule. Their function is to cushion the contact of the bone articulations, and to deepen the surfaces of the tibial condyles in order to receive the femoral condyles.

35.7 Lateral rotation of partially flexed leg (the knee is most stable in extension).

35.8 Fibrocartilage.

Station 36

36.1 A The greater trochanter

   B The ischial tuberosity

36.2 C Gluteus maximus

   E The hamstrings

36.3 D The natal cleft, intergluteal cleft, or vertical gluteal crease.

36.4 The sciatic nerve commences at the midpoint of a line joining the posterior superior iliac spine (at the sacral dimple) to the ischial tuberosity. The nerve curves laterally and inferiorly through a point midway between the greater trochanter and ischial tuberosity, and then continues vertically downwards in the midline of the posterior thigh.

36.5 Hilton's law states that nerves crossing a joint supply the muscles acting on that joint as well as the joint itself.

36.7 The superior and inferior gemelli are lateral rotators of the hip, and are supplied by branches of the sacral plexus (the nerve to quadratus femoris, and the nerve to obturator internus).

36.8 The hamstring group of muscles are outlined in **Table 2.24**.

36.9 *See answer to previous question.*

Table 2.24 The hamstring muscles

Muscle	Origin	Insertion	Nerve
Semitendinosus	Ischial tuberosity	Medial surface of tibia	Tibial
Semimembranosus	Ischial tuberosity	Medial tibial condyle	Tibial
Biceps femoris (long head)	Ischial tuberosity	Lateral side of head of fibula	Tibial
Biceps femoris (short head)	Lateral lip of linea aspera	Lateral side of head of fibula	Common peroneal

Station 37

37.1 This is the right hip (innominate) bone.

37.2 A Ischial spine

  B Ischial tuberosity

  C Anterior inferior iliac spine

  D Acetabular fossa

  E Superior pubic ramus

  F Pubic tubercle

  G Obturator foramen

  H Inferior pubic tubercle

37.3 A Ischial spine. Coccygeus muscle and sacrospinous ligament.

37.4 B Ischial tuberosity. Provides attachment for the adductor magnus, semimembranosus, biceps femoris, and semitendinosus. Also provides attachment to the sacrotuberous ligament.

37.5 C Anterior inferior iliac spine. The straight head of rectus femoris (**Figure 2.21**).

37.6 The pelvis is comprised of the innominate bones, the sacrum, and the coccyx. The innominate bones are: the ischium, the ilium, and the pubis.

37.7 Secondary cartilaginous (**Table 2.12**).

37.8 The male pelvis is heavier, thicker, with well-defined muscle attachments. The pelvic inlet is heart shaped in the male, and oval in the female. The false pelvis is much deeper in the male, and the pelvic canal is longer. The sacrum is long and narrow in the male, and short and flat in the female. In men, the angle between the inferior pubic rami (the subpubic angle) is about equal to the angle between the middle and index finger, whereas in women it is approximately the angle between

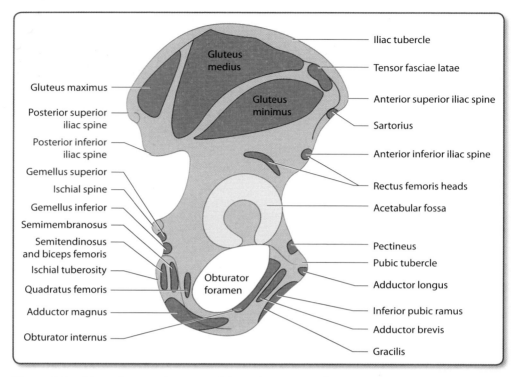

Figure 2.21 Muscular attachments of the pelvis viewed from its lateral surface.

the thumb and index finger. The male acetabulum is larger than the female. The ischial tuberosities are directed inwards in men and outwards in females.

37.9 The obturator internus originates from the medial surface of the obturator membrane, the ischium and the rim of the pubis. It leaves the pelvic cavity via the lesser sciatic foramen to insert on to the greater trochanter of the femur. It is supplied by the nerve to the obturator internus (sacral plexus), and acts as an external rotator of the femur.

37.10 The greater sciatic foramen is bounded anterolaterally by the greater sciatic notch of the ilium, posteromedially by the sacrotuberous ligament, and inferiorly by the sacrospinous ligament.

37.11 The lesser sciatic foramen is bounded anteriorly by the ischial tuberosity, superiorly by the spine of the ischium and the sacrospinous ligament, and posteriorly by the sacrotuberous ligament. It transmits: the tendon of obturator internus, the internal pudendal vessels, the pudendal nerve, and the nerve to obturator internus.

37.12 The sacroiliac joint.

37.13 The external iliac gives off inferior epigastric and deep circumflex iliac branches before continuing as the femoral artery (as it passes under the inguinal ligament).

37.14 **Table 2.25** lists the branches of the internal iliac artery.

Table 2.25 Branches of the internal iliac artery	
Anterior division	Umbilical (branching into the artery to the vas deferens and the superior vesical artery)
	Obturator
	Inferior vesical
	Middle rectal
	Internal pudendal
	Inferior gluteal
	Uterine (female)
	Vaginal (female)
Posterior division	Iliolumbar
	Lateral sacral
	Superior gluteal

Station 38

38.1 **A** Right common femoral artery

   B Right lateral circumflex femoral artery

   C Right superficial femoral artery

   D Left profunda femoris artery

38.2 Superficial epigastric, superficial circumflex iliac, superficial external pudendal, deep external pudendal, and profunda femoris (with its medial and lateral circumflex femoral branches). The common femoral artery continues as the superficial femoral artery after giving off the profunda femoris, and then as the popliteal artery as it emerges from the adductor canal.

38.3 The dorsalis pedis can be palpated between the tendons of flexor hallucis longus and extensor digitorum on the upper surface of the foot.

   The posterior tibial artery can be felt behind the medial malleolus.

38.4 Blood may reach the foot via collaterals from the profunda femoris. These travel via genicular vessels to provide flow to the popliteal artery.

38.5 The adductor canal contains the femoral artery and vein, the saphenous nerve, and the nerve to vastus medialis.

38.6 The femoral artery continues as the popliteal artery as it emerges from under the adductor hiatus.

38.7 The peroneal artery is usually evaluated by Doppler probe via its anterior perforating branch. This can be found by holding the probe in the lateral soft area above the ankle joint between the tibia and fibula.

Station 39

39.1 See **Figure 2.22**.

    A Tendon of extensor hallucis longus

    F The Achilles' tendon

39.2 B The head of the first metatarsal

    C The sustentaculum tali

    D The medial malleolus

    E The tuberosity of the calcaneum

39.3 The long saphenous vein.

    39.3a This vein forms from the medial end of the dorsal venous arch of the sole of the foot. It passes directly in front of the medial malleolus and ascends in the superficial fascia up the medial leg. It passes over the posterior parts of the medial condyles of the tibia and femur, and then curves forward to pass through the saphenous opening in the deep fascia to join the femoral vein about 4 cm below and lateral to the pubic tubercle.

    39.3b The saphenous nerve.

    39.3c Just before it joins the femoral vein, the saphenous vein receives three tributaries: the superficial circumflex iliac vein, the superficial epigastric vein, and the superficial external pudendal vein.

39.4 The short saphenous vein.

    39.4a The short saphenous arises from the lateral part of the dorsal venous arch of the foot. It ascends behind the lateral malleolus and then runs up the posterior aspect of the back of the leg in the midline. It pierces the deep fascia and passes between the heads of gastrocnemius in the lower part of the popliteal fossa to join the popliteal vein.

    39.4b The sural nerve.

39.5 The deep veins begin on the plantar aspect of the foot and follow the major arteries (i.e. the anterior and posterior tibial, and the peroneal). They drain into the popliteal and femoral veins. Most of the blood of the lower limbs is carried in these deep veins, hence high tie of the saphenous veins for treatment of varicose veins is usually a safe procedure.

39.6 As the deep venous system may be damaged by the previous deep vein thrombosis, the superficial veins may now be contributing significantly to the venous return. Ligating the superficial supply may then result in venous hypertension.

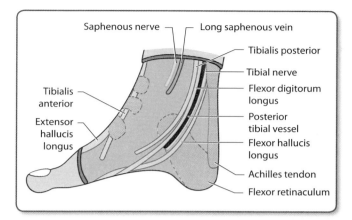

Figure 2.22 Structures at the medial ankle.

Labels in figure:
Saphenous nerve — Long saphenous vein — Tibialis posterior — Tibial nerve — Flexor digitorum longus — Posterior tibial vessel — Flexor hallucis longus — Achilles tendon — Flexor retinaculum — Tibialis anterior — Extensor hallucis longus

Station 40

40.1 See **Figure 2.23**.

  B L2

  D L4 or L5

40.2 B Lateral cutaneous nerve of the thigh (lumbar plexus)

  D Lateral sural nerve (common peroneal nerve)

40.3 The rectus femoris.

40.4 Vessels: the femoral vein, and the femoral artery

Nerves: the saphenous nerve, the nerve to vastus medialis, the medial femoral cutaneous nerve.

40.5 Saphenous nerve: numbness of the skin on the anteromedial surface of the leg.

Medial femoral cutaneous nerve: numbness of a patch of skin on the lower anteromedial thigh.

Nerve to vastus medialis: weakness of knee extension.

40.6 Hip flexion: L2, L3

Hip extension: L4, L5

40.7 **Table 2.26** lists the muscles responsible for movements of the hip (muscles which are the main contributors to the action are in bold):

40.8 The tensor fasciae latae originates from the iliac crest and inserts in to the iliotibial crest. It is supplied by the superior gluteal nerve and assists gluteus maximus in extending the knee.

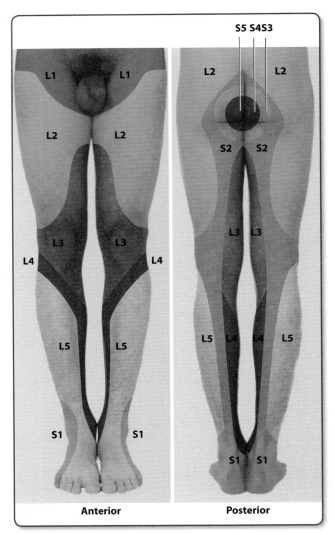

Figure 2.23
Dermatomes of the lower limb.

Table 2.26 Movements of the hip

Flexion	**Iliacus, psoas major**, rectus femoris, sartorius, pectineus.
Extension	**Gluteus maximus, hamstrings**
Adduction	**Adductor longus, brevis and magnus**, gracilis, pectineus
Abduction	**Gluteus medius and minimus, tensor fasciae latae**
Internal rotation	**Tensor fasciae latae, anterior fibres of gluteus medius and minimus**
External rotation	**Gluteus maximus**, obturators, gemelli, quadratus femoris

Station 41

41.1 A Medial plantar

B Lateral plantar

C Superficial peroneal

D Deep peroneal

E Sural

41.2 A L4/5

B S1/2

C L5

D L5

E S1

41.3 The plantar fascia is triangular and is attached to the tuberosity of the calcaneus and to the heads of the metatarsal bones.

41.4 The sustentaculum is an eminence on the medial surface of the calcaneus. It provides attachment for the flexor hallucis longus muscle. It also provides attachment to the plantar calcaneonavicular (spring) ligament, tibiocalcaneal ligament, the deltoid ligament, and the medial talocalcaneal ligament.

41.5 The medial longitudinal, the lateral longitudinal, and the transverse arches.

41.6 The medial cuneiform and first metatarsal.

41.7 The tuberosity at the base of the fifth metatarsal bone.

41.8 The base of the fifth metatarsal.

41.9 The peroneus tertius assists in dorsiflexion and eversion (in contrast to the peroneus longus and brevis that are plantar flexors and evertors of the foot).

Station 42

42.1 A Left medial malleolus

B Left calcaneus bone

C Left talus bone

D Left navicular bone

E Left cuboidal bone

42.2 The ankle joint is a synovial hinge joint. It has a capsule that is weak anteriorly and posteriorly, but is reinforced by strong ligaments laterally.

42.3 The articulation is between the tibia, the fibula, and the talus.

42.4 According to Hilton's law, the deep and superficial peroneal and tibial nerves supply the ankle joint.

42.5 The deltoid ligament (medial ligament of talocrural joint) has deep and superficial fibres, both attached to the medial malleolus. The deep fibres distally attach to the medial talus, and the superficial fibres attach to the talus, the sustentaculum tali, the plantar calcaneonavicular ligament, and the tuberosity of the navicular.

42.6 The tendons of peroneus longus and peroneus brevis run behind the lateral malleolus, bound by the superior and inferior peroneal retinacula.

42.7 A syndesmosis is an articulation united by an interosseous ligament, where a small degree of movement is allowed. Apart from the interosseous membrane, the tibiofibular joint is also connected by the anterior and posterior tibiofibular ligaments.

42.8 The Danis–Weber classification of ankle injuries is outlined in **Table 2.27**.

Table 2.27 Danis–Weber classification of fibular fractures

	Level of fibular fracture	Syndesmosis	Deltoid ligament	Medial malleolus	Stability
Type A	Below the ankle	Intact	Intact	Intact	Usually stable
Type B	At the ankle	Intact or partial injury	May be injured	May be injured	Variable stability
Type C	Above the ankle	Disrupted (widening of tibiofibular articulation)	May be injured	May be injured	Unstable and requires open reduction and fixation

Station 43

43.1 **A** The fifth metatarsal (head)

  B The intermediate (or second) cuneiform

  C The navicular

  D The medial (or first) cuneiform

  E The talus

43.2 Inferomedial surface of base of first metatarsal and the medial cuneiform.

43.3 The tuberosity of navicular bone and plantar surface of medial cuneiform.

43.4 Movements of the ankle, talocalcaneal and mid-tarsal joints (muscles which are the main contributors to the action are in bold) are outlined in **Table 2.28**.

43.5 Talocalcaneal, and mid-tarsal joints (calcaneocuboid and talonavicular).

43.6 See **Table 2.28**.

43.7 The big toe is flexed by flexor hallucis longus, and flexor hallucis brevis. It is extended by extensor hallucis longus, and extensor digitorum brevis.

Table 2.28 Muscles responsible for movements of the ankle	
Plantarflexion	**Gastrocnemius, soleus,** tibialis posterior, flexor hallucis longus, flexor digitorum longus, peroneus longus, peroneus brevis
Dorsiflexion	**Tibialis anterior,** extensor digitorum longus, extensor hallucis longus, peroneus tertius
Inversion	**Tibialis anterior and posterior,** long extensor and flexor tendons of the hallux
Eversion	**Peroneus longus, brevis and tertius**

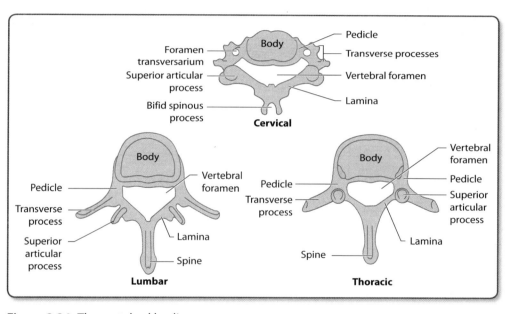

Figure 2.24 The vertebral bodies.

Station 44

44.1 This is a thoracic vertebra.

Differentiating features of the vertebra are given in **Table 2.29** and shown in **Figure 2.24**.

44.2 B Lamina

  C Vertebral foramen

  D Pedicle

Table 2.29 Differentiating features of the vertebra

Atlas	No body or spinous process
	Lateral mass on each side for articulation with occipital condyles, and mass on lower side of articulation with axis
Axis	Odontoid process
Cervical	Body is small
	Vertebral foramen large and triangular
	Transverse process has foramen transversarium containing the vertebral artery, vertebral vein, and a plexus of sympathetic nerves
	Spines are bifid
	The seventh process does not have a bifid spinous process; the foramen transversarium is small and only transmits the vertebral vein and sympathetic nerves.
Thoracic	Body is medium sized
	Vertebral foramen is small and circular
	Spines are long and inclined downwards
	Costal facets present on the transverse processes and bodies
	Superior articular processes have facets facing backward and laterally, and inferior articular processes have facets facing forwards and medially
Lumbar	Body is large and kidney shaped
	Vertebral foramens are triangular
	Transverse processes long
	Spines are short, flat, quadrangular, and project backwards
	Superior articular processes have articular processes that face medially, and inferior articular processes have processes facing laterally

44.3 A The superior articular process

    44.3a The superior articular processes articulates with the inferior articular process of the vertebra above.

    44.3b This is a synovial joint and as such is prone to osteoarthritis.

44.4 A Transverse costal facet, for articulation with the rib tubercles.

44.5 B Inferior costal demifacet, for articular with the head of the ribs.

44.6 The intervertebral discs have a peripheral region the anulus (or equally correctly 'annulus') fibrosus, and a central region the nucleus pulposus. The anulus fibrosus is formed from fibrocartilage, with the fibres arranged in concentric layers. The nucleus pulposus is a mass of gelatinous substance consisting of chondrocytes, collagen, and proteoglycan aggrecans.

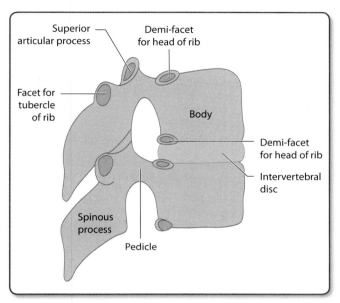

Figure 2.25 Articulations of the vertebral bodies.

The jelly-like nucleus pulposus allows the vertebra to accommodate sudden increases in compressive load. It also assists in flexion and extension of the vertebral column by allowing the vertebra to tilt forwards and backwards.

44.7 Skin, superficial fascia, supraspinous ligament, interspinous ligament, ligamentum flavum, areolar tiss ue (containing the internal vertebral venous plexus in the epidural space), dura mater, and arachnoid mater (**Figure 2.26**).

44.8 The pia mater ends at the lower border of the second sacral vertebra. Below this point the filum terminale continues, anchoring the spinal cord to the coccyx.

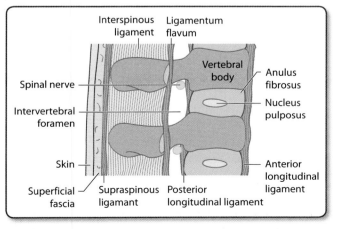

Figure 2.26 Sagittal section through the lumbar vertebral bodies.

44.9 A line joining the iliac crests passes through the 4th lumbar vertebra. The intervertebral spaces immediately above or below this line should be suitable for the procedure. The spinal cord ends at the L1/L2 vertebral level, forming the conus medullaris, therefore lumbar puncture is safe below this level.

44.10 Cervical vertebra. Observe the formamen transversarium, bifid spinous process and small body (**Figure 2.24**).

44.11 A Foramen transversarium. This carries the vertebral artery and vein in C1–C6, and just the vertebral vein in C7. It also transmits sympathetic nerves.

Station 45

45.1 **A** Teres major

45.2 The teres major arises from the inferior lateral border of the scapula and inserts in to the bicipital groove of the humerus. It medially rotates and adducts the arm.

45.3 Erector spinae (or extensor spinae).

45.4 There are three columns of the erector spinae muscle: the iliocostalis, the longissimus, and the spinalis. It is innervated by the dorsal rami of the spinal nerves. Its action is to extend the back and neck.

45.5 **C** Trapezius

45.6 The trapezius originates from the occipital bone, the ligamentum nuchae, and the spinous processes of C7–T12 vertebrae. Its upper fibres insert in to the upper lateral third of the clavicle, the middle and lower fibres in to the acromion and spine of the scapula. It is supplied by the spinal part of the accessory nerve. The upper fibres elevate the scapula, the middle fibres pull the scapula medially, and the lower fibres pull the medial border of the scapula downwards.

45.7 **D** T1/T2/T3

45.8 The posterior superior iliac spine.

Station 46

46.1 **A** L2 vertebral body

    B Intervertebral disc for L3/L4

    C Conus medullaris

    D Thecal sac containing cerebrospinal fluid

46.2 The L1/L2 vertebral level.

46.3 The spinal cord tapers off into the conus medullaris, from which continues a prolongation of pia mater termed the filum terminale, which is attached to the coccyx. The roots of the lumbar and sacral nerves below the termination of the spinal cord are called the cauda equina. There is also dura mater, arachnoid mater, and cerebrospinal fluid.

46.4 The spinal cord has three main blood sources. The anterior spinal artery originates from the fused vertebral arteries and runs within the anterior median fissure. The posterior spinal arteries arises directly or indirectly from the vertebral arteries and run down the sides of the spinal cord. There are also radicular arteries that enter the canal via the intervertebral foramina. These radicular arteries are branches of spinal arteries that in turn are branches of the posterior intercostal arteries.

46.5 The lateral spinothalamic tract transmits pain and temperature; the anterior tract transmits crude touch and pressure. Afferent fibres enter the dorsal spinal cord, ascend 1–2 vertebral levels, and decussate 1–2 spinal nerve segments above the entry point. They converge on the thalamus, before continuing to various parts of the brain

46.6 The posterior columns (or dorsal columns) carry fine touch and proprioception. There are two main tracts – fasciculus gracilis and fasciculus cuneatus. These ascend uncrossed until they reach the gracile and cuneate nuclei in the medulla, where they decussate ('the great sensory decussation') before reaching the thalamus.

46.7 The L3 spinal nerves emerge below the vertebral pedicle. There are 31 complementary paired spinal nerves. Each cervical spinal nerve emerges above its respective vertebra; each thoracic/lumbar/sacral spinal root emerges below its vertebra. Hence there is an 'extra' spinal nerve below C7 and above T1 – this is termed the C8 spinal nerve.

Station 47

47.1 A Inferior vena cava

   B Common iliac arteries

   C Right psoas major

   D Right exiting nerve root

   E Spinal cord

   F Right erector spinae

47.2 The scenario is suggestive of either sciatica or a herniated intervertebral disc.

47.3 The numbness is over the big toe and the anterior aspect of his shin so the affected dermatome is L5. This suggests nerve impingement is the L5 nerve root.

47.4 In the adult no arteries supply the intervertebral discs (they disappear about the age of 10). They are entirely dependent on diffusion from the anulus fibrosus and vertebral bodies.

47.5 This is via venous plexuses along the vertebral column both inside and outside the canal as well as anteriorly and posteriorly.

Station 48

48.1 A Anulus fibrosus (seen as an outer rim of reduced MRI signal on T2)

   B Nucleus pulposus (seen as a central portion of increased MRI signal on T2)

48.2 The anulus fibrosus (A) is composed of fibrous tissue and fibrocartilage and is arranged in multiple layers or 'laminae' around the nucleus pulposus.

48.3 The nucleus pulposus is a jelly-like material (consisting of collagen, proteoglycans and other substances). It offers a degree of 'cushioning' and shock absorbency for the vertebral bodies.

48.4 **C** Anterior longitudinal ligament

D Posterior longitudinal ligament

E Interspinous ligament

48.5 Apart from the three spinous ligaments labelled in the image there are (**Figure 2.28**):

- the ligamentum flavum: this is the strongest of the spinal ligaments. It is thickest within the lumbar spine and contributes to the posterior wall of the spinal canal running anterior to the posterior vertebral arches.
- the intertransverse ligament: running between the transverse processes of each vertebra these limit the extent of lateral flexion.
- the supraspinous ligament (sometimes considered with the interspinous ligament together as the interspinous ligament complex): connects the ends of the spinous processes between adjacent vertebrae.
- the iliolumbar ligament: this originates from the transverse processes of the L5 vertebra and attaches onto the posterior iliac crest to offer stability to the sacroiliac joint.

48.6 The anterior longitudinal ligament (C) runs along the anterior surface of the vertebral bodies beginning at the basi-occiput of the skull and anterior tubercle of the atlas (C1 vertebra) and inserting at to the anterior superior aspect of the sacrum.

The posterior longitudinal ligament (D) runs along the posterior surface of the vertebral bodies beginning superiorly at the back of the body of the axis and inserting into the superior aspect of the sacrum.

48.7 The muscles responsible for flexion and extension of the lumbar spine are given in **Table 2.30** below.

Table 2.30 Muscles responsible for flexion and extension of the lumbar spine

Flexion of the lumbar spine	Extension of the lumbar spine
Psoas major	Erector spinae
Iliacus Other extrinsic muscles that contribute to flexion include the abdominal muscles: - rectus abdominis - external oblique - internal oblique - transversus abdominis	There are a multitude of smaller muscles which also contribute, however the erector spinae is the largest contributor

Station 49

49.1 **A** Occipital bone

B Spinous process of C1 (atlas) vertebra

C Spinous process of C4 vertebra

D Hyoid bone

E Trachea

49.2 This can be achieved by:

- ensuring the patient is not suffering from any distracting injuries
- checking that the patient is not under the influence of any sedative or intoxicating drugs
- ensuring that the patient's Glasgow coma score (GCS) is 15
- examining the neck for tenderness of the spine.

If these four conditions are met and the mechanism of injury suggests a low probability of injury then the cervical spine can be mobilized gently.

49.3 **Table 2.31** is a non-exhaustive list of stable and unstable cervical spine fractures.

49.4 The first cervical vertebra is the atlas. Features which are unique to this vertebra (**Figure 2.27**) are:

Table 2.31 Demonstrating the stability of various cervical spine fractures		
Unstable	**Potentially unstable**	**Stable**
Flexion teardrop fracture	Anterior subluxation (mechanically stable but increased vertebral displacement may occur with flexion movements)	Simple wedge fracture without posterior column disruption
Bilateral facet joint dislocation (extremely unstable)	Extension teardrop fracture (unstable in extension, stable in flexion)	Clay shoveller's fracture (a fracture of the spinous process specifically at the C7/T1 level)
Atlantoaxial dislocation	Burst fracture of the vertebral body (only stable if no neurological impairment or retropulsion of fragments)	Unilateral facet joint dislocation.
Hangman's fracture (bilateral fractures through the pedicles of the C2 vertebra)	Burst fracture of the C1 vertebra (stable if no disruption of the transverse ligament)	Fracture of posterior arch of the C1 vertebra

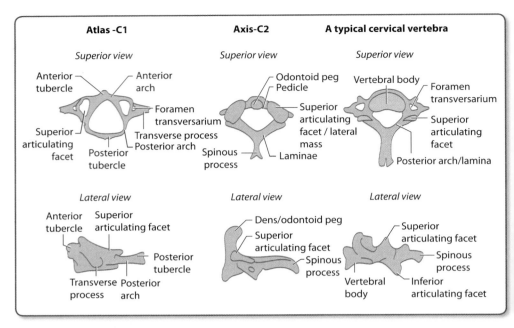

Figure 2.27 Features of the atlas, axis, and typical cervical vertebrae.

- no vertebral body
- very thick anterior arch
- prominent lateral masses which articulate with the occiput
- very thin posterior arch.

49.5 The absence of the posterior arch of the C1 vertebra does not make the cervical spine unstable. It is sometimes removed electively in addition to removal of part of the occipital bone to decompress cerebellar tonsil herniation through the foramen magnum. In some severe cases, the laminae of C2 and C3 may also be removed.

49.6 The second cervical vertebra (C2) is the axis. Features that are unique to this vertebra (**Figure 2.27**):

- possesses an odontoid peg
- deep anterior vertebral body
- broad pedicles bilaterally
- thickened laminae bilaterally
- large and flat superior articulating facet for articulation with the axis.

49.7 There are three main ligaments that confer stability to the atlantoaxial joint (**Figure 2.28**):

- anterior atlantoaxial ligament (which is continuous with the anterior longitudinal ligament inferiorly)
- posterior atlantoaxial ligament

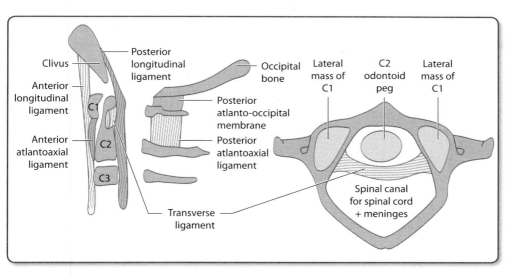

Figure 2.28 The atlantoaxial ligaments.

- transverse ligament (attached on both sides to the medial aspect of the lateral masses and keeps the odontoid peg in close contact to the anterior arch of the atlas.

49.8 There are five intervertebral discs between the C1 and C7 vertebral bodies. There is no intervertebral disc present between the atlas (C1) and the axis (C2). This is also true for the atlas and the base of the skull.

Chapter 3

Head and neck

Syllabus topics

The following topics are listed within the Intercollegiate MRCS Examination syllabus for head and neck anatomy. Tick them off as you revise these topics to ensure you have covered the syllabus.

General

- ❑ Branchial arches
- ❑ Face, scalp
- ❑ Cranial cavity, dural venous sinuses, pituitary gland
- ❑ Orbit, eyeball
- ❑ Ear
- ❑ Parotid gland
- ❑ Temporomandibular joint
- ❑ Nose and paranasal air sinuses
- ❑ Mouth, tongue
- ❑ Submandibular and sublingual glands
- ❑ Root of neck: thoracic duct
- ❑ Middle meningeal artery
- ❑ Neck blood vessels

- ❑ Central venous catheterisation
- ❑ Laryngeal structures
- ❑ Airway access
- ❑ Skull and cervical spine

Anterior triangle

- ❑ Anterior triangle
- ❑ Thyroid and parathyroid glands
- ❑ Larynx and trachea
- ❑ Pharynx and oesophagus
- ❑ Carotid sheath

Posterior triangle

- ❑ Spinal accessory nerve
- ❑ Cervical plexus

Station 1

A 35-year-old woman presents to the outpatient clinic with a 6-month history of a gradually enlarging, non-tender swelling in the middle of the anterior part of her neck. On examination, the mass is seen to move upwards during swallowing. Revise your knowledge of the anatomy of the region by answering the following questions based on the dissection shown on the following page.

This is a deep dissection of the anterior part of a normal neck, viewed from the front:

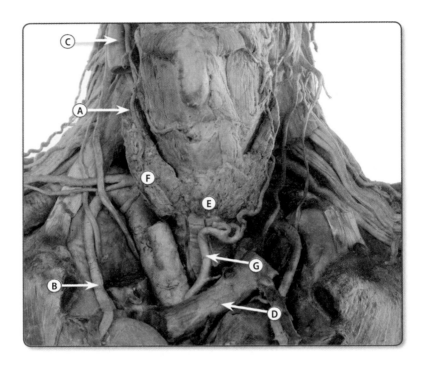

1.1 At which vertebral level is the cricoid cartilage situated?

1.2 What other important structures are found at this level?

1.3 At which vertebral level is the isthmus of the thyroid gland situated?

1.4 Explain why the patient's swelling ascends when she swallows.

1.5 Identify the structures labelled A to G.

1.6 What is the blood supply to the thyroid gland?

1.7 Where is an incision for thyroidectomy placed?

1.8 Name, in sequence, the tissue layers that must be incised during the approach to the thyroid gland.

1.9 List the complications of thyroidectomy.

Station 2

A 23-year-old woman presents with a small (2 cm), cystic, non-tender midline swelling of the neck just above the level of the thyroid notch. The lump is seen to ascend when the patient protrudes her tongue.

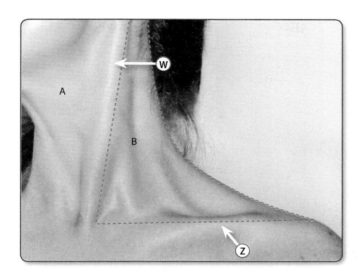

2.1 What are the boundaries of the region labelled A?

2.2 Which two neck muscles further subdivide this area of the neck?

2.3 Name the four subdivisions of the region labelled A.

2.4 Which structures are found in each of these regions?

2.5 What are the boundaries of the region labelled B?

2.6 What structures are found in this region?

2.7 What are the clinical consequences of severing the spinal accessory nerve?

2.8 What is the surface marking of the path of the spinal accessory nerve?

2.9 Identify the structures labelled W and Z.

2.10 What is the most likely diagnosis of this patient's lump?

2.11 Describe the embryology of the thyroid gland.

2.12 What is a thyroglossal cyst?

2.13 Why do thyroglossal cysts ascend on protrusion of the tongue?

Station 3

A 25-year-old man presents in the outpatient clinic with a midline neck swelling. At the previous appointment a computed tomography scan of his neck was arranged. Before calling the patient into the room you wish to familiarise yourself with the anatomical details in a normal scan.

The image below is an axial computed tomography slice from a normal subject's neck:

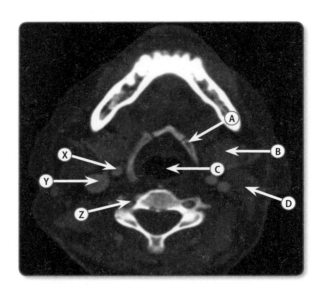

3.1 Identify the structures labelled A to D.

3.2 Approximately, at what vertebral level has the above image been taken?

3.3 Name the structures X and Y. What is the fascial layer that contains them?

3.4 Which other structures, not seen in this scan, are contained within this fascial layer?

3.5 What is the name of the vessel labelled Z?

3.6 What other muscle has the same motor innervation as the muscle labelled D?

Station 4

A 26-year-old woman presents to the emergency department with a 3-day history of otalgia and aural discharge following a recent upper respiratory tract infection.

The image on the following page shows the external aspect of a normal right ear.

4.1 Identify the structures labelled A to J.

4.2 What is the arterial supply to the external ear?

4.3 Describe the cutaneous innervation of the external ear?

4.4 What is the 'Ramsay Hunt' Syndrome?

4.5 What makes up the medial boundary of the outer ear?

4.6 What type of epithelium lines the outer aspect of the tympanic membrane?

4.7 What type of epithelium lines the inner aspect of the tympanic membrane?

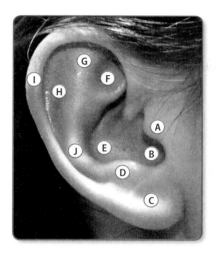

Station 5

A 75-year-old man attends the otolaryngology clinic complaining of an intermittently painful swelling in the cheek, just in front of the ear. This swelling tends to worsen around meal times and prevents him from enjoying his food. Your consultant suspects that the patient may have an inflammatory condition of a major salivary gland, and orders a sialogram. Not ever having seen a sialogram before you wish to familiarise yourself with normal sialographic anatomy.

The following image demonstrates a normal sialogram of one of the major salivary glands:

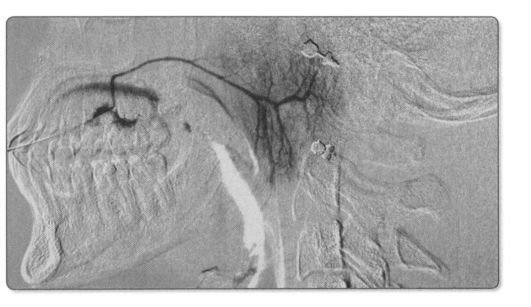

5.1 Into which salivary duct has contrast been administered?

5.2 Where is the opening of this duct within the oral cavity?

5.3 Describe the surface marking of this duct.

5.4 What are the surface markings of the gland to which this duct belongs?

5.5 Define the superficial and deep lobes of this gland.

5.6 Name three neoplasms that originate within this gland.

5.7 What important (non-glandular) structures lie within this gland?

5.8 What is Frey's Syndrome?

Station 6

An 89-year-old man presents to the emergency department. He has sustained a laceration to the top of his head and is bleeding profusely from his scalp.

This is a superficial dissection of the layers of the scalp and meninges:

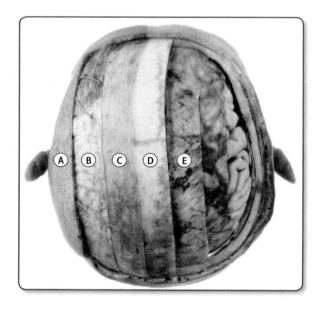

6.1 What are the five layers of the scalp from superficial to deep?

6.2 Identify the structures labelled A to E.

6.3 What is the arterial supply to the scalp?

6.4 Within which layer of the scalp do these vessels run principally?

6.5 Why do scalp lacerations bleed profusely? How can bleeding be controlled?

6.6 Why may scalp infections be life threatening?

6.7 Describe the cutaneous innervation of the scalp.

6.8 Describe the cutaneous innervation of the face.

Station 7

You are referred a 32-year-old man with sudden onset of unilateral periorbital oedema, proptosis, photophobia and a severe frontal headache. He has an infected skin lesion on his philtrum.

The image below is a coronal reconstruction of a normal computed tomography scan of the brain:

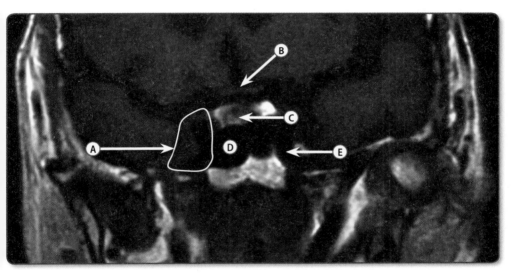

7.1 What is the venous drainage of the face?

7.2 What is the 'danger triangle' of the face?

7.3 What is the likely diagnosis in the patient described in the clinical scenario?

7.4 What may be the causative predisposing factors for this condition?

7.5 Identify the structures labelled A to E.

7.6 Which cranial nerves pass through (or in relation to) the cavernous sinus?

7.7 What neurological signs may be seen in a patient with a mass or tumour invading the cavernous sinus?

7.8 What is unique about the anatomy of the cavernous sinus?

Station 8

A 62-year-old man presents to the emergency department with tension headaches and double vision. You notice that the patient is unable to abduct his left eye on lateral gaze. He denies periorbital pain or swelling.

This photograph shows the orbits of a normal adult skull viewed from the front:

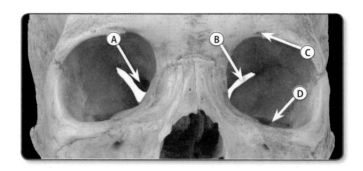

8.1 Identify the structures labelled A to D.

8.2 Name the bones which contribute to the walls of the orbit.

8.3 Which structures pass through A?

8.4 Which structures pass though D?

8.5 Which structures pass through B?

8.6 Which muscle is responsible for abduction of the eyeball and what is its innervation?

8.7 Describe the course of this nerve.

8.8 What clinical condition must be considered in a patient with a palsy of this nerve?

Station 9

You are called to the ward as a matter of urgency and find a 78-year-old gentleman looking very anxious and agitated. He is coughing, choking and is having difficulty in breathing. You suspect an upper airway obstruction.

On the following page a superficial dissection of a normal neck is viewed from its anterior aspect.

9.1 What is the narrowest part of the airway in the adult and in the child?

9.2 Which layers are traversed in superficial to deep sequence when performing a needle cricothyroidotomy?

9.3 Name, in sequence the layers which are incised when performing an elective surgical tracheostomy?

9.4 Name the structures labelled A to E in the image above.

9.5 What are the complications of a surgical tracheostomy?

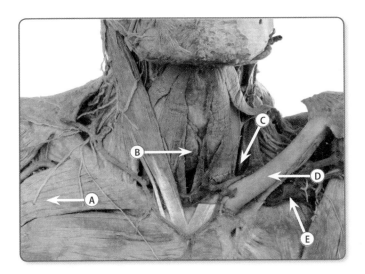

Station 10

A 19-year-old woman Hodgkin's lymphoma deteriorates rapidly on the ward and requires a central venous catheter. There are multiple palpable lymph nodes in the neck. Whilst inserting the catheter you consider the anatomy of the neck.

The image below is a deep dissection of the lower part of the neck in a normal adult:

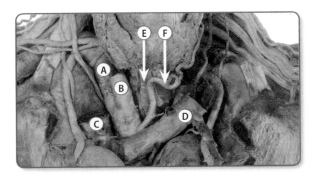

10.1 Identify the structures labelled A to F.

10.2 Into which two vessels are central venous catheters most commonly inserted?

10.3 On a plain chest radiograph where would you expect the tip of a correctly placed central venous catheter to lie?

10.4 What are the complications of central venous line catheterisation?

10.5 Name the groups of cervical lymph nodes.

10.6 Define the levels of the cervical lymph nodes.

10.7 How is this knowledge of the location of cervical lymph nodes used in clinical practice?

Station 11

A 69-year-old man is referred with hoarseness of the voice and dysphagia. You are due to assist your consultant performing his laryngectomy, and prior to surgery you revise the anatomy of this region.

Both images below are dissections of the normal larynx with the cervical vertebral column removed. Image (a) is a dissection of the larynx and pharynx viewed from the lateral aspect. Image (b) is a dissection of the larynx viewed from behind. In both images the cervical column has been removed.

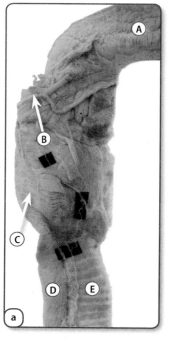
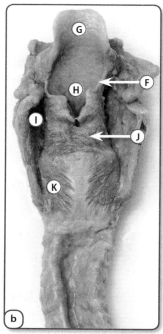

11.1 Identify the structures labelled A to K.

11.2 What are the functions of the larynx?

11.3 Name the intrinsic muscles of the larynx.

11.4 What is the innervation of these muscles?

11.5 How is the cricothyroid muscle different to the other intrinsic laryngeal muscles?

11.6 What structures do the left and right recurrent laryngeal nerves loop beneath, respectively?

11.7 What is the consequence of damage to the recurrent laryngeal nerve if the damage is:

   11.7a unilateral?

   11.7b bilateral?

11.8 Define the true and false vocal cords.

11.9 What is the lymphatic drainage of the larynx:

   11.9a above the true vocal cords?

   11.9b below the true vocal cords?

Station 12

An 85-year-old man attends outpatient clinic one month after left parotidectomy for malignancy. The patient complains of drooping of the left side of his face.

The image on the following page shows a superficial dissection of the left side of a normal adult face.

12.1 Identify the structures labelled A to F.

12.2 In the patient described in the scenario above, what neurological complication is very likely to have occurred as a result of the operation?

12.3 Describe the path of the nerve that may have been involved.

12.4 Name the branches that this nerve gives off:

   12.4a Within the facial canal.

   12.4b Distal to the stylomastoid foramen, before entering the parotid gland.

   12.4c Within the parotid gland.

12.5 Intraoperatively, how may this nerve be identified?

12.6 What is the clinical distinction between an upper motor neurone and lower motor neurone lesion of this nerve?

12.7 Which nerve is responsible for the motor innervation of the sternocleidomastoid muscle?

12.8 What are the insertion and origin points for this muscle?

12.9 How may one assess the function of this muscle on the right side?

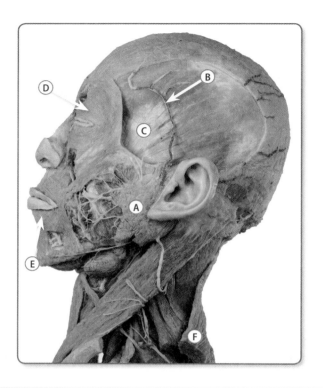

Station 13

A 30-year-old man sustains multiple facial injuries in a road traffic accident and is brought to the emergency department. During clinical examination he complains of blurred vision and diplopia.

The image below is an axial magnetic resonance image through the normal human orbits:

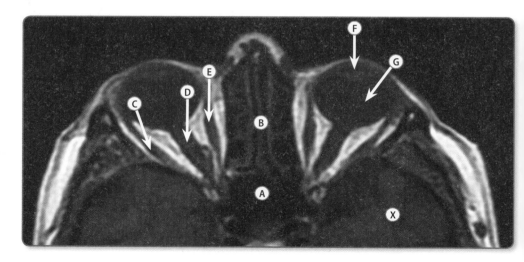

13.1 Identify the structures labelled A to E.

13.2 Which intracranial foramen does the structure labelled D traverse?

13.3 What are the attachments of the structure labelled E?

13.4 What is the name given for the intraorbital structures labelled F and G?

13.5 Explain the function of structure labelled G.

13.6 Identify the lobe of the brain labelled X.

Station 14

A 45-year-old man is taken to the emergency department following a road traffic accident in which his car is reported to have collided with another car.

The images below are computed tomography scans of the normal cervical spine. On the left is the sagittal reformat and on the right the coronal reformat.

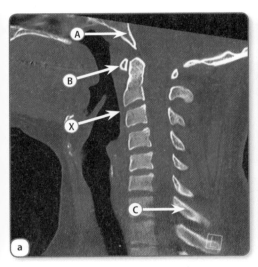 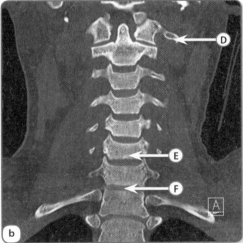

14.1 Identify the structures labelled A to F.

14.2 How does the prevertebral soft tissue margin, labelled X, differ above and below the C4 vertebral level? Give figures where appropriate.

14.3 Of what clinical relevance is this information when assessing a cervical spine radiograph in trauma?

14.4 State three morphological differences between cervical and lumbar vertebrae?

14.5 How many cervical vertebrae are there in the human vertebral column?

14.6 Which cervical vertebra is also known as the 'vertebra prominens' and why?

14.7 Name the spinal nerve which passes superior to the pedicles of the following vertebrae:

14.7a C1

14.7b C7

14.7c T1

14.7d T7

14.8 For what reason does the T7 spinal nerve not pass superior to the T7 pedicle?

Station 15

A 48-year-old female presents with a history of irregular periods, loss of libido and central headaches. She denies any visual problems but does report a lack of coordination recently.

These are magnetic resonance images of a normal brain. The upper radiograph is a coronal view through the suprasellar cistern. The lower radiograph is a mid-sagittal view of the brain.

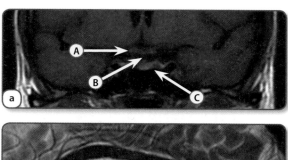

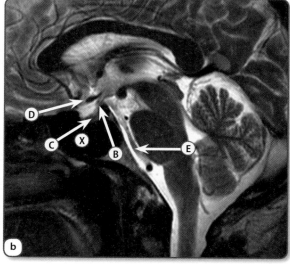

15.1 Identify the structures labelled A to E. (Structures B and C are the same in both images.)

15.2 Name the region labelled X. State how the knowledge of the proximity of X to the structure C is clinically relevant.

15.3 Name the lobes of structure C.

15.4 How do these lobes differ in their development?

15.5 List the secretions released by of each of the lobes.

15.6 What is the most common pathology to develop within the structure C? Which lobe does this commonly affect?

15.7 Describe the deficit in vision one would expect if the structure A were compressed.

15.8 Which vessels combine to form the structure labelled E and where does this confluence occur?

Station 16

A 28-year-old male motorcyclist is brought to the emergency department following a road traffic accident. In the secondary survey he complains of decreased sensation down the left side of his neck.

This is a prosection showing the anterior and lateral aspects of the neck:

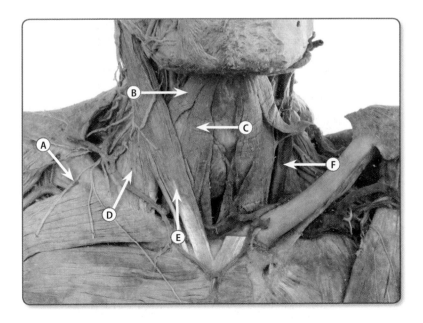

16.1 Identify the structures labelled A to F.

16.2 Which spinal nerves contribute to the cervical plexus?

16.3 Name the cutaneous branches of the cervical plexus.

16.4 Which muscles does the cervical plexus supply?

16.5 Where in the neck is the ansa cervicalis located?

16.6 Which muscles does the ansa cervicalis supply?

16.7 What is the innervation of the infrahyoid muscle that is not supplied by the ansa cervicalis?

Station 17

You are asked to examine a 31-year-old woman in the outpatient department who is complaining of pain down her neck and right arm. She has a past medical history of Raynaud's Syndrome and has been told by her general practitioner that she may be eligible for 'a nerve block' in her neck to help the symptoms.

The image below is an axial cadaveric dissection through the root of the neck at the T1 vertebral level:

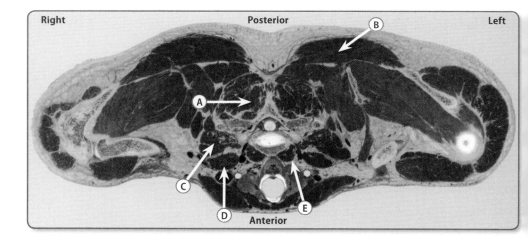

17.1 Identify the structures labelled A to E.

17.2 Which spinal cord segments contribute to the sympathetic nervous system?

17.3 What is the stellate ganglion, and what are the clinical effects of blocking it?

17.4 What are the indications for stellate ganglion block?

17.5 What are the anterior and posterior relations of the stellate ganglion?

17.6 In approximately what percentage of individuals is the stellate ganglion absent?

Station 18

A 21-year-old woman presents to the otolaryngology clinic with a hemispherical lump in the midline of his neck. The consultant evaluates the patient and sends her for an ultrasound scan.

The image below is a photograph of the anterolateral view of the neck of a normal individual:

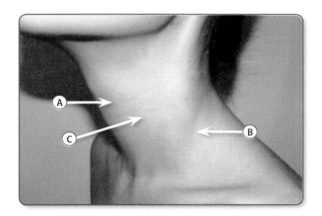

18.1 What is the differential diagnosis of a lump at A?

18.2 What is the differential diagnosis of a lump at C?

18.3 What is the differential diagnosis of a lump at B?

18.4 Name the infrahyoid 'strap' muscles.

18.5 What is the innervation and function of the infrahyoid 'strap' muscles?

18.6 What is a cystic hygroma and where is it usually located?

18.7 What is a branchial cyst and where is it usually located?

18.8 What is a chemodectoma and where is it usually located?

18.9 What is Ludwig's angina? In which tissue space does Ludwig's angina occur?

Station 19

A 44-year-old man presents to the emergency department with red, painful eyes. You are asked to assess him.

This image demonstrates the normal anatomy of the eyes:

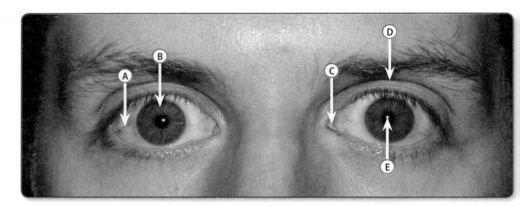

19.1 Identify the structures labelled A to E.

19.2 How many lacrimal glands drain each eye?

19.3 Where are the lacrimal glands located?

19.4 Describe the passage of tears from the lacrimal gland to the nasolacrimal duct.

19.5 What is the 'annulus of Zinn', and what structures arise from it?

19.6 Which cranial nerves are responsible for the efferent and afferent limbs of the pupillary light reflex?

19.7 How would this reflex be affected if the left optic nerve were completely transected?

19.8 How would this reflex be affected if the right oculomotor nerve were damaged?

Station 20 (Generic)

A 55-year-old man attends the otolaryngology clinic complaining of a permanently blocked nose, and intermittent episodes of facial pain.

The image on the following page shows an axial dissection through the head taken at a level just superior to the orbit. It demonstrates normal anatomy.

20.1 Identify the sinuses labelled A to C. What is D?

20.2 What are the boundaries of the nasal cavity?

20.3 What is the nasal vestibule?

20.4 Which structures drain into the superior meatus of the nasal cavity?

20.5 Which structures drain into the middle meatus of the nasal cavity?

20.6 Which structures drain into the inferior meatus of the nasal cavity?

20.7 What is the sphenoethmoidal recess?

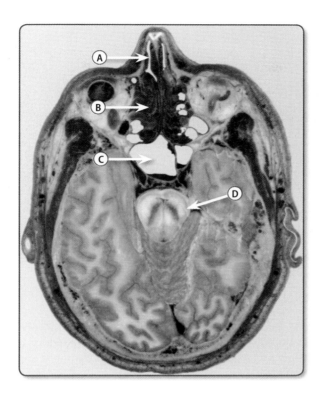

20.8 What type of epithelium lines most of the nasal cavity?

20.9 Which nerves supply sensation to the nasal cavity?

20.10 Why do patients with frontal sinusitis often also have maxillary sinusitis?

20.11 Why is maxillary sinusitis associated with dental infections?

Station 21

An 86-year-old woman in the emergency department has been fitted with a soft cervical collar after falling down the stairs. She complains of neck pain and on examination she is noted to have tenderness over the lower half of the cervical spine.

Images (a) and (b) on the following page are flexion and extension plain views of a normal cervical spine.

21.1 Which muscles are responsible for neck flexion and extension?

21.2 Within which fascial compartment in the neck does the Trapezius muscle lie?

21.3 What other structures are contained within this fascial compartment?

21.4 Name the other three major fascial compartments of the neck.

21.5 Which fascia is the prevertebral fascia continuous with?

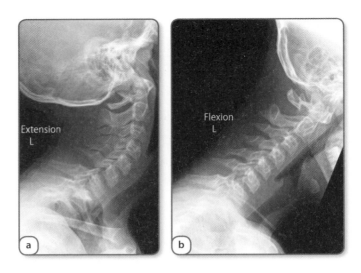

Station 22

You are referred a 66-year-old woman who presents with a 3-month history of repeated, very short-lived sharp paroxysms of pain over the right side of her face. The pain, which she describes as 'electric shock like,' is often brought on by trivial stimuli such as touching and scratching or even moving the right side of her face.

This is a superficial dissection of the normal face:

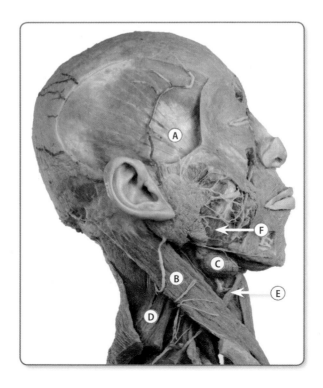

22.1 Identify the structures labelled A to F.

22.2 Which cranial nerve supplies the muscles A and F?

22.3 Which cranial nerve supplies the skin over the lower jawline?

22.4 What is the action of the structure labelled A?

22.5 What are the origin and insertion points of the muscle A?

22.6 How can you test the action of this muscle?

22.7 Where do the three sensory branches of the trigeminal nerve converge?

Station 23

A 63-year-old woman experiences two episodes of left-sided weakness over the course of a week, each lasting for less than 1 hour. She undergoes a carotid duplex scan, which demonstrates 80% stenosis of the left internal carotid artery, and 75% of the right internal carotid artery. She is booked for an urgent carotid endarterectomy.

The image below is an axial dissection of the head at the level of the maxillary sinuses and inferior brainstem viewed from below. It demonstrates normal anatomy.

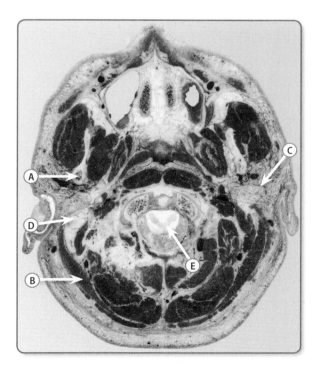

23.1 Identify the structures labelled A to E.

23.2 Which internal carotid artery should be operated on?

23.3 Name in sequence, the tissue layers which are incised in order to expose the carotid artery?

23.4 Describe the arrangement of the structures within the carotid sheath above the level of bifurcation of the common carotid artery.

23.5 How may the internal carotid artery be distinguished from the external carotid artery?

23.6 What would be the clinical consequences of damage to the superior laryngeal nerve?

23.7 What would be the clinical consequences of damage to the great auricular nerve?

23.8 What would be the clinical consequences of damage to the marginal mandibular branch of the facial nerve?

Station 24

A 35-year-old man presents to the emergency department with deep neck lacerations and profuse bleeding after suffering a knife attack outside a pub. The bleeding is being stopped by pressure but he is taken immediately to theatre for exploration.

The image below reveals the normal surface anatomy of the anterior aspect of the neck:

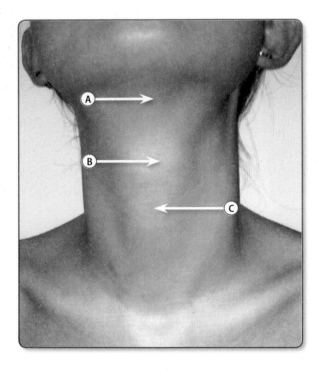

24.1 What structures are normally palpable at points A, B, C?

24.2 What is the origin and insertion of the anterior scalene muscle?

24.3 What is the origin and insertion of the posterior scalene muscle?

24.4 What structures run in front of the anterior scalene muscle?

24.5 What structures run between the anterior and middle scalene muscles?

24.6 What is the origin and insertion of the digastric muscle?

24.7 What is the origin and insertion of the mylohyoid muscle?

24.8 What is the origin and insertion of the platysma muscle?

Station 25

An 82-year-old man presents to the otolaryngology clinic with symptoms of chronic sinusitis and headaches. On inspection you notice that he has a partial ptosis of the left eyelid. He is a lifelong smoker and is frequently breathless but denies haemoptysis.

This is a coronal reconstruction of a normal computed tomography scan of the face:

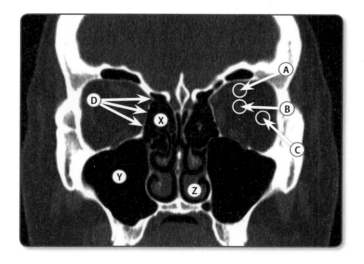

25.1 Identify the structures labelled A to C.

25.2 Which nerve is responsible for the innervation of the muscle labelled A?

25.3 Name the other muscles supplied by this nerve.

25.4 What clinical signs are found in a palsy of this nerve?

25.5 How would the clinical signs differ in Horner's syndrome?

25.6 Identify the structures labelled X, Y and Z.

25.7 What is the name given to the medial wall of the orbit labelled D? What must you consider when performing instrumentation of the nasal cavity near this region?

Station 26

You examine a 59-year-old man in the outpatient clinic who complains of a frontal headache with rhinitis. You suspect he is suffering from rhinosinusitis.

This is a sagittal reconstruction of a normal computed tomography scan of the paranasal sinuses. The windowing of the scan has been altered to demonstrate the bony anatomy.

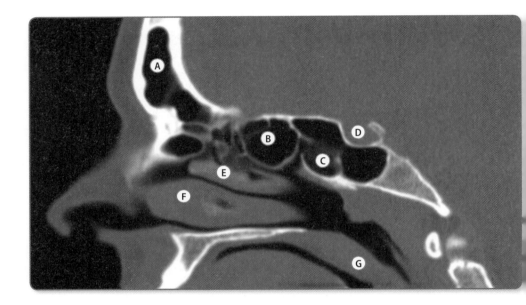

26.1 Identify the structures labelled 'A' to 'G'.

26.2 Where does each of the paranasal sinuses drain into the nasal cavity?

26.3 What is the osteomeatal complex and what is its clinical significance?

26.4 What are the functions of the paranasal sinuses?

26.5 Why do allergies predispose a patient to sinusitis?

26.6 To which lymph nodes do the lymphatics from the paranasal sinuses and nose drain?

26.7 Describe the arterial supply to the nasal cavity.

26.8 What is 'Kiesselbach's plexus'? Where is it located?

26.9 Where is 'Woodruff's plexus' located?

26.10 What is the venous drainage of the nose?

Station 27

You are referred a 45-year-old female patient with high calcium and low phosphate blood levels. The patient has also been complaining of backache and abdominal pain.

The image below is a dissection of the side of the face and neck of a normal subject:

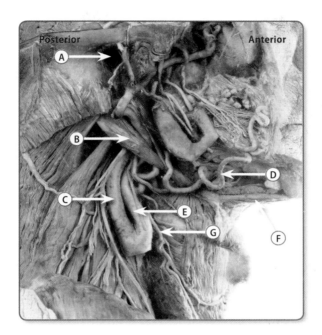

27.1 Identify the structures labelled A to G.

27.2 Which gland is responsible for this patient's symptoms?

27.3 Where in the neck are these glands located?

27.4 What is the blood supply to these glands?

27.5 What are the pharyngeal pouches and pharyngeal (branchial) arches? How many of each is present in the developing human?

27.6 From which pharyngeal pouch do the superior members of this gland arise?

27.7 From which pharyngeal pouch do the inferior members of this gland arise?

27.8 To which pharyngeal (branchial) arch does the facial nerve belong?

Station 28

A 72-year-old man presents with right-sided facial drooping and slurred speech. A diagnosis of cerebrovascular accident is made and the patient undergoes carotid artery angiography. As the junior resident in charge of the patient you wish to familiarize yourself with normal carotid angiographic anatomy.

The image on the following page is a normal carotid artery angiogram demonstrating the branches of the external carotid artery.

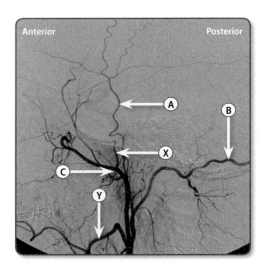

28.1 What are the origins of the right and left common carotid arteries?

28.2 At which vertebral level does the common carotid artery bifurcate?

28.3 Name vessels labelled A, B and C.

28.4 What are the names of the other branches of the external carotid artery not labelled above?

28.5 The artery labelled C is often subdivided descriptively into three parts by which muscle?

28.6 Identify the artery labelled X (a branch of C).

28.7 What may be the result of a traumatic rupture of the distal part of artery X?

28.8 What branch of C causes epistaxis at the back of the nasal cavity?

28.9 What is the name of the artery labelled Y?

28.10 Where can this artery be palpated?

28.11 Is it possible to ligate this artery without serious consequences?

Station 29

A 46-year-old woman complains of preprandial pain at the back of her lower jaw. A sialogram is obtained.

The image on the following page is a normal sialogram of one of the major salivary glands.

29.1 Into which salivary duct has contrast been administered?

29.2 Where is the opening of this duct within the oral cavity?

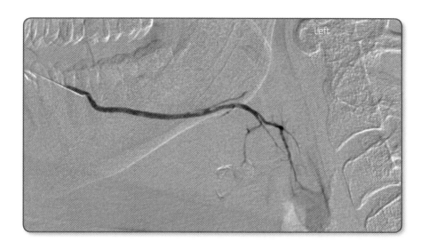

29.3 Describe the incision made during excision of this gland?

29.4 What structures may be damaged during excision of this gland?

29.5 What would be the clinical consequences of severing the lingual nerve?

29.6 Why is sialolithiasis more common in this than in any other salivary gland?

29.7 Name the minor salivary glands.

Station 30

You are asked in the otolaryngology clinic to examine a 6-year-old boy complaining of otalgia. After taking a clinical history and external examination of the ear, you proceed to inspect the external auditory canal with an otoscope:

The image below is a normal tympanic membrane as seen through the otoscope:

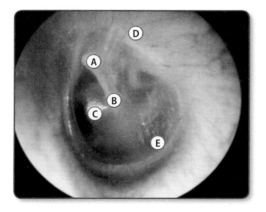

30.1 Identify the structures labelled A to E.

30.2 Is the above image from the right or left ear?

30.3 How does the sensory supply to the inner aspect of the tympanic membrane differ from that to the outer aspect?

30.4 Define the boundaries of the middle ear.

30.5 Within which bone are the ossicles contained?

30.6 Name the ossicles of the middle ear.

30.7 Which muscles are attached to the stapes and the malleus respectively?

30.8 What is the function and innervation of these muscles?

30.9 What channel connects the middle ear with the pharynx?

30.10 What epithelium lines this channel?

30.11 What connects the middle ear with the mastoid air cells?

Station 31

An 18-year-old man presents to the emergency department with multiple facial injuries. He remembers being punched across the chin and now has pain on opening his mouth and complains of a 'locked' jaw.

This is a 3D reconstruction of a computed tomography scan of the right lateral aspect of a normal adult skull:

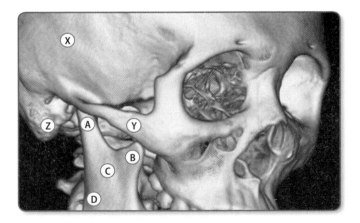

31.1 Identify the parts of the mandible labelled A to D.

31.2 Identify the parts of the skull labelled X, Y and Z.

31.3 Which nerve passes through the mandibular foramen?

31.4 What is the result of an anaesthetic block of this nerve?

31.5 Which part of the mandible is most frequently fractured?

31.6 Which bone does part 'A' articulate with?

31.7 What type of joint is the temporomandibular joint?

31.8 What type of cartilage lines its articulating surfaces?

31.9 What type of cartilage is the intra-articular disc of the temperomandibular joint composed of?

31.10 Name three ligaments associated with the temporomandibular joint.

31.11 List the muscles of mastication.

31.12 Which nerve innervates these muscles?

31.13 In an uncomplicated dislocation, in which direction is the temporomandibular joint likely to dislocate?

Station 32

A 19-year-old woman presents to the emergency department complaining of a high temperature and painful swallowing. She was told by her general practitioner 3 days ago to drink plenty of water and rest but was not prescribed any specific medification.

The image below is a sagittal dissection of the normal head and neck:

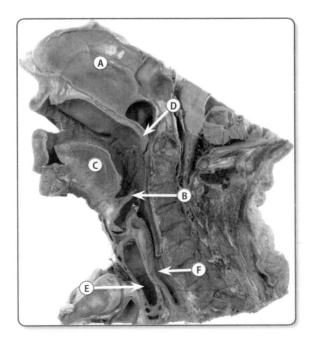

32.1 Identify the structures labelled A to F.

32.2 Name and define the boundaries of the three parts of the pharynx.

32.3 Within which subdivisions of the pharynx are the following located?

    32.3a The palatine tonsils

    32.3b The adenoids

    32.3c The Eustachian tube

32.4 List the pharyngeal constrictor muscles.

32.5 Where might you find a pharyngeal diverticulum?

32.6 What is the sole muscle in the pharynx to be innervated by the glossopharyngeal nerve?

32.7 What is the sensory innervation of the pharynx?

32.8 At which vertebral level is the hyoid bone located?

32.9 Name the muscles attached to the hyoid bone.

32.10 If a fracture of this bone is found at postmortem, what must be considered as the cause of death?

Station 33

A 39-year-old man is involved in a fight and sustains extensive bruising over his face especially in the periorbital region. You assess him in the emergency department.

This is the lateral aspect of a normal adult human skull. Different colours designate the various skull bones.

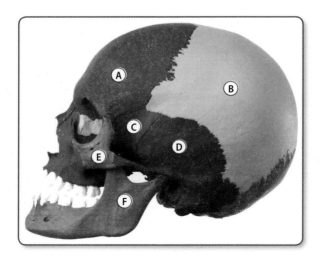

33.1 Identify the bones of the skull labelled A to F.

33.2 Which bone of the skull is most commonly fractured?

33.3 Which skull bones are involved in a 'tripod fracture'?

33.4 Why are tripod fractures associated with numbness of the ipsilateral cheek?

33.5 What are the other complications of a 'tripod fracture'?

33.6 What is a 'blow out' fracture and what is the usual mechanism of injury?

33.7 What sign is seen on a plain radiograph of the facial bones with 'blow out' fractures?

33.8 If the fracture is not adequately repaired what may be the resulting complication?

33.9 What is the commonest type of temporal bone fracture resulting from blunt trauma?

33.10 What is the commonest type of temporal bone fracture resulting from penetrating trauma?

33.11 What structures may be damaged in each of these two fractures?

Station 34

An 88-year-old man referred by his general practitioner, presents with a painless lump at the back of his tongue associated with persistent halitosis. He also complains of several 'lumpy' areas on his neck.

The images below demonstrate two sagittal dissections of the tongue. Image (a) demonstrates the tongue with surrounding structures and image (b) demonstrates the vessels supplying the tongue with the tongue muscles removed.

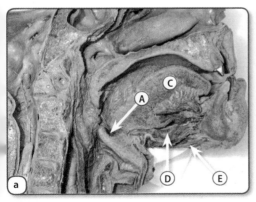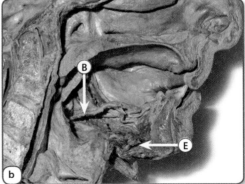

34.1 Identify the structures labelled A to E.

(the structure labelled E is the same structure in both images).

34.2 Name the four extrinsic muscles of the tongue and their actions.

34.3 What is the motor innervation of these muscles?

34.4 What nerves transmit taste sensation from the tongue?

34.5 Describe the lymphatic drainage of the tongue.

34.6 Why are malignant growths within the posterior third of the tongue usually more advanced at time of presentation than those in the anterior two-thirds?

34.7 What type of epithelium lines the tongue?

34.8 What is the commonest type of cancer to arise from the tongue?

Station 35

You review a 69-year-old woman in the otolaryngology clinic with a history of squamous cell carcinoma of the upper lip that was removed 6 months ago. Since the operation she has noticed numbness of the lower eyelid, upper lip and cheek on the same side as operation took place.

The image below is an axial computed tomography scan through base of the skull of a normal individual. The windowing of the image has been altered to display the bony anatomy.

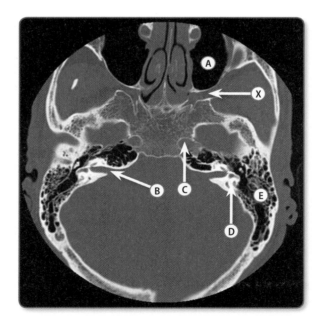

35.1 Identify the structures of the mandible labelled A to E.

35.2 Which cranial nerves traverse the foramen labelled B?

35.3 Which structures traverse the foramen labelled C?

35.4 Name the fossa labelled X.

35.5 What are the contents of X?

35.6 What are the boundaries of X?

35.7 Describe the pathways in which malignancy may spread via 'X'?

Station 36

You examine a 25-year-old woman in the emergency department who has sustained a laceration to her upper lip. You have been asked by the nurse in charge to suture the wound.

This is a photograph of the lower aspect of the face. It demonstrates normal anatomy:

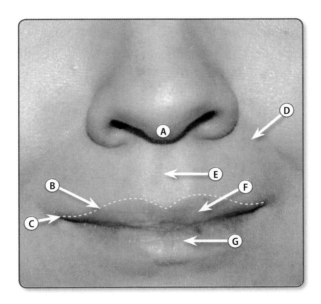

36.1 Identify the structures labelled A to G (note that the label B is referring to the dotted line).

36.2 Describe the embryological development of the upper jaw.

36.3 What is cleft lip? How does this deformity arise?

36.4 What is cleft palate? How does this deformity arise?

36.5 Classify the types of cleft palate.

Station 37

You review a 30-year-old man in the outpatients department who is keen to have rhinoplasty after a rugby injury left him with a deviated nasal septum and difficulty in breathing 1 year ago.

The image on the following page shows the inferior aspect of the normal nose.

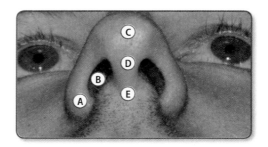

37.1 Identify the structures labelled A to E.

37.2 Which cranial nerve is responsible for the sense of smell?

37.3 Through which foramen (or foramina) does this nerve enters the cranial cavity?

37.4 Within which bone in the skull is this foramen contained?

37.5 List the common causes of unilateral anosmia?

37.6 Where in the human nasal cavity is the olfactory mucosa located?

37.7 What type of epithelium is the olfactory mucosa?

Station 38

A 6-year-old boy undergoes elective tonsillectomy for repeated episodes of tonsillitis. The operation is quite difficult and there is more than the usual amount of bleeding.

The image below demonstrates the normal anatomy of the oropharynx:

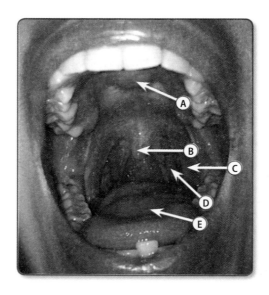

38.1 Identify the structures labelled A to E.

38.2 What comprises 'Waldeyer's ring' of lymphoid tissue?

38.3 What is the arterial supply to the palatine tonsils?

38.4 What comprises the anterior and posterior pillars of the palatine tonsils?

38.5 What forms the floor of the tonsillar fossa?

38.6 Describe the lymph drainage of the palatine tonsil.

38.7 Which major artery lies approximately 2–3 cm directly behind the palatine tonsil?

38.8 What is quinsy?

Station 39

A 35-year-old lady is diagnosed with a squamous cell carcinoma of the right forehead, 1.5 cm in diameter. She attends the day surgery unit for excision of the lesion.

The image below demonstrates a normal surface anatomy of the forehead:

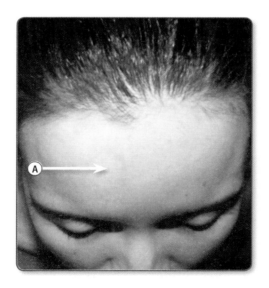

39.1 Which cutaneous nerves will be affected during the infiltration of local anaesthetic at the point labelled A?

39.2 What is the origin of these nerves?

39.3 Which arteries supply this region of the face?

39.4 What is the origin of these arteries?

39.5 Where would you palpate for lymphadenopathy in the patient described in the scenario?

39.6 What would you consider as an acceptable margin for excision of this lesion?

39.7 What muscles causes wrinkling of the skin of forehead skin?

Station 40

You review a 45-year-old woman in the otolaryngology clinic who is complaining of dizziness, poor balance and tinnitus.

This is a normal axial T2-weighted magnetic resonance image through the internal acoustic meatus:

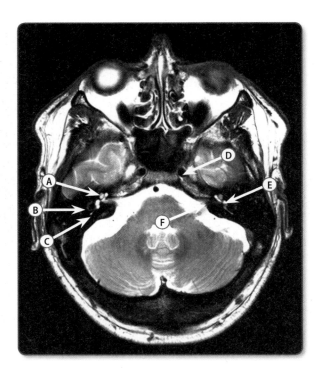

40.1 Identify the structures labelled A to E.

40.2 What is the name of the region labelled F and which nerves enter this area?

40.3 Describe the orientation of these nerves within the region labelled F.

40.4 Within which bone is the inner ear contained?

40.5 Name the semilunar canals.

40.6 Explain how the semilunar canals contribute to balance.

40.7 Describe the mechanism whereby the cochlea contributes to the sense of hearing.

Station 41

A 56-year-old man presents to the otolaryngology clinic with a 4-week history of hoarseness of voice. A barium swallow has been requested.

The images below are those of a normal barium swallow: (a) lateral view (b) anteroposterior view.

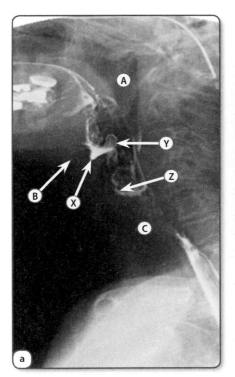 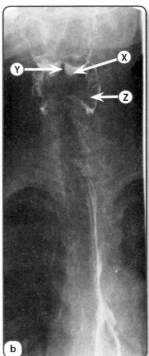

41.1 What do X, Y and Z indicate? (these are the same structures in both images).

41.2 What do A, B and C indicate?

41.3 At which vertebral level is B?

41.4 What type of tissue is structure Y composed of?

41.5 During laryngoscopy where is the tip of the laryngoscope blade placed in relation to the epiglottis?

41.6 Describe the boundaries of the area labelled Z.

41.7 What is the significance of area Z in relation to clinical practice?

Answers

Station 1

1.1 The inferior border of the cricoid cartilage is found at the C6 vertebral level.

1.2 Other important structures at the C6 vertebral level are:
- the superior parathyroid glands
- the junction of the larynx and the trachea
- the junction of the pharynx with the oesophagus
- the middle cervical sympathetic ganglion
- the inferior thyroid artery entering the thyroid gland
- the middle thyroid vein leaving the thyroid gland
- the omohyoid muscle (superior belly) crossing the carotid sheath
- the vertebral artery entering the foramen transversarium of C6 vertebra
- the level of the carotid tubercle (of Chassaignac).

1.3 The isthmus of the thyroid gland lies at the C7 vertebral level, which also corresponds to the level of the 2nd–4th tracheal rings. One way to remember this is to think of the rhyme: 'Rings 2,3,4 make the isthmus floor'. The isthmus is a midline structure lying inferior to the cricoid cartilage. The lobes of the thyroid extend from the level of the thyroid cartilage (C4 vertebral level) down to the level of the 6th tracheal ring inferiorly (T1 vertebral level).

1.4 The lump is almost certainly related to the thyroid. The thyroid gland is enveloped by the pretracheal fascia which in turn is attached to the trachea and larynx. This attachment causes the thyroid gland to move on swallowing, since the larynx and trachea move upwards during swallowing.

1.5 **A** Right superior thyroid artery

   B Right internal thoracic artery

   C Right common carotid artery

   D Left brachiocephalic vein

   E Thyroid isthmus

   F Right lobe of the thyroid gland

   G Thyroidea ima artery

1.6 The thyroid gland is supplied by three arteries as summarised in **Table 3.1**. All these arteries anastomose richly with each other.

   It is drained by three veins as shown in **Table 3.2**.

1.7 A transverse incision is made in the neck approximately 1 cm inferior to the cricoid cartilage and two finger breadths superior to the suprasternal notch. This is at the level of the thyroid isthmus and corresponds to the relaxed skin tension lines of the neck. The eventual scar is thin and cosmetically appealing.

Table 3.1 Arteries supplying the thyroid gland

Artery	Artery originates from
Superior Thyroid Artery (right and left)	External carotid artery
Inferior Thyroid Artery (right and left)	Thyrocervical trunk (a branch of the sub-clavian)
Thyroidea Ima Artery (only present in 2–5% of the population).	Usually aortic arch or brachiocephalic

Table 3.2 Veins draining the thyroid gland

Vein	Vein drains into
Superior Thyroid Vein (right and left)	Internal jugular vein
Middle Thyroid Vein (right and left)	Internal jugular vein
Inferior Thyroid Veins (multiple)	Brachiocephalic veins

1.8 The layers encountered in superficial to deep sequence are:
- skin
- subcutaneous fat
- superficial fascia (including platysma)
- investing layer of the deep cervical fascia
- strap muscles – first sternohyoid then sternothyroid
- pretracheal fascia
- thyroid isthmus.

1.9 Complications resulting from a thyroidectomy include:
- bleeding, e.g. from the middle thyroid vein, superior thyroid artery or branches of the inferior thyroid artery (note that part of the inferior thyroid artery supplying the parathyroid glands is preserved during the operation so as not to render the parathyroid glands ischaemic).
- inadvertent removal of the parathyroids leading to hypoparathyroidism.
- damage to the recurrent laryngeal nerve resulting in a hoarse voice if unilateral or aphonia and airway obstruction if bilateral. In unilateral nerve damage, the right recurrent laryngeal nerve is more commonly damaged as it runs a relatively more superficial course.
- injury to the external branch of the superior laryngeal nerve, resulting in paralysis of the ipsilateral cricothyroid muscle. The cricothyroid tenses the vocal fold and impairment of the muscle weakens the patient's voice.

Station 2

2.1 A The anterior triangle of the neck. Its boundaries are:

- anteriorly: the midline of the neck
- posteriorly: the anterior margin of the sternocleidomastoid muscle
- superiorly: the lower border of the body of the mandible and a line from the angle of the mandible to the mastoid process.

2.2 The digastric and omohyoid (superior belly) muscles subdivide the anterior triangle of the neck into four further subdivisions (**Figure 3.1**).

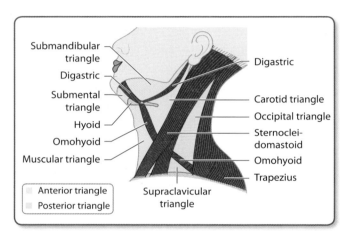

Figure 3.1 The anterior and posterior triangles of the neck and their boundaries.

2.3 The subdivisions of the anterior triangle are the submandibular, submental, muscular and carotid triangles.

2.4 Structures contained within each of these subdivisions are shown in **Table 3.3**.

2.5 B The posterior triangle of the neck. Its boundaries are:

- anteriorly: posterior border of sternocleidomastoid muscle
- posteriorly: anterior border of the trapezius muscle
- inferiorly: middle third of the clavicle
- floor: prevertebral fascia
- roof: investing layer of deep fascia.

The posterior triangle may also be further subdivided into two smaller triangles by the inferior belly of the omohyoid muscle into the occipital and supraclavicular triangles.

2.6 The contents of the posterior triangle of the neck are:

- nerves: branches of the cervical plexus, and spinal accessory nerve

Table 3.3 The anterior sub-triangles of the neck and their contents

Submandibular	Submandibular gland and duct and lymph nodes
	Facial artery and its submental branch
	Lingual nerve and submandibular ganglion
	Mylohyoid muscle and its nerve
	Hypoglossal nerve (CNXII)
Submental	Submental lymph nodes
	The mylohyoid muscle originates from the body of the hyoid bone on the floor of the submental triangle and inserts into the mylohyoid line on the inside of the body of the mandible.
Muscular	Strap muscles (sternohyoid, superior belly of omohyoid, sternothyroid, thyrohyoid)
	Thyroid gland and associated structures (e.g. superior and inferior thyroid vessels, recurrent laryngeal nerves, parathyroids, thyroid membrane, larynx
	Trachea
	Oesophagus
Carotid	Carotid sheath containing the upper portion of the common carotid artery and branches of the external carotid arteries
	Vagus nerve, ansa cervicalis
	Internal jugular vein and lymph nodes

- arteries: superficial cervical, suprascapular, occipital arteries
- veins: transverse cervical, suprascapular, external jugular veins
- muscle: omohyoid muscle with sling
- lymph nodes: supraclavicular, anterior and posterior chain lymph nodes.

The brachial plexus and subclavian artery being deep to the prevertebral fascia, the fascial floor of the posterior triangle, are strictly speaking not contents of the posterior triangle.

2.7 The spinal accessory nerve is an exclusively motor nerve. It arises from the spinal cord, ascends in the vertebral canal, crosses the foramen magnum and joins the cranial accessory nerve in the posterior cranial fossa. Together they leave the latter fossa through the jugular foramen, immediately after which the spinal accessory nerve parts company with the cranial accessory. The latter joins the vagus nerve and its fibres are distributed through the branches of the vagus.

The spinal accessory provides motor innervation to the trapezius and sternocleidomastoid muscles. Transection of the nerve in the anterior triangle will result in paralysis of the trapezius and sternocleidomastoid muscles, whereas section of the nerve in the posterior triangle will cause paralysis of the trapezius alone with sparing of sternocleidomastoid. There is weakness of rotating the head inwards on the ipsilateral side, and shrugging the ipsilateral shoulder.

2.8   The course of the spinal accessory nerve may be recalled using the rule of thirds. The nerve traverses the posterior triangle of the neck in the top third of the posterior border of the sternocleidomastoid muscle to the bottom third of the trapezius muscle (**Figure 3.2**).

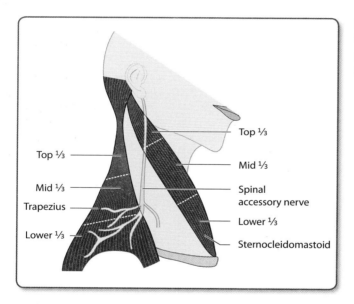

Figure 3.2 The superficial landmarks of the course of the spinal accessory nerve.

2.9   **W** Left sternocleidomastoid muscle

    Z   Left clavicle

2.10 A thyroid mass or thyroglossal cyst

2.11 The thyroid gland at the 4th week of gestation as a proliferation of cells at the back of the tongue known as the *foramen caecum* (**Figure 3.3**). These cells descend down the neck and a residual duct, the *thyroglossal duct,* is left behind connecting the developing thyroid cells to the foramen caecum. After reaching their final destination just inferior to the thyroid cartilage, the diverticulum becomes solidified and takes the shape of a bilobed structure as seen in the adult thyroid gland. The thyroglossal duct eventually obliterates. The thyroid is fully formed and descended by the 12th week in utero.

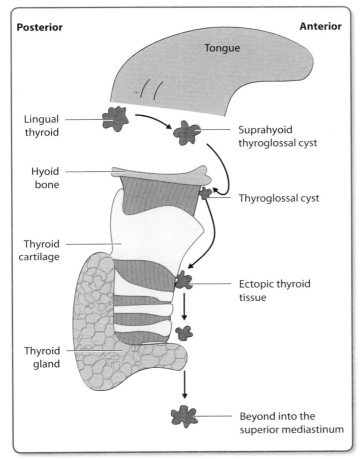

Figure 3.3 Schematic view of the pathway of descent of the thyroid gland. Ectopic thyroid tissue or a thyroglossal cyst may reside along any point of this pathway. In certain cases the descent of the thyroid tissue may continue inferior to the gland and reside within the superior mediastinum.

2.12 A thyroglossal cyst is a congenital abnormality that arises along the path of the thyroglossal duct. It is due to the persistence of part of this duct, which should normally involute in utero and not remain patent at birth. Thyroglossal cysts are usually below the level of the hyoid bone but may occur anywhere along the thyroglossal duct.

2.13 The cyst is rises on tongue protrusion as it lies along the path of the thyroglossal duct that has its origins at the posterior aspect of the tongue. This duct normally disappears during normal development, however in some cases (as in those where a thyroglossal cyst is present) a solid cord of cells representing the remnant of the duct may persist and the connection with the tongue is upheld.

Station 3

3.1 A Hyoid bone

    B Left parotid gland

C Oropharynx

D Left sternocleidomastoid

3.2 At this level in the scan you can visualise the hyoid bone and the top of the hyoid bone making this approximately C3–C4.

3.3 X Right common carotid artery

Y Right internal jugular vein

They are both contained within the carotid sheath.

3.4 The contents of the carotid sheath are:
- common carotid artery
- internal jugular vein
- vagus nerve
- deep cervical lymph nodes.

In CT imaging, the vagus nerve is not visualised and cervical lymph nodes are only seen if they are enlarged.

3.5 Z Right vertebral artery (lying within the foramen transversarium of the cervical vertebra)

3.6 The sternocleidomastoid muscle, D, is innervated by the spinal accessory nerve (CN XI). The trapezius muscle is the other muscle innervated by this nerve.

Station 4

4.1 A Tragus

B Intertragic notch

C Earlobe

D Antitragus

E Concha

F Triangular fossa

G Superior crus

H Scapha

I Helix

J Antihelix

4.2 The arterial supply to the outer ear is from branches (or sub-branches) of the external carotid artery:
- posterior auricular artery
- deep auricular artery (from the maxillary artery)
- auricular branch of the superficial temporal artery.

4.3 Sensory cutaneous nerve supply to outer ear
- great auricular and lesser occipital nerves, branches of the cervical plexus

- auriculotemporal branch of mandibular branch of the trigeminal nerve (CN V3)
- Auricular branch of the vagus nerve (C NX).

4.4 Ramsay Hunt syndrome is an acute facial neuropathy caused by the reactivation of the varicella zoster virus within the geniculate ganglion of the facial (CN VII) nerve. It commonly manifests as a deep pain within the ear and can include feelings of tinnitus, dizziness, facial drooping or vertigo. A vesicular rash over the external ear which can continue within the auditory canal is almost pathognomonic for this disease signifying the importance of closely examining the outer ear in all patients who complain with ear pain.

4.5 The outer ear consists of the pinna, concha laterally and extends to the outer aspect of the tympanic membrane at its most medial border.

4.6 The skin that covers the cartilage over the pinna and concha is continuous with the external acoustic meatus and lines the most superficial layer of the tympanic membrane. This consists of stratified squamous epithelium.

4.7 Simple cuboidal epithelium covers the inner aspect of the tympanic membrane.

Station 5

5.1 This is a parotid gland sialogram. Contrast has been administered via the parotid duct (also known as Stensen's duct).

5.2 The opening of the parotid duct is opposite the upper second molar tooth.

5.3 The parotid duct lies approximately 1.5 cm inferior to the zygomatic arch in the middle third of an imaginary line drawn from the intertragic notch to the philtrum. The duct arises from the anterior aspect of the parotid gland and pierces the buccinator muscle on its course before opening into the oral cavity.

5.4 The superficial landmarks of the borders of the parotid gland are:

- superiorly: the posterior two-thirds of the inferior border of the zygomatic arch
- anteriorly: the posterior border of the masseter muscle
- posteriorly: anterior to the external acoustic meatus and mastoid process
- inferiorly: an imaginary line drawn from the mastoid process to the greater cornu of the hyoid bone.

5.5 The parotid is divided into deep and superficial parts by the facial nerve (CN VII) (which runs through the gland substance) (**Figure 3.4**). The superficial lobe is much larger, comprising 80% of the gland's mass.

5.6 Salivary gland tumours are rare and represent only 2–4% of all head and neck malignancies. When present they are benign in over 80% of cases and the majority occur within the parotid. The three most common malignancies (in order of frequency) are listed below.

Pleomorphic adenoma: accounts for 85% of salivary gland neoplasms; benign in nature and of mixed cell type in origin.

Warthin's tumour (adenolymphoma): accounts for 15% of neoplasms. There is a strong association with smoking. They are usually situated in the tail of the parotid gland. In 10% of cases the tumour is bilateral.

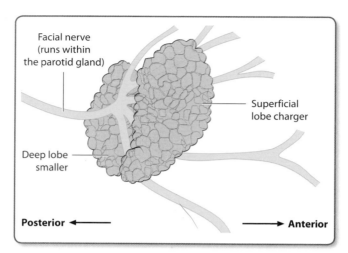

Facial nerve
(runs within
the parotid gland)

Superficial
lobe charger

Deep lobe
smaller

Posterior ←——————   ——————→ Anterior

Figure 3.4 The deep and superficial lobes of the parotid gland.

Mucoepidermoid cancer (in the parotid glands) or **adenoid cystic carcinoma (in the submandibular and sublingual glands)**: Although malignant, they are usually locally aggressive and slow to form distant metastases.

5.7 Important structures that lie within the parotid gland include (**Figure 3.5**):
- the facial nerve (the most superficial and also most prone to damage)
- the retromandibular vein
- the external carotid artery.

5.8 Frey's Syndrome is gustatory sweating. It can be congenital or acquired (usually after parotidectomy). The auriculotemporal branch of the mandibular nerve carries parasympathetic fibres which are secretomotor to the parotid gland. Sympathetic fibres on the other hand reach the face by accompanying facial blood vessels and various cutaneous nerves. Parotid surgery with its extensive subcutaneous dissection inevitably damages these autonomic fibres at a microscopic level. When these fibres regrow they make aberrant connections with each other (i.e. parasympathetic fibres connect with the stumps of sympathetic fibres). These connections take several months to develop. Once the connections are made however, parasympathetic stimulation (e.g. thinking about food) will cause sympathetic manifestations in addition to causing salivation: hence the facial sweating and tingling that are characteristic of gustatory sweating.

Station 6

6.1 The layers of the scalp can be remembered by assigning each letter in the word **SCALP** to a different layer, from superficial to deep:
- **S**: skin
- **C**: connective tissue
- **A**: aponeurosis
- **L**: loose connective tissue
- **P**: pericranium

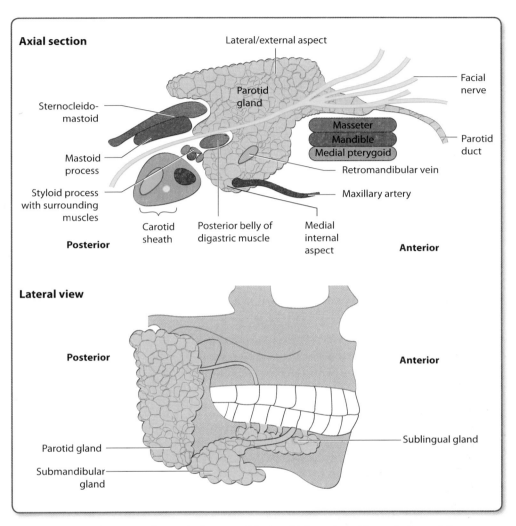

Figure 3.5 Axial section through the parotid gland (above) and lateral view of the parotid gland (below) demonstrating adjacent structures.

6.2 A Skin

  B Epicranial aponeurosis

  C Loose connective tissue and pericranium

  D Skull bone

  E Dura mater

6.3 The arterial blood supply to the scalp is predominantly from branches of the external carotid artery but there is also supply from the internal carotid artery:

- branches of external carotid artery: superficial temporal, posterior auricular and occipital arteries

- branches of the internal carotid artery: supratrochlear and supra-orbital arteries (branches of the ophthalmic artery (in turn a direct branch of the internal carotid artery)

6.4 The blood vessels of the scalp lie within the subcutaneous connective tissue layer.

6.5 Lacerations of the scalp bleed profusely because the vessels:
- are connected together via a dense anastomotic network thus giving the scalp a very rich and dense blood supply and
- are held in place by dense connective tissue that prevents them from contracting and retracting.

Haemorrhage can be halted by compressing the vessels against the skull circumferentially around the wound, or compressing them with artery forceps in the aponeurotic layer and suturing the laceration firmly both within the aponeurotic and subcutaneous layers.

6.6 The veins of the scalp are connected to veins that pierce the skull and connect with the intracranial venous sinuses (emissary veins). These veins do not contain valves and thus infections can spread rapidly through this connection leading to meningitis or venous sinus thrombosis (both potentially fatal conditions).

6.7 Cutaneous innervation to the scalp is from:
- Ophthalmic division (CN V1): via supraorbital and supratrochlear nerves
- Maxillary division (CN V2): via the zygomaticotemporal nerve
- Mandibular division (CN V3): via the auriculotemporal nerve
- C2 and C3 spinal nerves: via the greater and lesser occipital nerves and 3rd occipital nerve

6.8 Cutaneous innervation to the face is via the three branches of the trigeminal nerve (CNV) and the great auricular nerve as depicted (**Figure 3.6**). Note that the sensory supply from the ophthalmic branch of the trigeminal nerve (V3) extends to supply a large area of the scalp (up to the vertex and beyond) and does not end at the 'hairline'. This is a common misconception regarding the posterior limit of this nerve's territory.

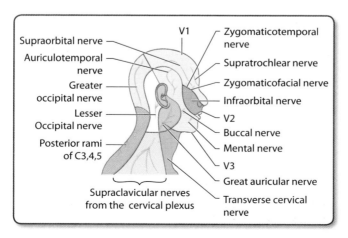

Figure 3.6 Sensory innervation of the head and neck.

Station 7

7.1 The venous drainage of the face follows the same pattern as its arterial supply:

- the supraorbital and supratrochlear veins run deep through the orbit terminating with the superior and inferior orbital veins.
- superficially the angular vein runs across the mandible becoming the anterior facial vein and contributing to the common facial vein.
- the superficial temporal vein becomes the retromandibular vein, which, together with the facial veins drain into the external and internal jugular veins.

7.2 The 'danger triangle' of the face is bounded by the lateral corners of the lips inferiorly and the nasal bridge superiorly (**Figure 3.7**). The veins draining this region of the face are connected indirectly to the cavernous sinus via the deep facial vein and pterygoid venous plexus. This provides a potential route for cutaneous infections to spread into the cranial cavity.

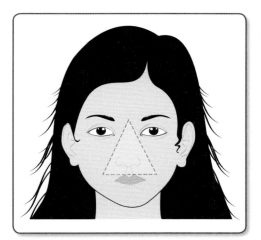

Figure 3.7 The danger triangle of the face, indicated by the shaded area.

7.3 Cavernous sinus thrombosis.

7.4 Causative factors may be bacterial infection within the danger area of the face (for example, skin infections, sinusitis, dental abscesses or gingivitis). Predisposing factors include diabetes, immunosuppression, and prothrombotic states (e.g. factor V Leiden).

7.5 A Right cavernous sinus

   B Optic chiasma

   C Pituitary gland

   D Right sphenoid sinus

   E Left cavernous portion of the internal carotid artery

7.6 See **Figure 3.8**. The cranial nerves travelling along or within the lateral wall of the cavernous sinus are (from superior to inferior):

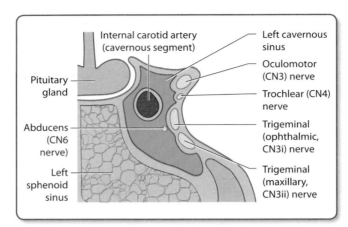

Figure 3.8 The arrangement of the contents of the left cavernous sinus.

Internal carotid artery (cavernous segment)

Left cavernous sinus

Oculomotor (CN3) nerve

Pituitary gland

Trochlear (CN4) nerve

Abducens (CN6 nerve)

Trigeminal (ophthalmic, CN3i) nerve

Left sphenoid sinus

Trigeminal (maxillary, CN3ii) nerve

- Oculomotor nerve (CNI II)
- Trochlear nerve (CN IV)
- Ophthalmic division of trigeminal nerve (CN V1)
- Maxillary division of trigeminal nerve (CN V2)

The abducens nerve (CN VI) is also found within the cavernous sinus but travels adjacent to the internal carotid artery rather than along the lateral wall of the cavernous sinus like the other nerves mentioned above.

7.7 Total ophthalmoplegia (a fixed, dilated pupil on the affected side) and loss of sensation over the region supplied by the ophthalmic and maxillary divisions of the trigeminal nerve (CN V1 and CN V2) may be seen.

7.8 The cavernous sinus is unique in that it is the only area of human anatomy where an artery (the cavernous portion of the internal carotid artery) travels within a venous structure.

Station 8

8.1 A Right optic canal

B Left superior orbital fissure

C Supraorbital foramen

D Left inferior orbital fissure

8.2 The bones which form the margins of the orbit are:
- superiorly: frontal bone
- medially: lacrimal, maxilla (frontal process) and frontal bones
- laterally: zygomatic bone and frontal bone (zygomatic process)
- inferiorly: maxilla, and zygomatic bones.

8.3 The optic canal transmits the optic nerve (CN II) and ophthalmic artery.

8.4 The inferior orbital fissure transmits the maxillary division of the trigeminal nerve (CN V2) and the infraorbital artery. The inferior orbital fissure allows communication of the orbit with the infratemporal and pterygopalatine fossae.

8.5 The superior orbital fissure allows communication between the orbit and middle cranial fossa. The structures passing through this fissure include:

    8.5a nerves: oculomotor nerve (CN III), trochlear nerve (CN IV), the ophthalmic division of the trigeminal nerve (CN V1) and abducens nerve (CN VI).

    8.5b veins: inferior and superior ophthalmic veins.

8.6 The lateral rectus muscle is responsible for abduction of the orbit and is supplied by the abducens nerve (CN VI).

8.7 The abducens nerve (CN VI) nucleus lies in the pons and emerges from the base of the brain to enter the cavernous sinus adjacent to the internal carotid artery. It exits the skull via the superior orbital fissure entering the orbit and piercing the deep surface of the lateral rectus muscle that it innervates.

8.8 The abducens nerve (CN VI) has the longest intracranial course of the cranial nerves. It is often the first nerve to be impaired in raised intracranial pressure.

Station 9

9.1 In adults the narrowest part of the airway is the glottis at the level of the true vocal cords. In children the narrowest part is the subglottis at the level of the cricoid.

9.2 The layers encountered (from superficial to deep) are:

- skin
- subcutaneous fat
- cricothyroid membrane.

9.3 The layers encountered (from superficial to deep) are:

- skin
- subcutaneous fat
- superficial fascia (including Platysma muscle)
- investing layer of the deep cervical fascia
- strap muscles (first sternohyoid then sternothyroid)
- pretracheal fascia
- thyroid isthmus
- trachea.

9.4 A Right pectoralis major muscle (clavicular part)

    B Isthmus of thyroid gland

    C Left internal jugular vein

    D Left clavicle

    E Left axillary vein

9.5 Complications from the creation of a tracheostomy include:
- bleeding from the thyroid isthmus or from anterior displacement of the tracheostomy tube (may lead to erosion into the brachiocephalic vein)
- infection around the tracheostomy site
- subcutaneous emphysema
- aspiration from blood tracking into the trachea
- tracheal stenosis from prolonged tracheostomy cuff use.

Station 10

10.1 **A** Right subclavian artery

    B Right common carotid artery

    C Right brachiocephalic vein

    D Left brachiocephalic vein

    E Trachea

    F Thyroidea ima artery

10.2 The two vessels that are commonly cannulated when inserting a central venous line are the subclavian vein and internal jugular vein. The right-sided vessels are more commonly used as they provide a shorter and less tortuous route into the superior vena cava.

10.3 The tip for a central venous catheter should lie within the cavoatrial junction (i.e. where the superior vena cava enters the right atrium). On a posteroanterior chest film this is just medial to the right superior aspect of the cardiac silhouette approximately at the level of the T6 vertebra and medial aspect of the anterior third rib.

10.4 Complications from central venous line insertion include:
- pneumothorax (more likely with the subclavian approach)
- haemorrhage from inadvertent arterial puncture (of the subclavian or common carotid arteries) and resultant haematoma or haemothorax formation
- malposition of the central line (either too proximal within in the brachiocephalic vein or too distal within the right atrium)
- arrhythmia (from a too distal tip placement within the right atrium or even right ventricle)
- line infection
- thrombosis within the line or air embolism.

10.5 There are 10 cervical lymph node groups (**Figure 3.9**):
- pre- and postauricular
- submental
- submaxillary
- occipital
- posterior cervical chain
- tonsillar
- deep and superficial cervical chain
- supraclavicular.

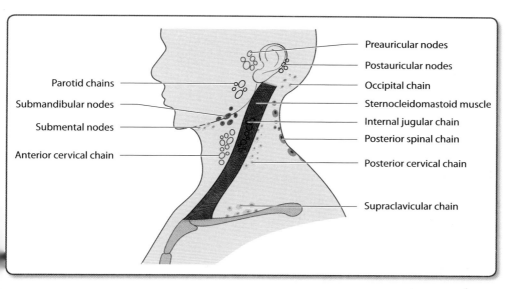

Figure 3.9 Cervical lymph node groups.

10.6 The cervical lymph node levels were defined by the Committee for Head and Neck Surgery and Oncology of the American Academy of Otolaryngology. These levels are demonstrated in **Figure 3.10** and **Table 3.4**.

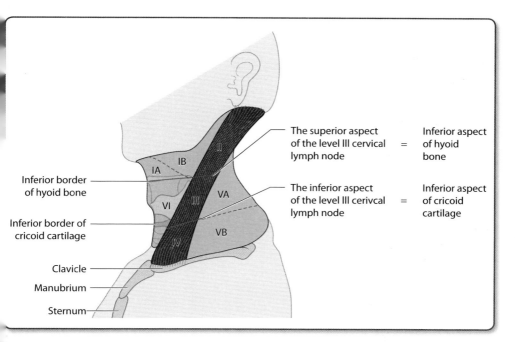

The superior aspect of the level III cervical lymph node = Inferior aspect of hyoid bone

The inferior aspect of the level III cerivcal lymph node = Inferior aspect of cricoid cartilage

Figure 3.10 Cervical lymph node levels.

Table 3.4 Cervical lymph node levels

Cervical lymph node level	Lymph node group
I	Submental (Ia) and submandibular (Ib) nodes
II	Upper jugular nodes
III	Middle jugular nodes
IV	Lower jugular nodes
V	Posterior triangle nodes • Va nodes: those associated with the spinal accessory nerve • Vb nodes: those associated with the transverse cervical and supraclavicular nodes.
VI	Anterior compartment nodes

10.7 This terminology is useful both in the understanding of the cervical lymph node drainage patterns and also in determining which nodes are to be dissected in a clearance operation.

Station 11

11.1 **A** Tongue

   B Hypoglossal nerve

   C Inferior constrictor muscle

   D Oesophagus

   E Trachea

   F Right aryepiglottic fold

   G Epiglottis

   H Vestibule

   I Piriform recess

   J Arytenoid muscles (the transverse and oblique parts of this muscle are difficult to identify from this specimen)

   K Left posterior cricoarytenoid muscle

11.2 The functions of the larynx include phonation, protection of the trachea and bronchial tree during ingestion of food and maintaining an open tract for respiration.

11.3 The intrinsic muscles of the larynx act to regulate the movements of the vocal cords. They are:
- lateral cricoarytenoid muscles
- posterior cricoarytenoid muscles
- cricothyroid muscles
- thyroarytenoid muscles.

11.4 The recurrent laryngeal nerve innervates all but one (the cricothyroid muscle) of the intrinsic laryngeal muscles. The cricothyroid muscle is innervated by the external branch of the superior laryngeal nerve. Other 'exceptions to the rule' within the head and neck are displayed in **Table 3.5**.

Table 3.5 'Exceptions to the rule' innervations of the face, tongue and larynx		
Muscles of	**Supplied by**	**Exceptions**
Facial expression	Facial (CN VII) nerve	Levator palpebrae superioris is supplied by the oculomotor (CN III) nerve
Tongue	Hypoglossal (CN XII) nerve	Palatoglossus is supplied by the pharyngeal plexus
Larynx	Recurrent laryngeal nerve (branch of vagus (CN X) nerve)	Cricothyroid is supplied by the external branch of the superior laryngeal nerve

11.5 The cricothyroid muscle is different to all other intrinsic laryngeal muscles:
- it is innervated by the external branch of the superior laryngeal nerve, not the recurrent laryngeal nerve
- it is the only tensor muscle of the larynx and therefore the only muscle to cause elongation of the vocal cords.

11.6 The left recurrent laryngeal loops underneath the arch of the aorta, posterior to the ligamentum teres, before ascending. The right recurrent laryngeal loops around the right subclavian artery (**Figure 3.11**).

11.7a Unilateral section results in the vocal cord assuming a position between abduction and adduction. Speech is not usually affected to a great extent but may be hoarse.

11.7b Bilateral section causes both the cords to assume this position, and breathing is made difficult due to closure of the rima glottides. Speech is not possible.

11.8 The true vocal cords consist of the vocal ligaments and an elastic membrane known as the *conus elasticus*, sitting between the vocal ligaments and cricoid cartilage (**Figure 3.12**). The false cords are located superiorly and laterally to the true and are also known as the 'vestibular folds'. They are not responsible for sound production.

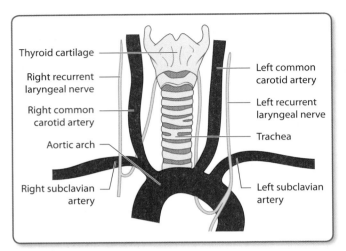

Figure 3.11 Pathways of the right and left recurrent laryngeal nerve.

Thyroid cartilage

Right recurrent laryngeal nerve

Right common carotid artery

Aortic arch

Right subclavian artery

Left common carotid artery

Left recurrent laryngeal nerve

Trachea

Left subclavian artery

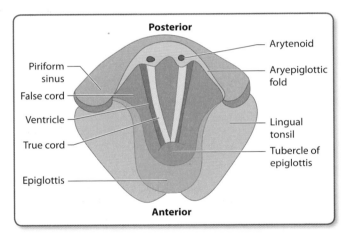

Figure 3.12 The false and true vocal cords viewed from above.

Posterior

Piriform sinus

False cord

Ventricle

True cord

Epiglottis

Arytenoid

Aryepiglottic fold

Lingual tonsil

Tubercle of epiglottis

Anterior

11.9a Above the vocal cords the larynx drains into the upper deep cervical lymph nodes (and further on to the mediastinal lymph nodes).

11.9b Below the vocal cords the drainage is to the lower deep cervical lymph nodes.

Station 12

12.1 A Left parotid gland

B Left superficial temporal artery

C Left temporalis tendon

D Left orbicularis oculi

E Left orbiculariss oris

F Left trapezius

12.2 The facial nerve has been damaged.

12.3 The facial nerve (CNVII) arises from the caudal aspect of the pons leaving the skull via the internal acoustic meatus with the vestibulocochlear (CNVIII) nerve. It travels through the facial canal within the petrous temporal bone to emerge from the stylomastoid foramen and dividing into its terminal branches within the parotid gland.

12.4a Within the facial canal, the facial nerve gives off the following branches:

- greater petrosal nerve
- nerve to stapedius
- chorda tympani
- auricular branch.

12.4b After leaving the stylomastoid foramen the facial nerve gives off:

- the posterior auricular nerve
- the nerve supplying the stylohyoid and posterior belly of the digastric.

12.4c Within the parotid gland the facial nerve gives off five branches which supply the muscles of facial expression:

- temporal
- zygomatic
- buccal
- mandibular
- cervical.

12.5 The facial nerve is first found at the stylomastoid foramen and then followed. Alternatively a peripheral branch of the facial nerve such as the marginal mandibular nerve can be traced proximally.

12.6 In lower motor neurone lesions there is complete unilateral impairment of facial movement. In upper lesions the weakness is only of the lower face because there is dual innervation of the muscles of the forehead (**Figure 3.13**).

12.7 Innervation of the sternocleidomastoid muscle is via the spinal accessory nerve (CNXI).

12.8 The origin of sternocleidomastoid is the mastoid process of the skull. As it descends anteromedially in the neck it divides into two heads. The medial head inserts into the sternum and the lateral head onto the superior aspect of the medial third of the clavicle.

12.9 Unilateral innervation of the sternocleidomastoid muscle tilts the head to the ipsilateral side and also rotates the face so that it looks to the other side of the muscle. In order to test the function of the right sternocleidomastoid muscle ask the patient to turn their head to the left and try to oppose this action.

Station 13

13.1 A Sphenoid sinuses

   B Nasal septum

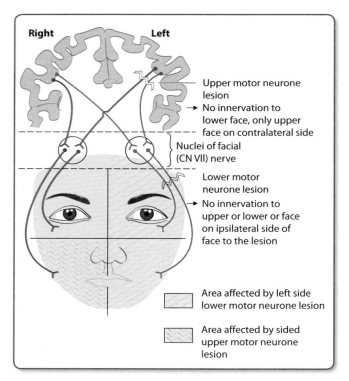

Figure 3.13 The motor innervation from the facial (CN VII) nerve to the upper and lower face.

Upper motor neurone lesion
→ No innervation to lower face, only upper face on contralateral side

Nuclei of facial (CN VII) nerve

Lower motor neurone lesion
→ No innervation to upper or lower or face on ipsilateral side of face to the lesion

Area affected by left side lower motor neurone lesion

Area affected by sided upper motor neurone lesion

Right   Left

     C Right lateral rectus muscle

     D Optic nerve

     E Right medial rectus muscle

13.2 D The optic nerve. This travels through the optic canal.

13.3 The right medial rectus muscle. The medial rectus originates from the annulus of Zinn (a tendinous ring of fibrous tissue surrounding the optic nerve at its entrance into the orbit) and inserts into the horizontal meridian, 0.5 cm from the limbus (the outer edge of the iris). It is the largest of the extraocular muscles.

13.4 F Lens

     G Vitreous humour

13.5 The vitreous humor is a clear gelatinous like substance within the eye that occupies the space between the lens and the retina. Its functions include maintaining the spherical shape of the eye and preventing retinal detachment by pressing against the retina. It also contains cells such as phagocytes that aid in the removal of cellular debris.

13.6 Left temporal lobe.

Station 14

14.1 A Clivus

B Anterior arch of C1 vertebra

C Spinous process of C7 vertebra

D Left transverse process of C1 vertebra

E Vertebral body of C6

F Intervertebral disc space of C7/T1

14.2 Above the C4 level the prevertebral soft tissue margin should measure less than 7 mm (or less than 50% the width of the adjacent vertebral body) and below this level it should not be more than 22 mm (or the width of the adjacent vertebral body).

14.3 This may be the only radiological clue that there is an underlying fracture to a cervical vertebra.

14.4 The ways in which the cervical vertebrae differ are listed below.

Size: the cervical spine vertebrae are smaller and broader in their lateral dimensions than in their anteroposterior dimensions.

Structure: cervical spine vertebrae consist of bifid spinous processes (non-bifid in the lumbar vertebrae) and their transverse processes contain 'foramen transversarium' which transmit the vertebral vessels and sympathetic supply. Their laminae are long and thin and give a triangular shape to the vertebral foramen in which the spinal cord is contained.

Number: there are seven cervical spine vertebrae whereas there are only five lumbar vertebrae.

14.5 There are seven cervical vertebrae.

14.6 The C7 vertebra is known as the *vertebra prominens* because of its long and prominently felt spinous process palpable under the skin at the base of the neck. It is the most prominent cervical vertebra in about 70% of people.

14.7 The following cervical nerves pass over the superior aspect of the following vertebrae:

14.7a C1 vertebrae – C1 nerve

14.7b C7 vertebrae – C7 nerve

14.7c T1 vertebrae – C8 nerve

14.7d T7 vertebrae – T6 nerve

14.8 There are eight cervical nerves but only seven cervical vertebrae. The cervical spinal nerves vertebra pass superior to their pedicles but those of the thoracic nerves pass underneath. Therefore there is a spare nerve between the C7 and T1 vertebra, and this is called the C8 spinal nerve (**Figure 3.14**).

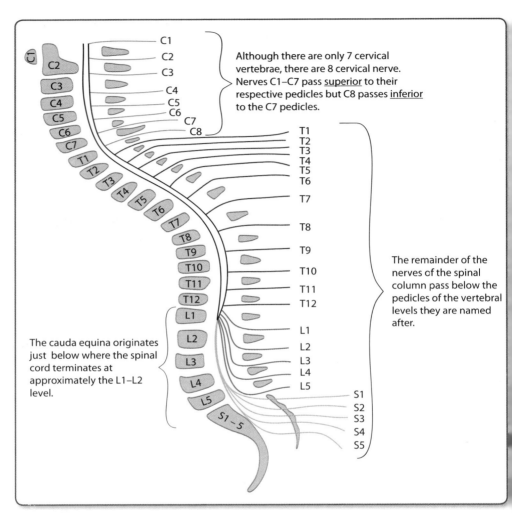

Figure 3.14 Schematic view of the spinal nerves.

Station 15

15.1 A Optic chiasm

    B Pituitary stalk (infundibulum)

    C Pituitary gland

    D Optic nerve

    E Basilar artery

15.2 X The sphenoid sinus. Its proximity to the pituitary gland is the reason why neurosurgeons are able to access the pituitary gland via the trans-sphenoidal route without requiring a more invasive intracranial course.

15.3 C The pituitary gland. It consists of two lobes: an *anterior* and a *posterior*. A third *intermediate* lobe is sometimes described however this is rudimentary in humans and has little function.

15.4 The embryology of the anterior and posterior pituitary differs considerably. The anterior pituitary gland originates from 'Rathke's pouch' (a pouch of ectoderm that begins in the midline from the developing mouth, the stomodeum). The infundibulum and posterior lobe are derived from the diencephalon (the posterior aspect of the forebrain). The anterior pituitary gland consists of secretory cells and is regulated via feedback mechanisms by the hypothalamus. The posterior pituitary gland does not create any hormones itself and only releases hormones produced by the hypothalamus.

15.5 The anterior pituitary lobe secretes the hormones prolactin (PRL), thyroid stimulating hormone (TSH), adrenocorticotrophic hormone (ACTH), growth hormone (GH), follicle stimulating hormone (FSH), luteinising hormone (LH). The posterior pituitary does not produce hormones however it releases hormones made by the hypothalamus (oxytocin and antidiuretic hormone, ADH).

15.6 The most common pathology of the pituitary gland (C) is a pituitary adenoma. This pathology commonly affects the anterior lobe of the gland and may either be hormone secreting or non-hormone secreting.

15.7 A The optic chiasm. Compression of this structure causes a bitemporal hemianopia (only the most medial aspect of vision is preserved).

15.8 E The basilar artery. This is formed from the right and left vertebral arteries at a level between the pons and the medulla.

Station 16

16.1 A Supraclavicular nerve(s)

B Right superior belly of omohyoid

C Right sternohyoid

D Right clavicular head of the sternocleidomastoid

E Right sternal head of the sternocleidomastoid

F Left internal jugular vein

16.2 The C1–C4 spinal nerves contribute to the cervical plexus. It lies in series with the brachial plexus on scalenus medius and is covered by the upper aspect of the sternocleidomastoid (**Figure 3.15**).

16.3 The cervical plexus has motor and sensory branches. The cutaneous branches of the plexus are:
- greater auricular nerve (C2, C3)
- lesser occipital nerve (C2)
- transverse cervical nerve (C2, C3)
- supraclavicular nerves (C3, C4).

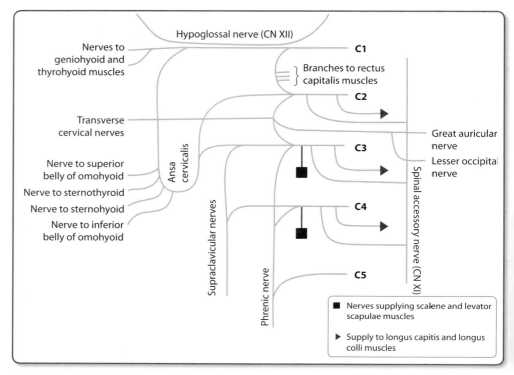

Figure 3.15 The cervical plexus.

16.4 The muscular branches of the cervical plexus and the structures which they supply is summarised in **Table 3.6**.

Table 3.6 The motor branches of the cervical plexus	
Muscular branches	**Structures innervated**
Ansa cervicalis (C1, C2, C3)	Most of the infrahyoid muscles (except for thyrohyoid muscle)
Phrenic nerve (C3, C4, C5)	Pericardium and diaphragm
Segmental branches (C1–C4)	Anterior and middle scalene muscles

16.5 The ansa cervicalis a nerve loop formed from the C1–C3 spinal nerves. It is located within the carotid sheath, lateral and superficial to the internal jugular vein, and is accompanied by the hypoglossal nerve (CN XII).

16.6 The ansa cervicalis supplies the sternothyroid, sternohyoid and omohyoid muscles (ipsilateral side).

16.7 The only infrahyoid muscle which the ansa cervicalis does not innervate is the thyrohyoid muscle which is innervated by the hypoglossal (CN XII) nerve.

Station 17

17.1 A Erector spinae

B Trapezius

C Middle scalene

D Anterior scalene

E Longus colli

17.2 The sympathetic nervous system has a thoracolumbar outflow from the T1–L3 spinal nerve roots. The parasympathetic nervous system has a craniosacral outflow from the spinal nerve roots of: C3,7,9,10 and S2–4.

17.3 The stellate ganglion is a sympathetic mass of nervous tissue formed by the fusion of the inferior cervical ganglion and first thoracic ganglion. Blocking results in the ipsilateral dilatation of the upper limb vasculature, decreased sweating and a mild reduction in left ventricular contractility.

17.4 Common indications include complex regional pain syndromes, hyperhidrosis and diseases causing vascular insufficiency (such as Raynaud's syndrome).

17.5 Posterior to the stellate ganglion are:
- the transverse process of the C7 vertebra
- the neck of the 1st rib
- the brachial plexus sheath
- longus colli
- the anterior scalene muscles.

Anterior to the ganglion are the vertebral artery and the sternocleidomastoid.

17.6 The stellate ganglion is absent in about 20% of the population.

Station 18

18.1 A lump at region A indicates a midline neck swelling. Differential diagnoses could include: subcutaneous abscesses, enlarged lymph nodes, sebaceous cyst, lipoma, dermoid cyst, thyroglossal cyst, thyroid mass.

18.2 A lump at region C indicates a mass in the anterior triangle. Differential diagnoses could include: subcutaneous abscesses, enlarged lymph nodes, sebaceous cyst, lipoma, branchial cyst, parotid tumour, laryngocele, carotid artery aneurysm/tumour.

18.3 A lump at region B indicates a mass in the posterior triangle. Differential diagnoses include: subcutaneous abscesses, enlarged lymph nodes, sebaceous cyst, lipoma, cervical rib, pharyngeal pouch, cystic hygroma, Pancoast's tumour, subclavian artery aneurysm.

18.4 The infrahyoid 'strap' muscles are: sternothyroid, thyrohyoid, sternohyoid, omohyoid.

18.5 They are supplied by the ansa cervicalis and their function is to fix the hyoid bone so that the suprahyoid muscles can contract against an immoveable base.

18.6 A cystic hygroma is a congenital multiloculated lymphatic lesion in the lower posterior triangle of the neck. It is benign but can be disfiguring and the treatment is excision.

18.7 A branchial cyst is a cystic mass filled with squamous or columnar epithelium. It is usually located along the anterior border of the sternocleidomastoid at the junction of the superior/middle third. It is thought to be a remnant of the branchial arches (usually the second), although another theory is it arises from squamous clefts in cervical lymph nodes.

18.8 A chemodectoma is a carotid body paraganglioma. It presents as a pulsatile mass along the anterior border of the sternocleidomastoid at the level of the hyoid. The mass can be moved from side to side but not up and down. It is associated with a small risk of malignancy.

18.9 Ludwig's angina is an acute bacterial infection of the submandibular fascial space, often associated with dental infection. It may cause life-threatening airway obstruction.

Station 19

19.1 **A** Right sclera

   B Right iris

   C Left caruncula lacrimalis

   D Left superior palpebral sulcus

   E Pupil of the left eye

19.2 Each eye is drained by one lacrimal gland. Each lacrimal gland consists of two lobes: the larger *orbital* and smaller *palpebral*.

19.3 Each lacrimal gland is located in the superotemporal aspect of the orbit (**Figure 3.16**).

19.4 The nasolacrimal duct drains tears from the lacrimal gland to the nasal cavity. The superior and inferior lacrimal puncta and papillae are located at the medial corner of the eyes and receive tears. They then pass in to the superior and inferior lacrimal canaliculi, and thence in to the lacrimal sac before entering the lacrimal duct (**Figure 3.16**).

19.5 The 'annulus of Zinn' is a fibrous ring that encircles the optic nerve and is continuous with the dura of the middle cranial fossa. The four recti muscles originate from this structure.

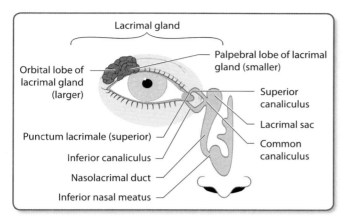

Figure 3.16 The lacrimal gland and nasolacrimal ductal system.

19.6 The afferent limb of the pupillary light reflex is the optic nerve (CN II). The efferent limb is the oculomotor nerve (CN III), which innervates the constrictor pupillae (**Figure 3.17**).

19.7 The direct pupillary reflex is lost but the consensual pupillary reflex is intact. This means that light shone in to the damaged eye would not cause pupillary constriction of either eyes, but light shone in to the undamaged eyes would cause constriction of both.

19.8 Damage to the right oculomotor (CN III) nerve would prevent constriction of the pupil of the right eye. Whether light was detected within the right or left eye, only

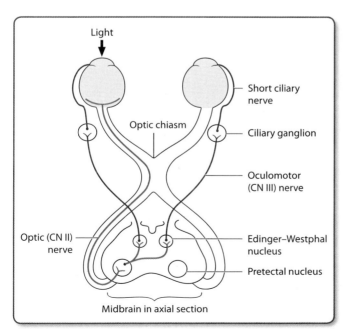

Figure 3.17 The afferent and efferent pathways of the pupillary light reflex.

the left eye would be able to demonstrate pupillary constriction. In other words the 'direct pupillary and consensual reflex' is lost.

Station 20

20.1 **A** Anterior ethmoid sinus

   B Posterior ethmoid sinus

   C Sphenoid sinus

   D Midbrain

20.2 Boundaries of the nasal cavity:
- anterior: the nostrils
- posterior: the posterior nasal apertures
- floor: the palatine process of the maxilla and the palatine bone
- roof: anteriorly is the nasal and frontal bones, in the middle is the cribriform plate of the ethmoid bone, and posteriorly is the sphenoid bone
- medial: nasal septum, made up of septal cartilage, the vertical plate of the ethmoid, and the vomer
- lateral: the ethmoid bone above, the medial surface of the maxilla and the perpendicular plate of the palatine bone below.

20.3 The nasal vestibule is the anterior part of the nasal cavity that is lined by stratified squamous keratinizing epithelium. It has small hairs, *vibrissae*, which filter the air.

20.4 The superior meatus receives the posterior ethmoidal air sinuses.

20.5 The middle meatus receives the openings of:
- the anterior (via the infundibulum) and middle ethmoidal air sinuses
- the frontal sinus (via the infundibulum and hiatus semilunaris)
- the maxillary sinus (via the hiatus semilunaris).

20.6 The inferior meatus receives the opening of the nasolacrimal duct.

20.7 The sphenoethmoidal recess is an area above the superior concha that receives the opening of the sphenoid air cells.

20.8 The nasal cavity proper is lined with ciliated pseudostratified columnar epithelium, containing mucous secreting goblet cells. The mucociliary escalator transfers material trapped by mucous cranially to be swallowed or expectorated.

20.9 Sensation is supplied via the ophthalmic and maxillary branches of the trigeminal nerve. The olfactory mucous membranes are innervated by the olfactory nerves, which travel through the cribriform plate to the olfactory bulbs.

20.10 The hiatus semilunaris is the common drainage pathway for the frontal and maxillary sinuses, and communication between the maxillary from the frontal is possible. Additionally, the drainage orifice of the maxillary sinus is situated near the roof of the sinus, and is therefore only effective when already full of fluid.

20.11 The floor of the maxillary sinus is closely approximated to the first and second molar teeth, and the apices of the roots sometimes protrude through and are occasionally dehiscent in to the space.

Station 21

21.1 **Table 3.7** describes the muscles responsible for the movements of the neck.

Table 3.7 Muscles responsible for the neck movements	
Neck action	**Muscles responsible**
Flexion	Sternocleidomastoid and scalene muscles
Extension	Trapezius, cervicis, splenius capitis, semispinalis capitis, semispinalis cervicis muscles
	Other contributing muscles include: spinalis capitis and longissimus cervicis
Rotation	Splenius capitis, sternocleidomastoid, levator scapula, suboccipitalis
Lateral flexion	Scalene muscles

21.2 The trapezius is contained within the investing layer of the deep cervical fascia.

21.3 Other structures within the investing layer of the deep cervical fascia are:
- sternocleidomastoid
- fibrous capsule of the parotid gland
- submandibular gland.

21.4 The three remaining fascial compartments (**Figure 3.18**) are:
- carotid sheath – containing the common carotid artery, vagus nerve (CN X) and the internal jugular vein
- prevertebral fascia – passing in front of the prevertebral muscles
- pretracheal fascia – containing the thyroid gland.

21.5 The prevertebral fascia is continuous with the axillary sheath inferior to the clavicles.

Station 22

22.1 A Temporalis muscle

   B Sternocleidomastoid muscle

   C Right submandibular gland

   D Right scalenus muscle (anterior and middle)

   E Right superior belly of omohyoid muscle

   F Right masseter muscle

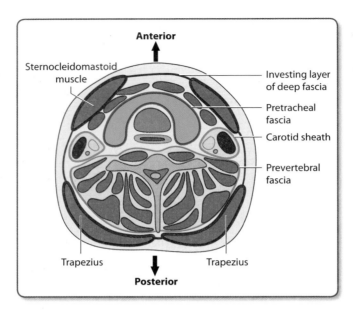

Figure 3.18
The fascial compartments of the neck.

22.2 The trigeminal (CN V) innervates the muscles of mastication which include the masseter and temporalis muscle.

22.3 The mandibular branch of the trigeminal nerve (CN V) innervates the skin over the lower jawline.

22.4 The temporalis muscle (A) elevates and retrudes the mandible.

22.5 The temporalis muscle (A) is a large fan shaped muscle originating from the temporal fossa on the external surface of the skull and inserting into the coronoid process of the mandible.

22.6 You can test the temporalis muscle by asking the patient to tightly clench their jaw whilst palpating the temples and feeling for contraction of the muscle.

22.7 The three sensory branches of the trigeminal nerve converge at the trigeminal ganglion within Meckel's cave (or the trigeminal cave) lateral to the cavernous sinus within the sphenoid bone.

Station 23

23.1 A Mandible

B Sternocleidomastoid

C Parotid gland

D Mastoid air cells

E Upper spinal cord

23.2 Left sided weakness indicates ischaemia of the right side of the brain, which is supplied by the right internal carotid artery. As this has significant stenosis it would be suitable for endarterectomy.

23.3 Skin, superficial fascia, platysma, investing layer of deep cervical fascia, and carotid sheaf. The incision is made along the anterior border of the sternocleidomastoid, from approximately the level of the lower border of the thyroid cartilage to the angle of the mandible.

23.4 The internal carotid artery is initially lateral to the external carotid but as they ascend it winds posterior to it. The jugular vein and vagus nerve have constant positions to the internal carotid: the former stays lateral and the latter runs behind and between the internal carotid and the jugular vein.

23.5 The internal carotid artery has no branches in the neck.

23.6 The superior laryngeal nerve has *internal* and *external* branches. The *internal* laryngeal supplies sensation to the piriform fossa and larynx above the level of the vocal cords. The *external* laryngeal supplies the cricothyroid muscle and division produces paralysis of the cricothyroid and weakness of the voice.

23.7 Section of the great auricular nerve results in numbness over the angle of the mandible, the parotid gland, and on both surfaces of the auricle.

23.8 Section of the marginal mandibular branch of the facial nerve results in drooping of the ipsilateral side of the lip and an asymmetrical smile.

Station 24

24.1 **A** Laryngeal prominence of the thyroid cartilage

B Hyoid bone

C Cricoid cartilage

24.2 The origin and insertion of the scalene muscles are shown in **Table 3.8**.

24.3 See above.

Table 3.8 The scalene muscles		
Muscle	**Origin**	**Insertion**
Anterior scalene	Anterior tubercles of transverse processes C3–6	Scalene tubercle of first rib
Middle scalene	Posterior tubercles of transverse processes of C2–7	Anterior to the tubercle of the first rip, on its superior surface
Posterior scalene	Posterior tubercles of transverse processes of C4–6	Posterolateral second rib

24.4 Anterior relations of the anterior scalene muscle:
- arteries: carotids, transverse cervical, suprascapular
- veins: internal jugular, subclavian
- nerves: vagus, phrenic
- lymph: deep cervical
- fascia: prevertebral layer of deep cervical fascia.

24.5 Structures between the anterior scalene and middle scalene muscles:
- arteries: subclavian (second part)
- nerves: brachial plexus
- fascia: pleura of the lung.

24.6 The digastric has two bellies: the origin of the *anterior* belly is the digastric fossa on the posterior surface of the symphysis menti, and the origin of the posterior is the base of the medial aspect of the mastoid process. The muscle inserts in to the lesser cornu of the hyoid bone.

24.7 The mylohyoid arises from the mylohyoid line on the internal aspect of the mandible. The middle and anterior fibres insert in to the midline raphe (extending from the symphysis menti to the hyoid bone). The posterior fibres insert in to the body of the hyoid bone.

24.8 The platysma arises from the skin and deep fascia over pectoralis major and deltoid. It inserts in to the inferior border of the mandible and overlying skin.

Station 25

25.1 A Superior rectus muscle

　　B Optic nerve

　　C Lateral rectus muscle

25.2 The oculomotor nerve (CN III).

25.3 Muscles supplied by the oculomotor nerve (CN III) are:
- superior rectus muscle
- inferior rectus muscle
- medial rectus muscle
- inferior oblique muscle
- levator palpebrae superioris.

25.4 The clinical signs of an isolated oculomotor (CN III) nerve palsy includes:
- deviation of the orbit 'down and out' (abducted and inferiorly deviated) due to the unopposed actions of the lateral rectus and superior oblique muscles not supplied by the same nerve
- ptosis of the ipsilateral eyelid
- dilatation of the ipsilateral pupil
- impairment of the accommodation reflex and consensual (not direct) light reflex on the affected side.

- In Horner's syndrome just the sympathetic pathway is disrupted. There is a ptosis of the upper eyelid, anhydrosis, but no deviation of the orbit. The pupil is constricted and slow to dilate but there is no impairment of the direct or consensual light reflex.

25.6 X Ethmoid sinus

    Y Right maxillary sinus

    Z Left inferior turbinate/concha

25.7 The medial wall of the orbit is also known as the 'lamina papyracea' that translates literally into to 'paper thin'. This wall of the orbit is easily damaged during instrumentation of the nasal cavity.

Station 26

26.1 A Frontal sinus

    B Posterior ethmoid sinuses

    C Sphenoid sinus

    D Pituitary fossa

    E Middle turbinate

    F Inferior turbinate

    G Soft palate

26.2 The paranasal sinuses drain into the nasal cavity via openings known as 'ostia'. The various openings of the sinuses and position of their ostia are demonstrated in **Table 3.9** and **Figure 3.19** below.

Table 3.9 The openings of the various paranasal sinuses within the nasal cavity

Paranasal sinus	Opening within the nasal cavity
Frontal	Frontal recess in the anterior middle meatus (via the frontonasal duct)
Sphenoid	Sphenoethmoidal recess (above the superior turbinate)
Maxillary	Hiatus semilunaris within the middle meatus
Anterior ethmoid	Hiatus semilunaris (via the ethmoid infundibulum) or the ethmoid bulla within the middle meatus
Middle ethmoid	Ethmoid bulla
Posterior ethmoid	Superior nasal meatus

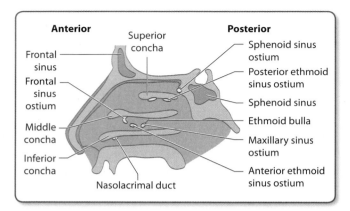

Figure 3.19 The openings of the various paranasal sinuses within the nasal cavity.

26.3 The osteomeatal complex is a region where the frontal, ethmoidal and maxillary sinuses drain through. The passage through which these various sinuses drain is very narrow and therefore any blockage at this region will cause stasis and obstruction of drainage of secretions from the involved paranasal sinuses. It is made up of the maxillary ostium, uncinate process, middle turbinate, ethmoidal bulla and ethmoidal infundibulum (**Figure 3.20**).

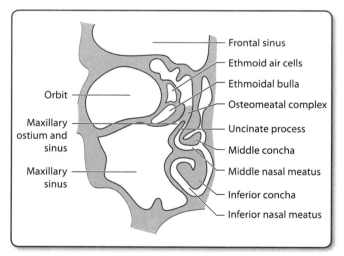

Figure 3.20 A coronal section of the orbit and paranasal sinuses demonstrating the osteomeatal complex.

26.4 The functions of the paranasal sinuses include:

- reduction of the weight of the skull
- increasing the area for olfactory input
- resonators for voice production
- production of mucus to humidify the nasal chambers
- providing a buffer between the skull and brain against trauma to the face.

26.5 Allergic reactions cause irritation and hyperplasia of the mucosal lining to the paranasal sinuses and can impair their drainage of mucus secretions. The build-up and stagnation of these contents provides a good medium for infective organisms to proliferate.

26.6 The lymphatics of the posterior paranasal sinuses drain into the retropharyngeal lymph nodes and the submental nodes anteriorly. Both of these lymph nodes eventually drain into the upper deep cervical nodes.

26.7 The arterial supply to the nasal cavity is via branches of the external and internal carotid arteries (**Figure 3.21**):

26.7a External carotid artery: via the superficial labial artery (facial artery) and the sphenopalatine artery (maxillary artery)

26.7b Internal carotid artery: via the anterior and posterior ethmoidal arteries (ophthalmic artery)

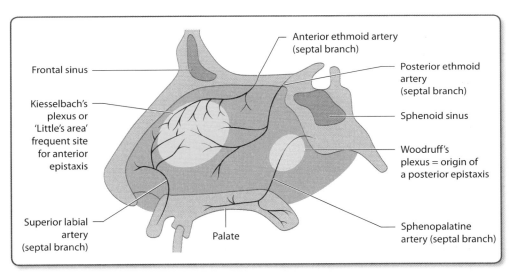

Figure 3.21 Blood supply to the nasal cavity.

26.8 Kiesselbach's plexus (Little's area) is located on the anteroinferior aspect of the nasal septum. Here, the external and internal carotid arteries anastomose. It is a frequent site for epistaxis.

26.9 Woodruff's plexus is the name given to the area where the sphenopalatine artery leaves the sphenopalatine foramen and enters the nasal cavity. It is situated at the posterior limit of the middle turbinate and the origin for a posterior epistaxis.

26.10 The venous drainage of the nose is named after the arteries:

- anterior and posterior ethmoidal veins drain into the ophthalmic vein
- sphenopalatine and greater palatine veins drain to the pterygoid plexus of veins
- the angular vein drains into the anterior facial vein.

The ophthalmic vein and pterygoid plexus of veins have connections with the cavernous sinuses and infection within the nasal cavity can spread intracranially via this route predisposing to a cavernous sinus thrombosis.

Station 27

27.1 A Right external acoustic meatus

B Posterior belly of the right digastric muscle

C Right internal carotid artery (note the lack of arteries given off in the neck)

D Right facial artery

E Right external carotid artery

F Anterior belly of the right digastric muscle

G Right superior thyroid artery

27.2 The parathyroid glands.

27.3 There are normally four parathyroid glands, two superior and two inferior, although this number may vary. The superior parathyroid glands are found constantly at the superolateral aspect of the superior pole of the thyroid gland. The position of the inferior parathyroid glands is more varied. During embryological development they have a shared migration path with the thymus gland. They are often found at the level of the inferior pole of the thyroid gland but may also be within the superior mediastinum or even the carotid sheath.

27.4 The parathyroid glands are supplied by the inferior thyroid artery. Branches of this artery are carefully preserved during thyroidectomy to prevent ischaemia to the glands and rendering the patient hypocalcaemic.

27.5 The branchial apparatus is a set of metameric structures in early development that develops into structures within the head and neck. Each 'apparatus' consists of:
- branchial (or pharyngeal) arch
- groove
- pouch
- membrane.

In total there are five branchial arches labelled 1, 2, 3, 4 and 6 (the 5th branchial arch only exists transiently and fails to develop in utero). The same nerve innervates structures that arise from each arch. The pharyngeal (or branchial) pouches develop between the branchial arches. There are four pairs of pharyngeal pouches, the 5th is usually absent or very small.

27.6 The superior parathyroid glands are derived from the fourth pharyngeal pouch (**Table 3.10**). The parafollicular cells of the thyroid gland (which secrete calcitonin) are also derived from this same pouch.

27.7 The inferior parathyroid glands are derived from the third pharyngeal pouch. Other structures which are also derived from this pouch include the thymus gland.

27.8 Pharyngeal (branchial) arch derivatives and their innervation are given in **Table 3.11**.

Table 3.10 The derivatives of the pharyngeal pouches

Pharyngeal pouch	Derivatives
First	Tubotympanic recess contributing to development of the tympanic membrane, external acoustic meatus, mastoid antrum and tympanic cavity
Second	Contributes to formation of the palatine tonsils
Third	Inferior parathyroid glands and thymus gland
Fourth	Superior parathyroid glands and parafollicular cells of the thyroid gland

Table 3.11 The branchial arches

Branchial arch		Artery	Nerve	Muscle	Skeletal
1	Mandibular	Maxillary	Mandibular division of trigeminal (Vc)	Muscles of mastication (masseter, temporalis), digastric (anterior belly), mylohyoid, tensor tympani, tensor veli palatini	Incus, malleus, Mandible (as a model for the mandible), Meckel's cartilage
2	Hyoid	Stapedial	Facial (VII)	Stylohyoid, stapedius (posterior belly), muscles of facial expression (including buccinator, platysma)	Hyoid: lesser cornu and superior part of body, styloid process, stapes, Reichert's cartilage
3	Thyrohyoid	Internal carotid	Glossopharyngeal (IX)	Stylopharyngeus	Hyoid: greater cornu and inferior part of body
4		Part of right subclavian, left aortic arch	Vagus (X) and superior laryngeal branch	Intrinsic muscles of soft palate (including levator veli palatini), cricothyroid, pharyngeal constrictors	Thyroid cartilage, epiglottic cartilage
6		Ventral pulmonary artery, dorsal ductus arteriosus	Vagus (X) and recurrent laryngeal branch	Intrinsic muscles of larynx (except cricothyroid)	Cricoid cartilage, arytenoid cartilage, corniculate cartilage

Station 28

28.1 The right common carotid artery originates from the brachiocephalic artery. The left common carotid artery is the second branch of the aortic arch.

28.2 The common carotid bifurcate into its internal and external branches at the C4 vertebral level.

28.3 **A** Superficial temporal artery

   B Occipital artery

   C Maxillary artery

28.4 The branches of the external carotid artery are, from inferior to superior (**Figure 3.22**):

- superior thyroid artery
- ascending pharyngeal artery
- lingual artery
- facial artery
- occipital artery
- posterior auricular artery
- maxillary artery
- superficial temporal artery.

A mnemonic that may help you to remember these branches is 'Some Anatomists Like Flirting with Obliging Pretty Medical Students'. In order to help identify the

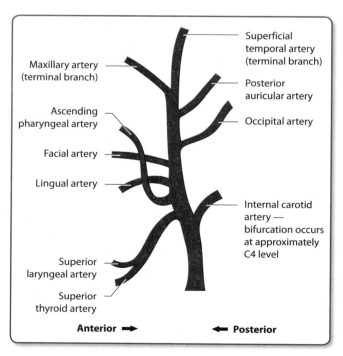

Figure 3.22 The branches of the external carotid artery.

vessels on an angiogram it is useful to remember that the occipital and posterior auricular arteries arise from the posterior aspect of the external carotid artery.

28.5 This is divided into three parts by the lateral pterygoid muscle.

28.6 X The middle meningeal artery. It is a branch of the first part of the maxillary artery.

28.7 The distal part of this artery runs beneath the pterion of the skull and can bleed profusely forming an extradural haematoma.

28.8 The sphenopalatine artery. This is also known as the 'artery of epistaxis' and is one of the terminal branches of the maxillary artery. This artery causes bleeding in the posterior nasal cavity, making it more difficult to control than an anterior bleed.

28.9 Y The facial artery

28.10 The facial artery runs along a line drawn from the corner of the mouth to the angle of the mandible. It can be felt in front of the masseter muscle on the lower border of the body of the mandible. It can also be felt at the angle of the mouth.

28.11 Yes, the facial artery is often ligated during removal of the submandibular gland.

Station 29

29.1 Contrast has been administered via the submandibular duct (also known as Wharton's duct) to obtain a submandibular gland sialogram.

29.2 The opening of the submandibular duct is in the floor of the mouth, lateral to the frenulum of the tongue.

29.3 The surgical incision for submandibular gland removal is approximately 2 cm below the angle of the mandible, to avoid damage to the marginal mandibular branch of the facial nerve. This nerve provides innervation to the muscles of the lower lip and chin and ligation would result in drooping of the ipsilateral corner of the lip.

29.4 During excision of the submandibular gland the following structures are at risk:

- lingual nerve
- marginal mandibular nerve
- nerve to mylohyoid muscle
- hypoglossal nerve.

29.5 The lingual nerve is a branch of the mandibular) portion of the trigeminal nerve (CN V3). It supplies sensation to the floor of the mouth, the lingual gingival and anterior two-thirds of the tongue. It also supplies taste to anterior two-thirds of the tongue (via the chorda tympani, a branch of the facial nerve).

29.6 Sialolithiasis (salivary gland calculi) affects the submandibular gland in 80% of cases followed by the sublingual gland and then the parotid gland. The postulated reasons are:

- the submandibular gland produces viscous saliva composed of mucinous and serous secretions.

- the submandibular duct forms a steep up-sloping angle to the floor of the mouth promoting stasis of its contents and stone formation.

29.7 Minor salivary glands, which are scattered throughout the oral mucosa and submucosa, include:
- labial glands
- buccal glands
- palatoglossal glands
- palatal glands
- lingual glands

(The major salivary glands are the sublingual gland, the parotid gland and the submandibular gland.)

Station 30

30.1 A Malleolar prominence

B Umbo (tip of the malleus)

C Cone of light

D Pars flaccida

E Pars tensa

30.2 It is possible to tell which ear is being examined by looking at just the image of the tympanic membrane as the handle of the malleus always points posteriorly with its lateral process situated anteriorly. In the image provided, the left ear is being examined.

30.3 The innervation of the tympanic membrane:
- outer surface: the auriculotemporal branch of the trigeminal nerve (CN V3) and the auricular nerves (from the cervical plexus)
- inner surface: the tympanic branch of the glossopharyngeal nerve (CN IX)

30.4 The boundaries of the middle ear are:
- laterally: the tympanic membrane
- medially: the lateral wall of the inner ear
- superiorly: the tegmen tympani (a part of the petrous temporal bone)
- inferiorly: the jugular fossa and thin plate of bone
- anteriorly: the carotid canal.

30.5 The petrous part of temporal bone.

30.6 There are three bones of the ossicular chain (from external to internal): the malleus, incus and stapes. Their purpose is to transmit sound vibrations from the tympanic membrane to the oval window (**Figure 3.23**).

30.7 Stapes: the stapedius.

Malleus: the tensor tympani.

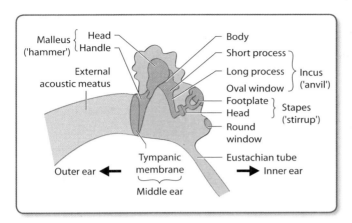

Figure 3.23 The ossicles of the middle ear.

30.8 The stapedius is innervated by the facial nerve (CN VII) and the tensor tympani is innervated by the mandibular branch of the trigeminal nerve (CN V3). Their function is to dampen loud sounds to avoid damage to the inner ear stereocilia, to expand the range of sounds heard and to reduce the volume of self-generated noises such as chewing and vocalisation.

30.9 The Eustachian tube or canal.

30.10 The first third of the eustachian tube is cartilaginous and the remaining two thirds are lined by ciliated columnar epithelial cells containing numerous mucous glands and lymphoid tissue. Infection may cause inflammation of these tissues resulting in blockage of the tube. This can manifest as otalgia and deafness.

30.11 The middle ear is connected to the mastoid antrum by an entrance called the *aditus*. This may serve as a portal through which infection can spread into the middle ear from the mastoid cells.

Station 31

31.1 A Condyle of the mandible

B Coronoid process of mandible

C Ramus of the mandible

D Angle of the mandible

31.2 X Temporal bone

Y Zygoma bone

Z Mastoid process of the temporal bone

31.3 Inferior alveolar nerve.

31.4 The inferior alveolar nerve is a branch of the mandibular nerve (CN V3) and is sometimes known as the 'dental nerve'. An anaesthetic block of this nerve gives total loss of sensation of the lower teeth of the ipsilateral half of the mandible.

31.5 The commonest regions, decreasing order of frequency, are the body, angle, condyle and symphysis. Just as in the pelvis when one part breaks often too does another.

31.6 The condyle of the mandible (A) articulates with the glenoid fossa of the temporal bone.

31.7 The temporomandibular joint is a synovial joint that allows 'hinge' and 'sliding' movements at the joint.

31.8 As with all synovial joints, hyaline cartilage lines the articulating surfaces.

31.9 The temporomandibular joint is one of only two synovial joints in the body (the other is the sternoclavicular joint) that have an articulating disc. This is made of fibrocartilaginous tissue.

31.10 Three ligaments which are related to the temporomandibular joint include:
  • the lateral temporomandibular ligament
  • the sphenomandibular ligament
  • the stylomandibular ligament.

31.11 The muscles of mastication are responsible for the movements of the temporomandibular joint as given in **Figure 3.24** and **Table 3.12**.

31.12 The mandibular branch of the trigeminal nerve (CN V3) innervates the muscles of mastication.

31.13 In an uncomplicated dislocation the mandible is most likely to dislocate in the anteriorly.

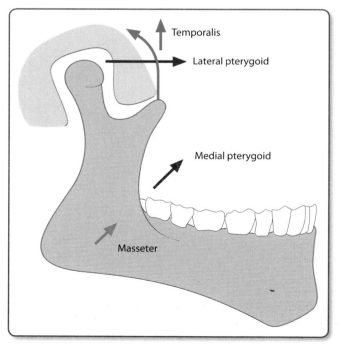

Figure 3.24 The movements of the muscles of mastication.

Table 3.12 Movements of the various muscles of mastication

Muscle	Origin	Insertion	Action
Masseter	Inferior and medial border of zygomatic arch	Lateral surface of ramus and angle of mandible	Closure and retraction of the mandible
Medial Pterygoid	Medial surface of lateral pterygoid plate	Medial surface of angle and ramus of mandible	Closing and protrusion of the mandible
Lateral Pterygoid	Superior head: infratemporal surface of sphenoid bone Inferior head: Lateral surface of the lateral pterygoid plate	Superior head: Articular disc and capsule of the TMJ	Opening and protrusion of the mandible
Temporalis	Floor of temporal fossa	Coronoid process and ramus of mandible	Retraction and closure of the TMJ

Station 32

32.1 A Nasal septum

   B Epiglottis

   C Tongue

   D Soft palate

   E Trachea

   F Oesophagus

32.2 The three parts of the pharynx are as follows:
- nasopharynx: lying behind the nasal fossae above the soft palate to the anterior pillars of fauces
- oropharynx: originating from the anterior pillars of fauces to the tip of the epiglottis
- laryngopharynx: originating from the tip of the epiglottis to the junction of the pharynx and oesophagus at the C6 vertebral level.

32.3a The palatine tonsils are found within the oropharynx.

32.3b The adenoids are located in the nasopharynx.

32.3c The Eustachian tube is located in the nasopharynx.

32.4 There are three pharyngeal constrictor muscles: the *superior*, *middle* and *inferior constrictors*. There function is to initiate pharyngeal peristalsis, enabling a food bolus to pass into the oesophagus. This is under autonomic control.

32.5 A pharyngeal diverticulum is commonly found within the fibres of the inferior pharyngeal constrictor muscle between its upper oblique and lower transverse portions. This area of weakness is termed *Killian's dehiscence* (**Figure 3.25**). A diverticulum at this position is called *Zenker's diverticulum*.

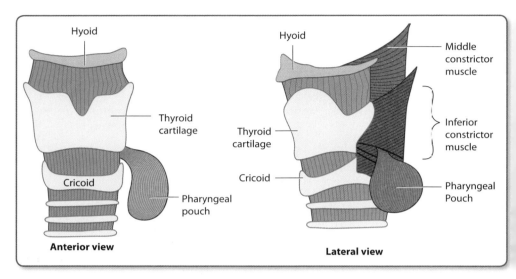

Figure 3.25 Zenker's diverticulum.

32.6 The stylopharyngeus muscle

32.7 The pharyngeal branches of the glossopharyngeal (CN IX) nerve provide sensory supply and the vagus (CN X) nerve provides motor supply of the pharynx. Sensory innervation to the nasopharynx is also provided by the maxillary division of the trigeminal (CN V) nerve.

32.8 The hyoid bone (X) is at the C3 vertebral level.

32.9 Muscles attached to the hyoid bone may be classified as the suprahyoid and infrahyoid (the 'strap muscles') groups. These muscles are all found within the anterior triangle of the neck (**Table 3.13**).

| Table 3.13 The suprahyoid and infrahyoid muscles of the neck ||
Suprahyoid	Infrahyoid
Digastric	Sternohyoid
Mylohyoid	Sternothyroid
Geniohyoid	Thyrohyoid
Stylohyoid	Omohyoid

Muscles which are not referred to as being within this supra- or infrahyoid group of muscles but which are also attached to the hyoid bone are the middle pharyngeal constrictor, hyoglossus and genioglossus.

32.10 It is extremely rare to fracture the hyoid bone and this suggests that the patient was strangled.

Station 33

33.1 A Frontal bone

   B Parietal bones

   C Sphenoid bone

   D Temporal bone

   E Zygoma bone

   F Mandible bone

33.2 The nasal bones.

33.3 In a tripod fracture (zygomaticomaxillary fracture) the areas disrupted are the zygomaticofrontal suture, the zygomatic arch and the zygomaticomaxillary suture (**Figure 3.26**). This combination of fractures commonly occurs together (even more often than an isolated fracture of the zygomatic arch).

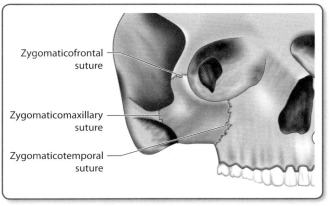

Figure 3.26 Fractures sites in a tripod fracture.

Zygomaticofrontal suture

Zygomaticomaxillary suture

Zygomaticotemporal suture

33.4 A tripod fracture cause damage to the infraorbital nerve, a branch of the maxillary division of the trigeminal nerve (CN V2). This nerve supplies the lower eyelid, upper lip and side of the nose (**Figure 3.27**).

33.5 Other complications of a tripod fracture may include:
- chronic maxillary sinusitis from poor drainage of the sinus.
- diplopia and enophthalmos, due to damage of the inferior orbital wall and trapping of the extraocular muscles

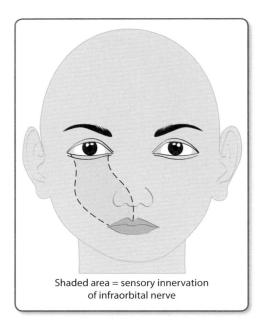

Figure 3.27 The sensory distribution of the infraorbital nerve. Shaded area denotes the sensory innervation.

Shaded area = sensory innervation of infraorbital nerve

- poor cosmetic outcome and facial deformity
- restricted range of motion of the mandible.

33.6 A 'blow out fracture' is a fracture of the walls of the orbit (without damage to the orbital rim) caused by blunt trauma (**Figure 3.28**). This occurs secondary to the sudden increase in the intraocular pressure brought about by the impact of the non-penetrating object that dissipates in to the orbital walls. The inferior and medial orbital walls are commonly involved.

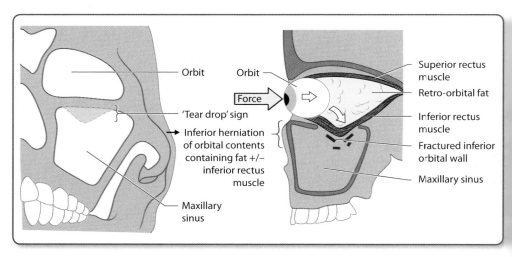

Orbit

Orbit

Force

Superior rectus muscle

Retro-orbital fat

'Tear drop' sign

Inferior rectus muscle

Inferior herniation of orbital contents containing fat +/– inferior rectus muscle

Fractured inferior orbital wall

Maxillary sinus

Maxillary sinus

Figure 3.28 The 'tear drop' sign and the mechanism of a blow out fracture.

33.7 On a plain film of the facial bones the 'tear drop' sign is seen. This shadow looks like a polypoid mass arising from the superior wall of the maxillary sinus but is in fact herniation of the orbital contents, periorbital fat and the inferior rectus muscle through the inferior orbital wall (**Figure 3.28**).

33.8 Failure to repair a blow out fracture may result in continued herniation of the orbital contents causing decreased visual acuity, diplopia on upward gaze (due to the entrapment of the inferior rectus muscle), periorbital haematoma formation and enophthalmos.

33.9 Longitudinal temporal bone fracture (the most common type of all temporal bone fractures). This classically extends from the thin squamous part of the temporal bone, through the middle ear and along the long axis of the petrous temporal bone.

33.10 Transverse temporal bone fracture, classically originating from the foramen magnum and running perpendicular to the long axis of the petrous temporal bone.

33.11 Knowledge of the structures traversed in each of these types of fractures allows prediction of the potential complications (**Table 3.14**).

Table 3.14 Complications of temporal bone fractures

Longitudinal fracture	Transverse fracture
Conductive hearing loss due to middle ear ossicular disruption	Sensorineural hearing loss and vertigo due to disruption of the facial nerve and vestibulo-cochlear apparatus
CSF otorrhea (due to disruption of the tympanic membrane)	CSF rhinorrhoea (there is not usually disruption to the tympanic membrane and CSF leakage is more usually through the nasal cavity via the Eustachian tube)
Meningitis	Meningitis
Facial nerve injury	Facial nerve injury (higher incidence than in longitudinal fractures)
Perforation of the tympanic membrane	

Station 34

34.1 **A** Vallecula

　　B Lingual artery

　　C Tongue

　　D Geniohyoid

　　E Mylohyoid

34.2 The extrinsic muscles of the tongue are:
- genioglossus
- hyoglossus
- styloglossus
- palatoglossus.

34.3 The motor innervation of the extrinsic muscles of the tongue is the hypoglossal nerve (CN XII) except for the palatoglossus, which is innervated by the vagus nerve (CN X) via the pharyngeal plexus.

34.4 Taste from the anterior two-thirds of the tongue is transmitted via the lingual nerve (a branch of the trigeminal nerve) and also by the chorda tympani (a branch of the facial nerve). For the posterior third of the tongue, taste is transmitted via the glossopharyngeal nerve (CN IX). The very posterior aspect of the tongue is also supplied by the internal laryngeal nerve.

34.5 The tip of the tongue drains to the submental nodes, the anterior two-thirds of the tongue drains to the submental and submandibular nodes (then to the lower nodes of the deep cervical chain) and the posterior one-third drains to the upper nodes of the deep cervical chain.

34.6 There is more drainage across the midline of the posterior-third compared to the anterior two-thirds.

34.7 The tongue is lined with stratified squamous epithelium.

34.8 Squamous cell carcinoma is the commonest type of tongue cancer.

Station 35

35.1 A Left maxillary sinus

  B Right internal acoustic meatus

  C Left carotid canal

  D Left cochlea

  E Left mastoid air cells

35.2 The nerves which exit via the internal acoustic meatus are the:
- superior and inferior vestibular nerves (CN VIII)
- cochlear nerve (CN VIII)
- facial nerve (CN VII)

35.3 C The carotid canal. This transmits the internal carotid artery and sympathetic fibres.

35.4 X The pterygopalatine fossa

35.5 Contents of the pterygopalatine fossa are:
- pterygopalatine ganglion

- maxillary artery
- maxillary branch of the trigeminal (CN V2) nerve.

35.6 The pterygopalatine fossa is located posterior to the trigeminal cave and inferior to the orbit. Its boundaries are:

- anteriorly: infratemporal surface of maxilla
- posteriorly: root of the pterygoid process and greater wing of sphenoid bone.
- inferiorly: palatine bone (pyramidal part)
- laterally: pterygomaxillary fissure
- medially: palatine bone (perpendicular plate and orbital sphenoidal processes)

35.7 The connections of the pterygopalatine fossa are given in **Figure 3.29** and **Table 3.15**.

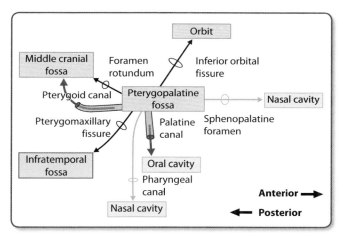

Figure 3.29 Pathways from the pterygopalatine fossa to other sites within the head and neck.

Table 3.15 Connections of the pterygopalatine fossa

Connection from pterygopalatine fossa to:	Via	Orientation of connection
Orbit	Inferior orbital fissure	Anteriorly/superiorly
Middle cranial fossa	Foramen rotundum, pterygoid canal	Posteriorly
Nasal cavity	Pharyngeal canal	Posteriorly
	Sphenopalatine foramen	Medially
Infratemporal fossa	Pterygomaxillary fissure	Laterally
Oral cavity	Palatine canals	Inferiorly

Station 36

36.1 **A** Nasal tip or columella

　　　　B Upper vermilion border (Cupid's bow)

　　　　C Right labial commissure

　　　　D Left nasolabial groove

　　　　E Philtrum

　　　　F Upper lip

　　　　G Lower lip

36.2 Knowledge of the embryology of the upper jaw is necessary in understanding the pathology of cleft lips and palates (**Figure 3.30**). The upper jaw is formed during the 4th to the 8th week in utero from the fusion of five different outgrowths of tissue that originate from the first branchial arch. These five tissue outgrowths are arranged around the primitive mouth and are named the *frontonasal* (consisting of the medial and lateral nasal prominences), *maxillary* (right and left) and *mandibular* (right and left) prominences.

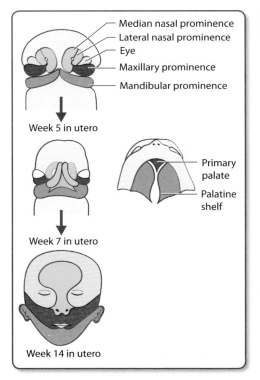

Figure 3.30 The embryology of the upper lip and palate.

Between the 5–6th weeks the maxillary prominences and medial nasal prominences fuse to form the upper lip and primary palate. The secondary palate forms slightly later after the sixth week from two 'palatal shelves' of the posterior aspects of the maxillary prominences. After the 'shelves' have descended they begin to fuse in the midline and also anteriorly with the primary palate. The mandibular prominences fuse to form the lower jaw and lower lip.

36.3 Cleft lip is a defect within the upper lip that appears as a vertical split. It occurs where there is a failure of fusion from the either the medial, lateral and maxillary nasal processes during embryological development. Like cleft palates, these deformities can occur spontaneously, due to environmental factors in utero, or from a genetic deformity (for example, Pierre Robin syndrome).

36.4 Cleft palate can occur in isolation or in conjunction with a cleft lip. It consists of failure of fusion of soft or hard palates.

36.5 Two common classifications are used for cleft palates. The 'Veau classification' provides a quick overview of four different types of deformity and is illustrated in **Figure 3.31**.

- Type A is cleft of the soft palate only
- Type B is cleft of the soft and hard palate extending anteriorly towards the incisive foramen

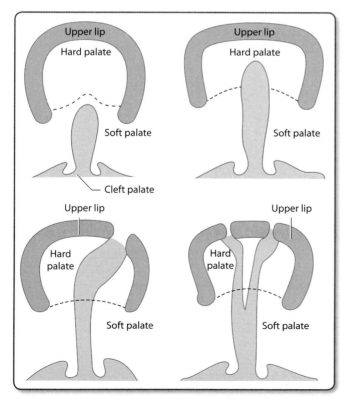

Figure 3.31 The 'Veau classification' for cleft palate.

- Type C is a unilateral cleft of the soft palate, hard palate and lip
- Type D is a bilateral cleft lip with cleft palate.

The 'Kernahan and Stark classification' is more detailed and relies on knowledge of the embryology of the defect. There are two categories, each of which is further subdivided based on whether the defect is complete, incomplete, total or subtotal.

- Category 1 defects involve the primary palate and structures anterior to the incisive foramen
- Category 2 defects involve the secondary palate and structures posterior to the incisive foramen.

Station 37

37.1 A Right nasal alar/sidewall

  B Right nostril

  C Infratip lobule or nasal tip

  D Columella

  E Columella-labial junction

37.2 Olfactory nerve (CN I).

37.3 The cribriform fossa.

37.4 The cribriform plate is part of the ethmoid bone and has the appearance of a sieve. It has multiple foramina allowing the olfactory nerves to pass to the olfactory bulb, which lies on the surface of the plate.

37.5 Anosmia can be unilateral or bilateral, and partial or complete. Unilateral anosmia is due to blockage of the nostril, or disruption of the olfactory pathway from the olfactory mucosa to the anterior commissure of the temporal lobe. There are many causes of unilateral anosmia and these include: nasal obstruction from a deviated septum, increased mucosal secretions from an upper respiratory tract infection, growths in the nasal cavity (for example, polyps), and intracranial lesions.

37.6 The olfactory mucosa is located in the roof of the nasal cavity, in close proximity to the olfactory bulb of the olfactory nerve (CN I).

37.7 The olfactory mucosa is comprised of pseudostratified columnar epithelium that containing olfactory cells and receptors. It has the potential to regenerative if damaged by noxious agents.

Station 38

38.1 A Hard palate

  B Uvula

  C Anterior pillar of the fauces (or palatoglossal arch)

  D Palatine tonsils

  E Tongue

38.2 Waldeyer's ring is a group of lymphoid tissue surrounding the openings of the respiratory and digestive systems. The ring consists of:
- pharyngeal tonsils (adenoids): located in the roof of the nasopharynx
- tubal tonsils: located at the opening of the eustachian tube in to the lateral wall of the nasopharynx
- palatine tonsils: located on the lateral wall of the oropharynx
- lingual tonsils: located on the posterior third of the tongue.

38.3 The palatine tonsil is supplied by branches of the external carotid artery. The lower pole is supplied by the dorsal lingual artery, the ascending palatine artery, and the tonsillar branch of the facial artery. The latter being the principle supply. The upper pole is supplied by the ascending pharyngeal artery and the lesser palatine artery. The veins drain into the internal jugular vein via the lingual and pharyngeal veins.

38.4 The anterior pillar is formed by the projection of the palatoglossus muscle (delimiting the buccal cavity from the oropharynx), and the posterior pillar is formed by the projection of the palatopharyngeal muscle.

38.5 The tonsillar fossa is formed by the superior constrictor muscle of the pharynx. The tonsil is separated from the muscle by the tonsillar capsule and a layer of loose areolar tissue.

38.6 The lymph drainage is via the jugulodigastric node (a deep cervical lymph node), below the angle of the mandible. This may be palpable during episodes of tonsillitis.

38.7 The internal carotid artery.

38.8 Quinsy is a peritonsillar abscess, caused by spread of infection during an episode of tonsillitis outside the capsule of the palatine tonsil in to its surrounding areolar tissue.

Station 39

39.1 The supratrochlear and supraorbital nerves.

39.2 They are both branches of the frontal nerve, which is a branch of the ophthalmic division of the trigeminal nerve. The supraorbital nerve passes through the supraorbital foramen and ends in medial and lateral branches that supply the skin of the forehead as far back as the lambdoidal suture line. It additionally supplies the conjunctiva, the skin of the upper eyelid, and the frontal sinus. The supratrochlear nerve runs more medially than the supraorbital nerve and supplies the skin of the lower forehead close to the midline, the conjunctiva and the skin of the upper eyelid.

39.3 The arteries are identically named: the supratrochlear and supraorbital arteries.

39.4 The common origin is the ophthalmic artery. The ophthalmic artery is a branch of the internal carotid and passes through the optic canal within the optic nerve's dural sheath.

39.5 Lymph from the forehead and anterior face, including the region in which this lesion is present, drains into ipsilateral submandibular nodes via the buccal nodes. However lymph from the lateral face drains to the ipsilateral parotid nodes. Lymph from the lower lip chin drains to submental nodes. After passing to all of these destinations the lymph from these regions then drains to the deep cervical nodes.

39.6 4 mm margins are sufficient for squamous cell carcinoma.

39.7 The corrugator supercilii and occipitofrontalis muscles. The occipitofrontalis muscle has an *occipital* belly that originates from the highest nuchal line of the occipital bone, and a *frontal* belly originates from the superficial fascia and skin of the eyebrows. Both bellies insert into the epicranial aponeurosis. The muscle is supplied by the facial nerve.

Station 40

40.1 A Right cochlea

　　　B Right lateral semilunar canal

　　　C Right posterior semilunar canal

　　　D Left internal carotid artery

　　　E Left vestibule

40.2 F The internal acoustic meatus. Entering this region are the superior and inferior vestibular nerves, the cochlear nerve and the facial nerve. The sensory division of the trigeminal and glossopharyngeal nerves are also nearby.

40.3 The orientation of the nerves is illustrated in **Figure 3.32**. Think of them as each occupying a quadrant within the canal with the superior and inferior vestibular nerves occupying the posterior compartments in the inferior and superior aspects respectively. Within the anterior compartments, the facial nerve (CN VII) lies superiorly and the cochlear (CNVIII) nerve lies inferiorly. A way of remembering this orientation is to think of '7up' i.e. '7' referring to the facial nerve being the seventh cranial nerve.

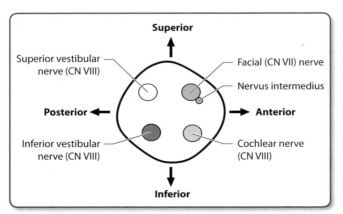

Figure 3.32 The arrangement of the cranial nerves within the internal acoustic meatus, as viewed through the inside of the meatus outwards.

40.4 The inner ear is contained within the petrous temporal bone.

40.5 There are three semilunar canals in the inner ear, *lateral, posterior* and *superior*. These are interconnected and perpendicular to each other (**Figure 3.33**).

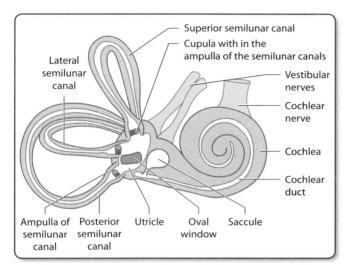

Figure 3.33 The inner ear.

40.6 Each semilunar canal contains a fluid-like substance, *endolymph*, as well as a small structure, the *cupola*, near its base. The cupola consists of thicker gelatinous fluid with multiple small microcilia. During rotational or vertical movements, the endolymph is disturbed bending the cilia. This action causes electrical stimulation of the vestibular nerve. The combination of electrical stimulation from the different semicircular canals is experienced as balance.

40.7 The cochlea is a shell shaped bony structure within the inner ear that contains endolymph and sensory epithelium consisting of numerous cilia upon a basilar membrane. As sound hits the tympanic membrane the waves are transmitted via ossicles within the middle ear to the inner ear. The vibrations cause disruption of the endolymph of the cochlea and disrupt the basilar membrane and cilia. This disruption causes neural impulses along the cochlear nerve which travel to the auditory cortex. Cilia within different positions along the spiral shaped cochlea convey different frequencies of sound. Violent disruptions of the basement membrane due to loud noises may result in the destruction of the hair cells and cause sensorineural deafness.

Station 41

41.1 X Vallecula (or pre-epiglottic region)

Y Epiglottis

Z Piriform fossa

41.2 A Oropharynx

B Hyoid bone

C Trachea

41.3 The hyoid bone corresponds to the C3 vertebral level.

41.4 The body of the epiglottis is composed of elastic cartilage but its surface is lined by two different cell types. The superior aspect of the body and the superior aspect of the laryngeal surface are lined by stratified squamous epithelium. The laryngeal aspect (its undersurface) is lined by ciliated columnar epithelium.

41.5 During laryngoscopy it is important to visualise the vallecula as this is where the tip of the laryngoscope blade is placed.

41.6 Z The piriform fossa. These are located either side of the laryngeal fossa. Medial to each fossae are the aryepiglottic folds and laterally are the lateral aspects of the thyroid cartilage and hyothyroid membranes.

41.7 The piriform fossa is a common area for malignancy. Its rich lymphatic supply means that early metastases are common to the cervical lymph nodes.

Chapter 4

Neurosciences

Syllabus topics

The following topics are listed within the Intercollegiate MRCS Examination syllabus for Neurosciences (Anatomy). Tick them off as you revise these topics to ensure you have covered the syllabus.

Central nervous system

- ❏ Cerebral hemispheres
- ❏ Ventricles
- ❏ Cerebellum, brainstem
- ❏ Spinal cord
- ❏ Meninges

Peripheral nervous system

- ❏ Cranial nerves
- ❏ Spinal nerves
- ❏ Peripheral nerves

Autonomic nervous system

- ❏ General organization

Surface anatomy

- ❏ Basic aspects

Imaging anatomy

- ❏ Arteriography
- ❏ CT/MRI

Station 1

A 79 year-old man is brought into the emergency department with weakness and decreased sensation within his left arm. He has a past medical history of atrial fibrillation. You examine him and are concerned that the patient may be suffering from an ischaemic neural event.

The image below is an axial MRI of a normal brain at the level of the midbrain demonstrating the circle of Willis:

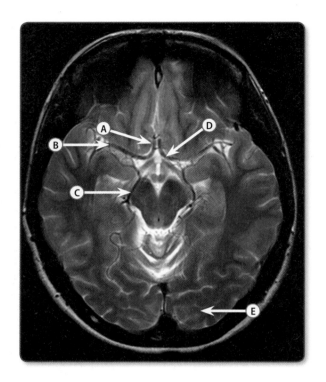

1.1 Identify the structures labelled A to D.

1.2 Which lobe of the brain is indicated by the arrow labelled E?

1.3 Which lobes (or parts of the lobes) of the brain are supplied by:

   1.3a the anterior cerebral artery?

   1.3b the middle cerebral artery?

   1.3c the posterior cerebral artery?

1.4 Given the clinical scenario above, which cerebral artery is most likely to have been affected by a thrombus?

1.5 Which gyrus contains the primary motor cortex? Which side of the body (contralateral or ipsilateral) do lesions or disruptions within this cortex affect?

1.6 What is meant by the 'motor homunculus'?

1.7 Within which lobes of the brain do the primary motor and primary somato-sensory cortices lie? What is the blood supply to these regions?

1.8 Which side of the body do lesions or disruptions of the primary somatosensory cortex affect?

Station 2

A 56-year-old man presents to the emergency department with non-specific symptoms of vomiting, nausea, and poor co-ordination. A CT scan of the brain performed after admission shows gross hydrocephalus.

Test your knowledge of cerebral anatomy with this axial MRI of a normal brain at the level of the lateral ventricles.

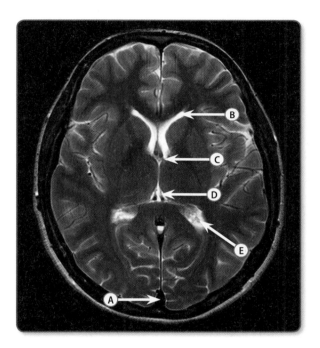

2.1 Identify the structures labelled A to E.

2.2 Where is cerebrospinal fluid produced and where is it resorbed?

2.3 Describe the flow of cerebrospinal fluid within the brain.

2.4 What is the normal volume of cerebrospinal fluid you would expect in an adult patient?

2.5 Classify the different types of hydrocephalus.

2.6 Give two causes for each of the various types of hydrocephalus you have listed.

2.7 Explain what is meant by the term 'cistern' in relation to neuroanatomy.

Station 3

A 12-year-old boy is struck by a ball to the right side of his head whilst playing field hockey. He appears alert initially, however, within a few minutes he starts to become confused and drowsy. He is taken to hospital immediately and diagnosed with a large intracranial haematoma. He is referred to the neurosurgeons and taken to theatre.

The image below is of a normal skull viewed from the left side:

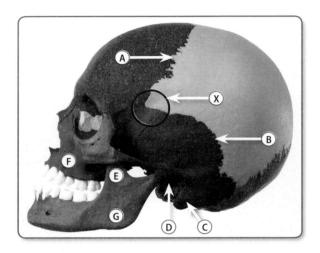

3.1 Identify the structures labelled A to G.

3.2 Which skull bones converge and meet at the region marked X?

3.3 Why is the area marked X clinically significant in this scenario? Which vessel is located deep to this structure?

3.4 What are the surface anatomical landmarks for locating the:

　3.4a anterior branch and

　3.4b posterior branch of this vessel?

3.5 What type of intracranial haematoma is the patient in this scenario likely to be suffering from?

3.6 Between which meningeal layers is this haematoma likely to be situated?

3.7 What are the superficial landmarks for siting a temporal burr hole?

3.8 Why is the site of the burr hole not located directly at the region X?

Station 4

You are asked by your consultant to give some anatomy teaching to a group of medical students. You decide to start with demonstrating the anatomy of the base of the skull.

The image on the next page is the inferior view of the base of the skull. It demonstrates normal anatomy.

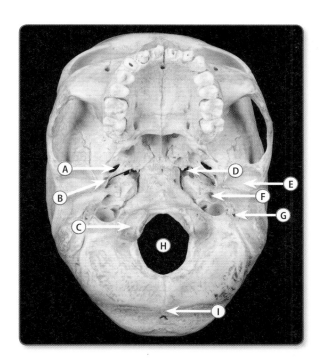

4.1 Identify the structures labelled A to I.

4.2 Through which foramen do the vertebral arteries enter the cranial cavity?

4.3 Which vascular structure is transmitted though B?

4.4 With which structure does the area labelled C articulate?

4.5 Which structures are transmitted through the foramen labelled D?

4.6 Which bone articulates at the region labelled E?

4.7 Which muscle attaches to the region labelled I?

Station 5

In the second half of your medical student teaching session, you show the students a different view of the base of the skull.

The image on the next page is the internal view of the normal base of the skull.

5.1 Identify the structures/areas labelled A to F.

5.2 To which skull bone does the structure labelled B belong?

5.3 Which vascular structure enters the skull through the area labelled C?

5.4 Which cranial nerve exits through the hypoglossal canal?

5.5 What structures pass through the foramen labelled D?

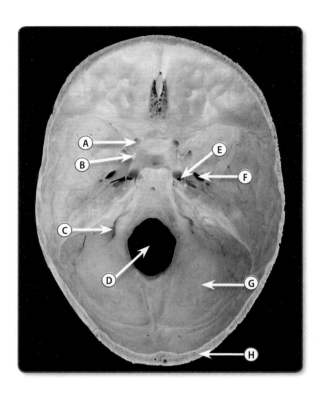

5.6 What clinical signs would you expect a patient to display if they were to suffer a fracture of the base of skull?

5.7 Which intracranial structure is situated in the indentation indicated by label G?

5.8 Which skull bone does the label H indicate?

Station 6

You attend to a patient in the neurosurgical outpatient clinic who is accompanied by his relatives and has been suffering a slow decline in cognitive function and increasing confusion. Before examining the patient you wish to review a normal MRI scan and refresh your knowledge of functional neuroanatomy.

The image on the next page is a sagittal MRI image of a normal brain taken through the midline of the head.

6.1 Identify the structures labelled A to G.

6.2 Name the four different lobes of the cerebral hemisphere.

6.3 How are these lobes demarcated anatomically?

6.4 Within which lobe are each of the following located?

    6.4a Auditory cortex

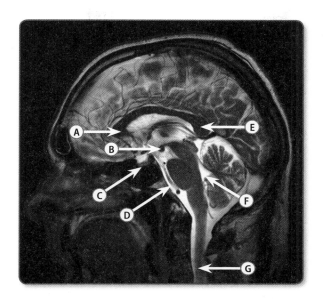

6.4b Visual cortex

6.4c Olfactory cortex

6.5 What is the function of the structure labelled A?

6.6 What are the different anatomical parts of this structure?

6.7 Which system in the brain does the structure labelled B belong to?

6.8 What is the function of this system?

6.9 Which vessels contribute to form the structure labelled D?

Station 7

You are asked to examine a 36-year-old woman in the emergency department who complains of a 1-week history of severe worsening headache accompanied by vomiting. Apart from being 1 week post partum she has no other medical history of note and is not on any medication. She does not complain of any neurological deficit.

The images on the next page are sagittal (a) and anteroposterior (b) views taken during a normal cerebral angiogram in the venous phase.

7.1 Identify the structures labelled A to G.

7.2 What is meant by the term 'Torcular Herophili'?

7.3 Into which sinus do the superficial cranial veins drain?

7.4 Into which sinus do the deep cerebral veins drain?

7.5 Which sinuses drain into the internal jugular vein?

7.6 What would be the clinical presentation of a patient who sustains a thrombus within the structure labelled A?

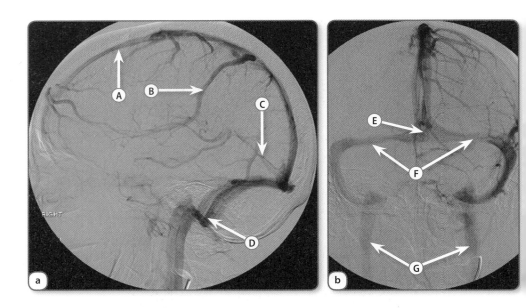

7.7 How are the dural venous sinuses connected to the extracranial veins? Why is this information clinically relevant?

Station 8

You are referred a 26-year-old man from the emergency department who is complaining of decreased sensation down the right side of his body. He reports having been in a car accident the day before which involved a head on collision with another vehicle. He did not sustain any obvious external injuries and only complains of some whiplash at the time. This is the first time he has sought any medical attention since the incident.

The image on the next page is a reconstruction from a cerebral CT angiogram of the main neck and intracranial vessels. There are no abnormalities demonstrated in this image.

8.1 Identify the structures labelled A to H.

8.2 From which vascular structure does the vessel labelled F arise? Is this the same on the left as it is on the right?

8.3 Apart from vessel labelled F, what other vascular branches does this vessel give rise to?

8.4 Describe the course of the artery labelled B from its origin to where it forms the artery labelled E.

8.5 Into which foramen in the base of the skull does the vessel labelled A enter?

8.6 Where is the most common location for a dissection of the vessel A? What is the presumed anatomical reason for this?

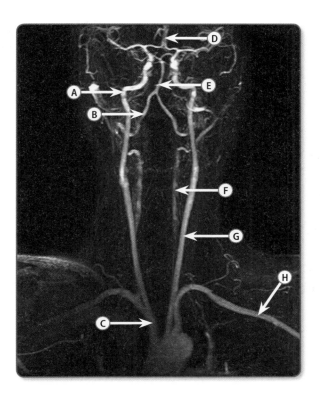

Station 9

An 84-year-old woman is taken to hospital after complaining of a left-sided headache after a fall in her nursing home. She is confused and a little drowsy but will not allow you to examine her. She does not appear to have sustained any open wounds on her head. Her carers are not able to tell you much about her past medical history. They do mention however that she is on warfarin.

The image on the next page is a dissection of the normal human brain demonstrating the dural reflections and base of the skull. The cerebral hemispheres have been removed.

9.1 Identify the structures labelled A to E.

9.2 Name the meningeal layers that surround the brain starting with the most superficial.

9.3 In the image above, structures A and B are reflections of which meningeal layer?

9.4 Which venous sinuses lie within the structures A and B?

9.5 What does the attached border of structure A adhere to? Where does its free border lie?

9.6 What does the attached border of structure B adhere to? Where does it free border lie?

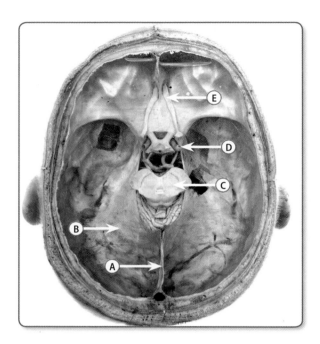

9.7 You want to rule out an intracranial haematoma in this patient and request a head CT. What is the most likely intracranial injury this patient has sustained given her age and clinical history?

9.8 Between which two meningeal layers would the blood accumulate in this type of haematoma?

9.9 Between which two meningeal layers is the subarachnoid space?

Station 10

You are referred a 50-year-old woman complaining of sudden, short-lived, sharp 'electrical shock' like episodes of pain down the right side of her face. Her general practitioner (GP) suspects trigeminal neuralgia.

The image on the next page is a dissection demonstrating the normal anatomy of the base of the skull. The cerebral hemispheres have been removed but the cranial nerves remain intact.

10.1 Identify the structures labelled A, B, D, and E.

10.2 What are the names of the three fossae that the base of the skull is divided into?

10.3 What are the borders of these anatomical divisions?

10.4 Which lobe of the brain occupies the space labelled C?

10.5 Name the vascular structure which is situated in the region labelled G.

10.6 Which foramen does the cranial nerve labelled D traverse?

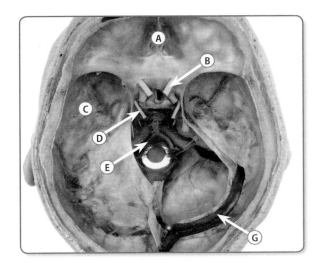

10.7 Where is the ganglion of this cranial nerve located?

10.8 Where is the sensory nucleus of this cranial nerve located?

10.9 Where is the motor nucleus of this cranial nerve located?

Station 11

A 63-year-old man, referred to you by the local GP, has been complaining of decreased sensation in both of his upper limbs. The GP's letter states that the patient's proprioception and light touch sensation are intact but pain and temperature are blunted. He has arranged for the patient to have a MRI scan of his cervical spine. Before viewing the patient's scan, you wish to familiarise yourself with the appearances on a normal scan.

The image on the next page is a sagittal MRI scan of a normal cervical and upper thoracic spine.

11.1 Identify the structures labelled A to F.

11.2 Which ascending pathway carries sensation of light touch and proprioception? Where is this pathway located within the spinal column?

11.3 Which ascending pathway carries sensation of temperature and pain? Where is this pathway located within the spinal column?

11.4 Where in the spinal column are the descending pathways that contribute to motor movement?

11.5 What would be the symptoms in a patient with a total transaction at level T2.

11.6 What is Brown–Sequard syndrome?

11.7 What symptoms and signs would you expect in a patient with Brown–Sequard syndrome due to a right sided defect at the level of T2?

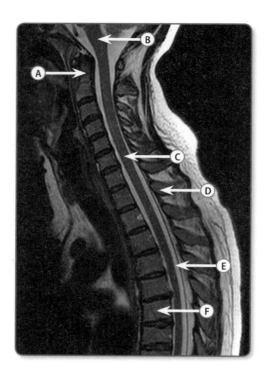

Station 12

A 23-year-old woman presents to the emergency department complaining of severe, sudden onset, occipital headache. Although she has no neurological signs and is fully alert, she appears very anxious and tells you that her mother died of an intracerebral haemorrhage when she was 35 years old.

The image on the next page is of a normal cerebral angiogram.

12.1 Identify the structures labelled A to F.

12.2 What type of intracerebral haemorrhage might the patient's mother have sustained given the history above?

12.3 What is the most likely cause for such a haemorrhage? In which vessel would you most expect the cause to manifest?

12.4 In what syndrome would you expect a patient to develop such a pathology, especially given a possible family inheritance?

12.5 Given the scenario above, what would be the first line investigation you would request to confirm your clinical suspicion? What investigation would you then proceed to if this first test were negative?

12.6 What is the 'blood brain barrier'? What is its function?

12.7 Are all areas of the brain 'protected' by the blood brain barrier? If not, which areas lack a blood brain barrier?

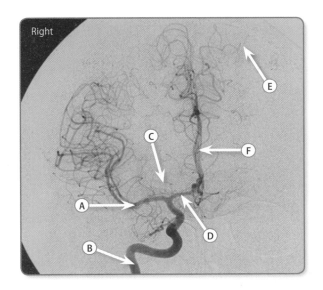

Station 13

You are a neurosurgical resident working in a large teaching hospital. Your consultant is performing a transsphenoidal operation on a 38-year-old woman suffering with a pituitary macroadenoma. Before joining him in theatre, you revise your anatomy of the relevant region.

The photographs below and overleaf show one of the bones of the skull. Photograph (a) is an anterior view and (b) is a posterior view of this bone. No pathology is demonstrated within these images.

13.1 Which bone is being demonstrated?

13.2 Identify the structures labelled A to E.

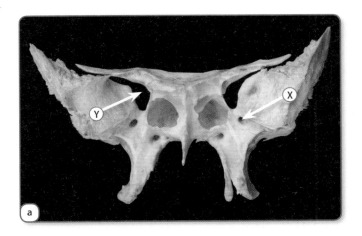

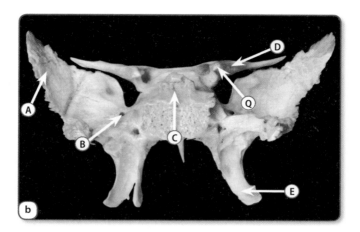

13.3 Which cranial nerves are transmitted via the foramina labelled X and Y respectively?

13.4 Which dural attachment does the structure labelled Q give rise to?

13.5 Name the other bones that articulate with the bone in the picture.

13.6 To which cranial fossa do the superior aspects of the greater wings of this bone contribute?

13.7 Within which area of the bone shown above does the pituitary gland sit?

13.8 Which lobe of the brain sits upon the lesser wings of this bone?

Station 14

You are referred a 50-year-old man with symptoms of ataxia and slurred speech. Although he admits to a former history of alcohol addiction, he adamantly denies any recent intake.

The images on the next page are of a dissection of the cerebellum viewed from the side (a) and from the front at a slight inferior angle (b).

14.1 Identify the structures labelled A to I.

14.2 Within which of the cranial fossae would you expect the cerebellum to be located?

14.3 What connects the cerebellum to the brainstem?

14.4 What intervenes between the cerebellum and the pons, in the median plane?

14.5 What are the functions of the cerebellum?

14.6 Are there any sensory functions attributable to the cerebellum?

14.7 After examining your patient, you find he has mainly right-sided symptoms. Within which cerebellar hemisphere would you expect a cerebellar lesion to be present?

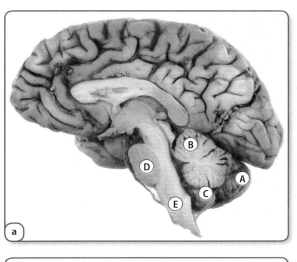

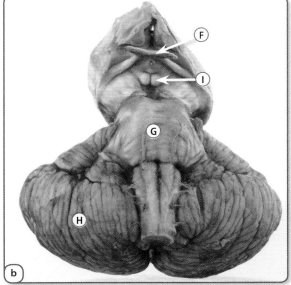

14.8 What features of cerebellar dysfunction would you expect with a lesion in this area?

14.9 How would these symptoms differ if the lesion or abnormality was situated within the midline of the cerebellum and not localised to either hemisphere?

Station 15

You are asked to review a 72-year-old man on the ward, who alongside other presenting features, displays features of cerebellar dysfunction secondary to a previous stroke. As a resident looking after the patient, you wish to familiarise yourself with the appearances of a normal MRI before viewing the patient's MRI scan.

The image below is an axial MRI image of a normal brain taken at the level of the cerebellum:

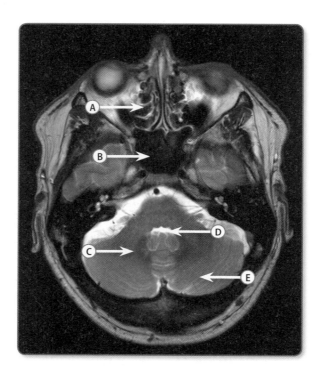

15.1 Identify the structures labelled A to E.

15.2 What are the gross anatomical subdivisions of the cerebellum?

15.3 How else is the cerebellum divided when considering its functional subdivisions?

15.4 How do each of these subdivisions contribute to the function of the cerebellum?

15.5 Name the four paired nuclei within the cerebellum. Where are they located?

15.6 During periods of raised intracranial pressure, through which foramen could the cerebellar tonsils herniate?

15.7 What are the clinical signs and symptoms of raised intracranial pressure?

15.8 Which anatomical landmark seen on axial imaging would help you determine whether or not the cerebellar tonsils are herniated?

15.9 What is the name given to the malformation where in the cerebellar tonsils are low lowing without there necessarily being any evidence of raised intracranial pressure?

Station 16

A 69-year-old woman presents to the emergency department complaining of sudden onset right-sided blindness. She denies any past medical history of diabetic retinopathy or ophthalmic disease or trauma, but has suffered a transient ischaemic attack within the last month. She has no other neurological symptoms.

The image below is of a normal cerebral angiogram:

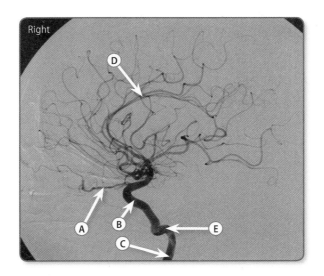

16.1 Which principal vessel is being highlighted in the image above?

16.2 Which area of the brain is supplied by this artery?

16.3 What neurological signs would you expect with a total occlusion of the principal vessel shown above?

16.4 Which vessel connects the vessel shown above to its left sided counterpart?

16.5 Identify the vascular structures labelled A to E.

16.6 Vessel C is descriptively divided into 'segments' or 'parts'. Name the segments.

16.7 Why is knowledge of the different segments of vessel C important?

16.8 Within which vascular structure would you most expect an occlusion to be present given the patient's symptoms?

Station 17

You review a 79-year-old man who has a past medical history of Parkinson's Disease. He had a seizure 3 weeks ago and has undergone an MRI scan.

The image below is an axial MRI of a normal brain through the level of the lateral ventricles:

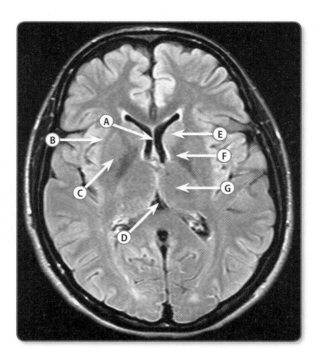

17.1 Identify the structures labelled A to G.

17.2 Which structures comprise the basal ganglia?

17.3 What is the function of the basal ganglia?

17.4 Which side of the body would you expect an abnormality to present if there was a lesion within the right basal ganglia?

17.5 Should the amygdala be included in the description of the basal ganglia? What is its function?

17.6 What structures comprise the corpus striatum?

17.7 Which structures comprise the lentiform nucleus?

17.8 Which structure within the lentiform nucleus has a midbrain extension?

17.9 What are the different anatomical parts of the structure labelled E and which structure does it follow closely?

Station 18

You attend a multidisciplinary meeting where radiologists and clinicians are discussing a patient on the ward who has sustained right-sided weakness from a brainstem haemorrhage.

The image below is a normal axial MRI slice at the level of the midbrain with the midbrain magnified:

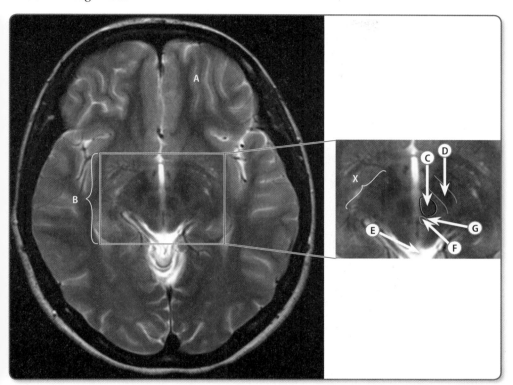

18.1 Identify the structures labelled A to G.

18.2 The region labelled G is sometimes implicated in multiple sclerosis through demyelination. What is the function of this region?

18.3 How does a deficit in this structure manifest itself? How do you examine for this?

18.4 Which structures are usually referred to by the term 'brain stem'?

18.5 Which cranial nerves arise from the brain stem?

18.6 Within which part of the brainstem do the corticospinal descending pyramidal tracts decussate?

18.7 Where do the first, second and third order fibres lie within the ascending dorsal sensory column? Where does this pathway decussate?

18.8 Where do the first, second and third order fibres lie within the ascending lateral spinothalamic sensory column? Where does this pathway decussate?

18.9 How is the knowledge regarding the pathways of the dorsal column fibres and lateral spinothalamic fibres clinically useful?

18.10 What clinical signs and symptoms would you expect in a patient with a unilateral brain stem lesion?

18.11 How do these differ in a patient with bilateral brain stem lesions?

Station 19

A 63-year-old woman is admitted to the emergency department with sudden loss of function in the right upper and lower limbs. She has multiple cardiovascular risk factors including atrial fibrillation and diabetes. You suspect an occlusion of the middle cerebral artery and lose no time in contacting the interventional neuroradiologists with a view to intra-arterial thrombolysis.

The image below is a coronal dissection of a normal brain seen from the front:

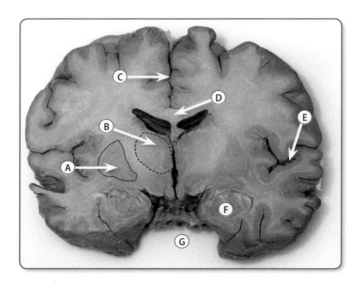

19.1 Identify the structures indicated by the labels A to F.

19.2 What is the blood supply to the basal ganglia?

19.3 How is this knowledge clinically significant in situations where there is an occlusion to the middle cerebral artery?

19.4 Which vessel lies within the region labelled E?

19.5 What is the function of the region labelled F and in which condition is this area seen to atrophy?

19.6 Where is the 'massa intermedia' located and to which structure does it refer?

19.7 Which part of the brain stem would you expect to be located in the region labelled 'G'?

19.8 Which cranial nerve nuclei arise from the pons?

19.9 How is the pons important in the function of respiration?

Station 20

You are called urgently to review a 76-year-old woman in the emergency department who is suffering from sudden onset paralysis of all extremities accompanied by aphasia. Despite early imaging and treatment she is pronounced dead within 1 hour of admission, the cause of death being basilar artery thrombosis.

The image below is of a normal cerebral angiogram demonstrating the posterior circulation:

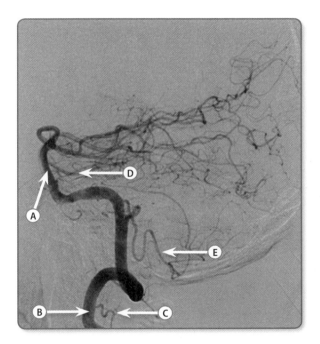

20.1 Identify the structures labelled A to E.

20.2 How many parts are there to the vessel labelled B? Describe what marks the transition point between these different divisions.

20.3 What are the branches of the vessel labelled B prior to its formation of the vessel A?

20.4 Anatomically, where is the origin of the vessel labelled A?

20.5 Describe the course of the vessel labelled A. Where does it terminate and what does it divide into?

20.6 What is the blood supply to the cerebellum?

Station 21

A 32-year-old man is admitted after a road traffic accident, having suffered a severe brain injury. He is ventilated and neurological testing has not been able to demonstrate any brain function.

The image below is a dissection of the inferior aspect of the base of the brain (demonstrating normal anatomy):

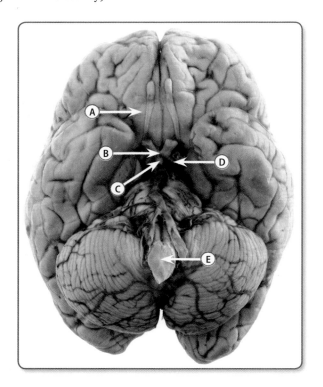

21.1 Identify the structures labelled A to E.

21.2 What do you understand by the 'brainstem death'?

21.3 What is the difference between the term 'persistent vegetative state' and 'brainstem death'?

21.4 State any three preconditions (criteria) that must be present and verified before the diagnosis of brain stem death is made.

21.5 What are the efferent and afferent cranial nerves responsible for mediating:

    21.5a the pupillary light reflex?

    21.5b the corneal reflex?

    21.5c the gag reflex?

21.6 Apart from the absence of the above reflexes, what other clinical tests (and their findings or lack of) are required for the diagnosis of brainstem death?

Answers

Station 1

1.1 A Right anterior cerebral artery (A2). This region of the anterior cerebral artery originates at the level of the anterior communicating artery just up to the level where the anterior cerebral artery divides to give off pericallosal and callosomarginal arteries.

    B Right middle cerebral artery

    C Right posterior cerebral artery

    D Left anterior cerebral artery (A1). This is the region of the artery that originates from the internal carotid artery to the level of the anterior communicating artery.

1.2 E Left occipital lobe

1.3 The areas of the brain which are supplied by the various cerebral arteries are described and shown in **Figure 4.1** and **Table 4.1**.

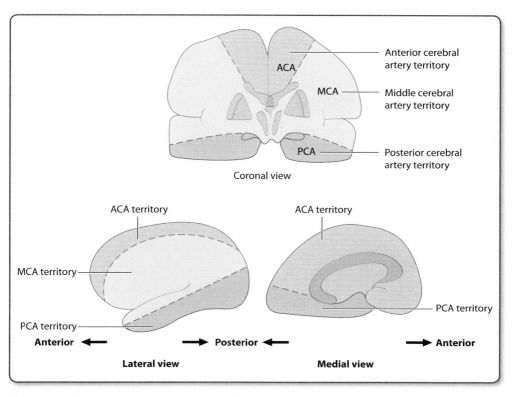

Figure 4.1 The regions of the brain supplied by the cerebral arteries.

Table 4.1 The arterial blood supply to the various lobes of the brain

Artery	Anatomy supplied
Anterior cerebral	Medial surface of the frontal and parietal lobes
	Anterior portions of the basal ganglia
	Anterior limb of the internal capsule
	The majority of the corpus callosum
Middle cerebral	Majority of the lateral surfaces of each cerebral hemisphere except the area supplied by the anterior cerebral artery
	Deep branches of the middle cerebral artery contribute to the blood supply to the basal ganglia and internal capsule
Posterior cerebral	Occipital lobes and posteromedial aspect of the temporal lobes

1.4 Given the signs and symptoms suffered by the patient in the clinical scenario, a thrombotic event within the right middle cerebral artery would be the most likely diagnosis.

1.5 The motor cortex is situated at the pre-central gyrus. Lesions affecting the pre-central gyrus within the left cerebral hemisphere would produce right-sided motor symptoms due to the decussation of the descending pathways within the medulla.

1.6 The motor (or cortical) homunculus is the representation of various anatomical regions within the motor cortex. Each part of the cortex is responsible for the

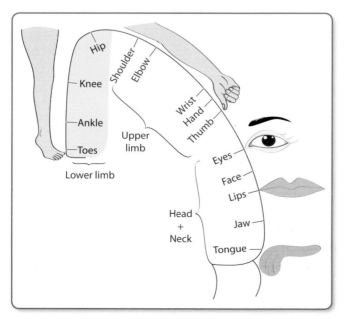

Figure 4.2 The motor homunculus.

innervation of different body parts and the homunculus represents diagrammatically how these areas within the cortex are distributed. The greater the proportion of the cortex dedicated to a particular body part relates to how richly innervated or how many muscle units are within that region (not necessarily the size of the region).

1.7 The primary somatosensory cortex is located within the post central gyrus within parietal lobe, and the pre-motor cortex is located within the pre-central gyrus of the posterior aspect of the frontal lobe (**Figure 4.3**). The primary somatosensory cortex and pre-motor cortex are both supplied by the middle cerebral artery (apart from the most medial aspect of these cortices which is supplied by the anterior cerebral artery).

1.8 Lesions within the primary somatosensory cortex would result in symptoms on the contralateral side of the body.

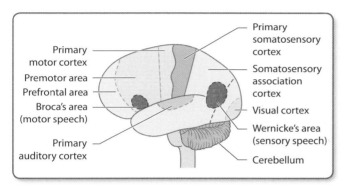

Figure 4.3 Regions of the premotor and somatosensory cortices.

Station 2

2.1 A Superior sagittal sinus

B Anterior horn of the left lateral ventricle

C Left foramen of Monro

D Third ventricle

E Left lateral ventricle (trigone)

2.2 Cerebrospinal fluid (CSF) is made by the choroid plexus (which consists of ependymal cells) and drains via the arachnoid granulations, small protrusions of arachnoid mater within the dura that allow the fluid to exit the ventricular system and drain into the venous sinus system of the brain.

2.3 The various regions of the ventricular system are demonstrated in **Figure 4.4**. The flow of CSF is as follows:

- CSF is made by the choroid plexus that mainly occupies the lateral ventricles, but also part of the third ventricle.

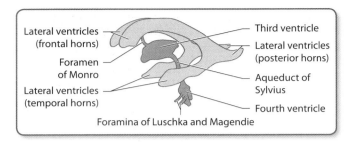

Figure 4.4 The ventricular system of the brain.

- CSF flows from the lateral ventricles via the foramen of Monro to the third ventricle.
- from the third ventricle, it flows via the cerebral aqueduct (also known as the aqueduct of Sylvius) to the fourth ventricle.
- from the fourth ventricle, the CSF flows via the foramen of Magendie and foramina of Luschka through to subarachnoid space that bathes the brain and spinal cord.
- fluid within the subarachnoid space is then exposed to the arachnoid granulations and exits these areas into the dural venous sinuses of the brain.

2.4 The average volume of CSF within the adult human body is approximately 150 mL. Approximately 500 mL of CSF is produced daily meaning that the cerebrospinous fluid is replenished 3–4 times daily.

2.5 Hydrocephalus can be classified as:

- communicating (where an obstruction in the system is not grossly obvious)
- non-communicating (where there is an obstruction to the flow of the CSF).

The condition can also be classified by pathological processes:

- Overproduction of CSF (communicating hydrocephalus).
- Failure of resorption of the CSF (communicating hydrocephalus).
- Blockage of the circulation of the CSF without problems in the production or resorption (non-communicating hydrocephalus).

2.6 Examples of communicating hydrocephalus include meningitis, subarachnoid haemorrhage, and intraventricular haemorrhage. A choroid plexus tumour that does not cause obstruction but results in an overproduction of CSF would also be a potential cause.

Non-communicating hydrocephalus is caused by obstruction within a ventricle or obstructed connection between ventricles, for example: malignancy, colloid cysts, atresia of the ventricular foramina, ependymitis, or haemorrhage.

2.7 The term 'cistern' (Latin, 'box') is easily confused with 'ventricle' as they both contain CSF even though they are not identical structures. Cisterns are areas of subarachnoid space within the brain created by the separation of pia and arachnoid mater. The important cisterns to know about are listed in **Table 4.2** and illustrated in **Figure 4.5**.

Table 4.2 The cerebral cisterns

Cistern	Also known as	Location and notes
Cisterna magna	Cerebellomedullary cistern	• The largest subarachnoid cistern • Lies inferior to the cerebellum and posterior to the medulla. Is filled with cerebrospinal fluid from the fourth ventricle via lateral and median apertures.
Cisterna pontis	Pontine cistern	• Situated anterior to the lower pons and upper medulla
Cisterna inter-peduncularis	Interpeduncular cistern	• Located anterior to the cerebral peduncles
Superior cistern	Quadrigeminal cistern	• Located posterior to the tectal or quadrigeminal plate
Cisterna ambiens	Ambient cistern	• Consists of thin sheet like projections that are dorsally continuous with the quadrigeminal cistern

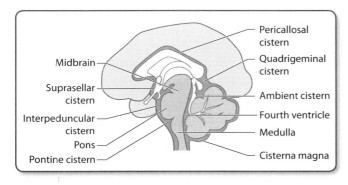

Figure 4.5 The cerebral cisterns.

Station 3

3.1 A Coronal suture

B Squamous suture

C Mastoid process

D External acoustic meatus

E Coronoid process of mandible

F Maxilla bone

G Angle of mandible

3.2 The area marked X is the junction between the frontal, parietal, temporal and sphenoid bones.

3.3 The area marked X is also known as the 'pterion'. This region is clinically relevant as the middle meningeal artery lies deep to the skull at this region and can be easily damaged leading to an extradural haematoma. It is a thin region of the skull that can be easily fractured.

3.4 The anatomical landmarks for the various branches of the middle meningeal artery are:

3.4a the anterior branch of the middle meningeal artery can be found approximately 3 cm above the midpoint from the zygomatic arch, just inferior to the pterion and

3.4b the posterior branch of the middle meningeal artery lies posterior to the anterior branch above, just at the level where a horizontal line from the outer canthus of the eye intersects a vertical line from the mastoid process.

3.5 An extradural haematoma for the reasons outlined above and also because of the classic history and symptoms of trauma and eventual decline in conscious level with an intermittent 'lucid' interval.

3.6 The blood in this scenario is extradural blood that collects between the cranium and the dura mater.

3.7 The superficial anatomical landmarks for siting a temporal burr hole are halfway between the outer canthus of the eye and external acoustic meatus. This is approximately 2 cm above the zygomatic arch.

3.8 The pterion is avoided when creating a burr hole in case the burr hole needs re-sizing or widening and is thus safely away from disrupting the middle meningeal artery which lies underneath the pterion.

Station 4

4.1 A Foramen ovale

B Foramen spinosum

C Occipital condyle

D Foramen lacerum

E Mandibular fossa

F Carotid canal

G Stylomastoid foramen

H Foramen magnum

I External occipital protuberance

4.2 The vertebral arteries enter the skull via the foramen magnum. Other important structures that are transmitted through the foramen magnum include: the medulla oblongata, spinal accessory nerve (CN XI), and the anterior and posterior spinal arteries.

4.3 The middle meningeal artery is transmitted via the foramen spinosum (B).

4.4 The occipital condyle (C) articulates with the superior articulating facets of the C1 vertebrae (also known as the atlas).

4.5 The foramen lacerum (D) is an irregularly shaped opening in the base of the skull that is covered by fibrocartilage along its inferior aspect and therefore does not actually transmit any vessels or nerves. The upper part, however, is traversed by the internal carotid artery and greater and deep petrosal nerves before they enter the pterygoid canal.

4.6 The condyle of the mandible (E) articulates with the mandibular fossa. It is here that the temporomandibular joint is located.

4.7 The trapezius muscle attaches at this site (the external occipital protuberance, I) and inserts into the posterior lateral third of the clavicle, the acromion, and the spine of the scapula.

Station 5

5.1 A Optic canal

   B Anterior clinoid process

   C Jugular foramen

   D Foramen magnum

   E Foramen lacerum

   F Foramen ovale

5.2 The anterior clinoid process (B) is part of the sphenoid bone

5.3 As the name suggests, the jugular bulb of the internal jugular vein is transmitted through the jugular foramen (C).

5.4 Again, as the name suggests, the hypoglossal nerve (CN XII) is transmitted through the hypoglossal canal.

5.5 The foramen magnum transmits the vertebral arteries, medulla oblongata, anterior and posterior spinal arteries, and the spinal accessory nerve (CN XI). The foramen magnum is the largest foramen of the skull. **Table 4.3** outlines the structures that are transmitted through the various skull foramina.

5.6 There are several signs associated with a base of skull fracture:
- leakage of the CSF either via the nose (CSF rhinorrhoea) or ears (CSF otorrhoea)
- blood may be seen to collect behind the tympanic membrane or if this is ruptured, the blood could drain out via the external acoustic meatus
- bruising may also develop, typically situated behind the ears ('Battle's sign) or around the eyes ('raccoon eyes').

Table 4.3 Foramina within the base of the skull

Foramen	Contents
Cribriform plate	Olfactory nerve fibres (CN I)
Optic canal	Optic (CN II) nerve
	Ophthalmic artery
	Sympatheticus from internal carotid plexus
Superior orbital fissure	Oculomotor (CN III) nerve
	Trochlear (CN IV) nerve
	Abducens (CN VI) nerve
	Ophthalmic division of the trigeminal (CN V1) nerves
	Superior ophthalmic vein
	Sympatheticus from the internal carotid plexus
Foramen rotundum	Maxillary division of the trigeminal (CN V2) nerve
Foramen ovale	Mandibular branch of the trigeminal (CN V3) nerve
	Accessory meningeal artery
	Lesser petrosal nerve and emissary veins
Internal acoustic meatus	Facial (CN VII) nerve
	Vestibulocochlear (CN VIII) nerve
	Labyrinth artery
Jugular foramen	Jugular bulb of the internal jugular vein
	Inferior petrosal sinus
	Glossopharyngeal (CN IX) nerve
	Vagus (CN X) nerve
	Accessory (CN XI) nerve
Hypoglossal canal	Hypoglossal (CN XII) nerve
Foramen magnum	Spinal cord and meninges
	Ascending rootlets of the accessory (CN XI) nerve
	Vertebral arteries
	Anterior and posterior spinal arteries
Supraorbital foramen	Supraorbital artery, vein and nerve
Infraorbital foramen	Infraorbital artery, vein and nerve
Inferior orbital fissure	Infraorbital and zygomatic nerves from the maxillary division of the trigeminal (CN V2) nerve
	Veins from orbit to pterygoid plexus
	Infraorbital artery and vein

Contd...

Table 4.3 cont.

Foramen	Contents
Foramen spinosum	Middle meningeal artery Nervous spinosus from the mandibular nerve Posterior trunk of the middle meningeal vein
Foramen lacerum	Largely filled by fibrocartilage
Pterygopalatine fossa	Maxillary division of trigeminal (CN V2) nerve Pterygopalatine ganglion Maxillary artery and vein branches

5.7 G Posterior cranial fossa. The cerebellum and brainstem are both contained within this fossa and the left cerebellar hemisphere sits within the indentation within the skull.

5.8 The occipital bone.

Station 6

6.1 A Genu of corpus callosum

   B Mammillary body

   C Pituitary gland

   D Basilar artery

   E Splenium of the corpus callosum

   F Fourth ventricle

   G Cervical spinal cord

6.2 The four lobes of the brain are the:
- frontal lobe
- temporal lobe
- parietal lobe
- occipital lobe.

6.3 **Table 4.4** and **Figure 4.6** define the lobes of the brain.

6.4 The cortices mentioned above are contained within the following lobes:

   6.4a auditory cortex: within the temporal lobe in the superior temporal gyrus, inferior to the lateral fissure.

   6.4b visual cortex: within the occipital lobe below the calcarine sulcus.

   6.4c olfactory cortex: within the medial aspect of the temporal lobes.

6.5 The corpus callosum is formed of neural fibres that help to facilitate communication between the right and left cerebral hemispheres. In congenital conditions where

Table 4.4 The boundaries of the various cerebral lobes	
Lobe of the brain	**Anatomical boundaries**
Frontal lobe	Anterior: frontal pole
	Posterior: central sulcus
Temporal lobe	Anterior: lateral fissure
	Posterior: the line connecting the top of the parieto-occipital sulcus and the pre-occipital notch
	Superior: lateral fissure
	Inferior: temporal pole
Parietal lobe	Anterior: central sulcus
	Posterior: parieto-occipital sulcus (seen on the medial surface of the cerebral hemispheres)
	Inferior: lateral fissure
Occipital lobe	Anterior: parieto-occipital sulcus (seen on the medial surface of the cerebral hemispheres)
	Posterior: occipital pole

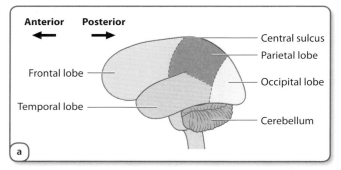

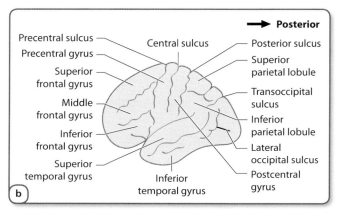

Figure 4.6 The boundaries of the different cerebral lobes (a); (b) shows the lateral and (c) the medial view of the left cerebral hemisphere.

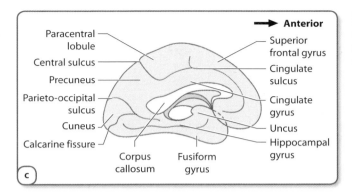

Figure 4.6 The boundaries of the different cerebral lobes, *continued.*

Labels: Paracentral lobule, Central sulcus, Precuneus, Parieto-occipital sulcus, Cuneus, Calcarine fissure, Corpus callosum, Fusiform gyrus, Anterior, Superior frontal gyrus, Cingulate sulcus, Cingulate gyrus, Uncus, Hippocampal gyrus

c

there is an absence of the corpus callosum, this is not fatal however individuals display delayed development and frequent seizure activity.

6.6 The different regions of the corpus callosum are best displayed when viewing the structure in sagittal section (**Figure 4.7**). The anterior portion of the corpus callosum is called the genu with the rostrum projecting inferiorly. The posterior portion is called the splenium and the section in between is called the body of the corpus callosum.

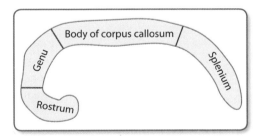

Labels: Body of corpus callosum, Genu, Rostrum, Splenium

Figure 4.7 The regions of the corpus callosum seen in sagittal section.

6.7 The mammillary bodies, (B), are considered part of the limbic system and thought to play a role in learning and memory.

6.8 The function of this system is to regulate human emotion, mood, and memory. Three structures make up the limbic system. These are contained within the medial aspect of the temporal lobe and consist of the hippocampus, amygdala, and olfactory cortex.

6.9 The basilar artery, (D), is formed by the right and left vertebral arteries.

Station 7

7.1 A Superior sagittal sinus

  B Cortical vein

   C Straight sinus

   D Sigmoid sinus

   E Confluence of sinuses

   F Transverse sinuses

   G Internal jugular veins

7.2 The 'Torcular Herophili' is another name for the 'confluence of sinuses' (where the sagittal, transverse and straight sinuses converge).

7.3 The superficial cranial veins drain into the superior sagittal and cavernous sinuses.

7.4 The deep cerebral veins drain into the great cerebral vein that is continuous with straight sinus.

7.5 The inferior petrosal and the sigmoid sinuses drain into the bulb of the internal jugular vein.

7.6 Superior sagittal sinus thrombosis can present with rather nonspecific symptoms including: generalized headaches, nausea, vertigo, seizures, and decreased conscious level.

7.7 The superficial veins that drain the scalp are connected to the dural venous sinuses via the emissary veins (**Figure 4.8**). Superficial scalp infections may therefore cause meningitis via this route.

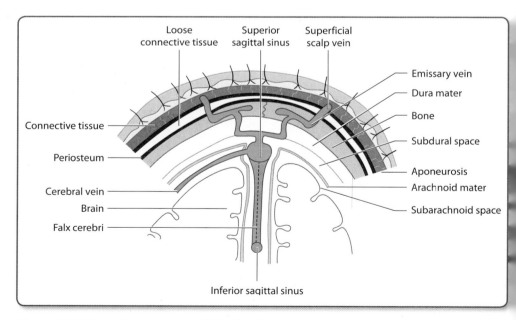

Figure 4.8 The emissary veins and the dural venous sinuses.

Station 8

8.1 **A** Right internal carotid artery

B Right vertebral artery (V4)

C Brachiocephalic artery

D Anterior cerebral artery

E Basilar artery

F Left vertebral artery (V2)

G Left common carotid artery

H Left subclavian artery

8.2 Vessel 'F' is the left vertebral artery and arises from the left subclavian artery. The right vertebral artery also originates from the right subclavian artery. Conversely, the subclavian arteries do not show this symmetry. The right subclavian artery is a branch of the brachiocephalic (or innominate) artery and the left subclavian artery originates from the arch of the aorta (**Figure 4.9**).

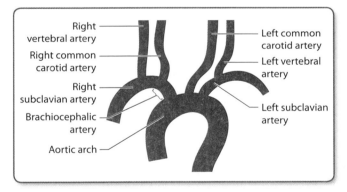

Figure 4.9 The origin of the subclavian and vertebral arteries.

8.3 The branches of the subclavian artery can be remembered using the mnemonic 'VIT **C** and **D**':

- **V**ertebral artery
- **I**nternal thoracic artery
- **T**hyrocervical trunk
- **C**ostocervical trunk
- **D**orsal scapular artery.

8.4 The vertebral artery can be divided into four parts, V1–V4 (**Figure 4.10**):

- the first part, V1, begins at the origin of the vertebral artery (from the subclavian artery) and ends at the foramen transversarium at the level of the C6 vertebra
- the second part, V2, continues from this point and emerges from the transverse process of C2.

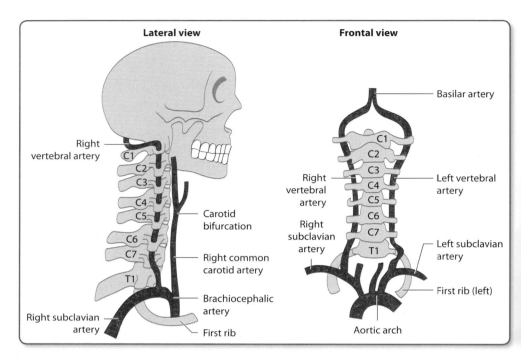

Figure 4.10 The course of the right vertebral artery.

- the third part, V3, is the most tortuous and loops posteriorly around the lateral mass of C1 before piercing the dura mater via the foramen magnum.
- the fourth part, V4, terminates where the vertebral artery joins its contralateral counterpart to form the basilar artery.

8.5 Vessel 'A' is the right internal carotid artery and enters the skull via the carotid canal. Other structures that also traverse this foramen include the sympathetic plexus of nerves from the internal carotid nerve.

8.6 The most likely area for carotid artery dissection is just before it pierces the dura of the brain. Here the distal segment is relatively more fixed than its proximal portion and at risk of damage during flexion-extension injuries.

Station 9

9.1 **A** Falx cerebri (the cut base is shown in the photograph)

B Left tentorium cerebelli

C Midbrain

D Right middle cerebral artery

E Right olfactory nerve (CN I)

9.2 Dura, pia, arachnoid mater.

9.3 The dura mater is a tough fibrous membrane that loosely covers the brain. In some areas, this fibrous layer forms reflections, greatest of which are the falx cerebri and tentorium cerebelli.

9.4 Superior sagittal sinus, transverse sinuses, and straight sinus lie within the falx cerebri and tentorium cerebelli.

9.5 The falx cerebri is formed by a vertical sheath of dura mater which extends from its fixed edge along the cranial roof (on the internal surface) in the midline to its free border which occupies the Interhemispheric fissure and terminates just above the corpus callosum.

9.6 The tentorium cerebelli is formed by a horizontal 'shelf' of dura mater with its fixed border along the inner surface of the skull at the occipitotemporal region and extends to its free border lying in the transverse cerebral fissure and encircling the midbrain. This fissure is situated superior to the cerebellum and inferior to the occipital lobe of the brain. In the midline, the tentorium cerebelli is continuous with the falx cerebri (**Figure 4.11**).

9.7 Subdural haematoma.

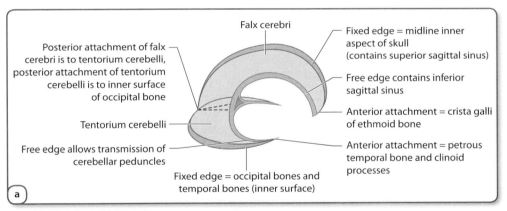

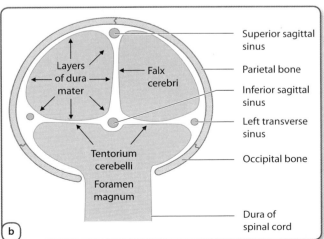

Figure 4.11 The tentorium cerebelli and falx cerebri. (a) Attachments of the falx cerebri and tentorium cerebelli. (b) Cross-sectional coronal diagram demonstrating the position of the cerebral sinuses within the dural reflections.

9.8 Blood in a subdural haematoma accumulates between the dura and pia mater.

9.9 The subarachnoid space is between the pia and arachnoid mater.

Station 10

10.1 **A** Cribriform plate

B Right optic nerve

D Left trigeminal (CN V) nerve

E Left vertebral artery

10.2 The anterior, middle, and posterior fossae.

10.3 The boundaries of the three fossae are given in **Table 4.5**.

10.4 The temporal lobe occupies the area labelled C, the temporal fossa.

10.5 The right transverse sinus occupies the region labelled G.

Table 4.5 The boundaries of the cranial fossae		
	Boundaries	**Important contents (this list is not exhaustive)**
Anterior fossa	Anterior: posterior wall of the frontal sinus Lateral: frontal bone Posterior: posterior border of the lesser wing of sphenoid, anterior clinoid processes Floor: orbital plate of the frontal bone, anterior border of the lesser wing of the sphenoid bone and anterior body of sphenoid bone	Frontal lobes of the brain Olfactory bulb and tract Cribriform plate Anterior aspects of the superior and inferior sagittal sinuses
Middle fossa	Anterior: greater wing of the sphenoid bone Posterior: clivus bone Lateral: greater wing of the sphenoid bone, squamous portion of the temporal bone, anteroinferior portion of the parietal bone Floor: greater wing of the sphenoid bone anteriorly and the petrous portion of the temporal bone posteriorly	Temporal lobes Pituitary gland Trigeminal ganglion Intracranial portion of the internal carotid artery Cavernous sinuses Greater superficial petrosal nerve

Contd...

Table 4.5 cont.

	Boundaries	Important contents (this list is not exhaustive)
Posterior fossa	Anterior: clivus	Cerebellum
	Posterior: occipital bones	Brainstem
	Floor: occipital bones with the foramen magnum occupying the central aspect of the floor	(CN 7–12 exit via the posterior fossa)

10.6 The nerve labelled D is the trigeminal nerve and is transmitted through the superior orbital fissure.

10.7 The trigeminal ganglion is located in Meckel's cave (otherwise known as the 'trigeminal cave'). This is immediately posterolateral to the cavernous sinuses within the middle cranial fossa.

10.8 The trigeminal sensory nucleus consists of three subnuclei and occupies a large area of the brainstem extending from the midbrain down to the upper cervical cord. It is the largest of the cranial nerve nuclei.

10.9 The motor nucleus of trigeminal nerve occupies a separate and distinct area just medial to its sensory counterpart within the superior aspect of the pons (in the pontine tegmentum). It is smaller than the sensory trigeminal nucleus.

Station 11

11.1 **A** Odontoid peg

B Medulla oblongata

C Cervical spinal cord

D Spinous process of T1 vertebra

E CSF fluid surrounding the spinal cord within the thecal sac

F Vertebral body of T6

11.2 The dorsal column transmits light touch, vibration, and proprioception. This is an ascending spinal tract and located within the dorsal (posterior) aspect of the spinal canal (**Figure 4.12**).

11.3 The spinothalamic tract transmits crude touch, pain, and temperature. It is located in the ventrolateral aspect of the spinal cord and is sometimes known as the 'anterolateral tract'.

11.4 Motor descending pathways include the pyramidal (corticospinal tracts) and the extrapyramidal tracts (rubrospinal, reticulospinal, olivospinal, vestibulospinal tracts). The lateral corticospinal tract is found in the dorsolateral region of the spinal cord, the anterior corticospinal tract is found anteromedially within the spinal cord. The extrapyramidal tracts can be seen to also occupy the anteromedial and dorsolateral regions and are better visualized in the diagram below.

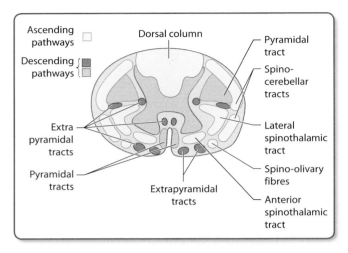

Figure 4.12 The ascending and descending pathways within the spinal cord.

11.5 A total transection of the spinal cord at T2 would prevent any motor or sensory innervation from the level of T2 downwards. At the level of T1, the exiting motor tracts will have left the spinal cord and the sensory information from the dorsal column fibres will be transmitted. The information from the spinothalamic tract fibres at the T1 level may not have yet decussated across the cord but would have entered above the transection level and would still be transmitted.

As the transection occurs below the level of innervation to the upper limbs sensation and motor function to the upper limbs is spared, however there will be lack of motor or sensory function from the superior aspect of the thorax downwards, including no innervation to the lower limbs.

11.6 Brown–Sequard syndrome results from a lateral hemisection of the spinal cord.

11.7 The signs that would result from a right hemitransection of the spinal cord at the level of T2 include:

- Loss of motor function on the right side of the body from the T2 vertebral level downwards. This results in an upper motor neuron lesion leading to spastic paralysis.
- Loss of transmission of sensory information from the dorsal column tract (i.e. no vibration, proprioception or light touch sense) from the right side of the body at the level of T2 downwards.
- Normal transmission of sensory information from the spinothalamic tract (i.e. crude touch, temperature and pain) on the right but loss of such sensory information from the contralateral side beginning approximately one or two vertebral levels inferiorly; in this example loss of information from T4 downwards on the left.

Station 12

12.1 A Right middle cerebral artery (MCA)

   B Right internal carotid artery

    C Lenticulostriate branches of MCA

    D Anterior cerebral artery (ACA) A1

    E Cortical branches of the anterior cerebral artery

    F Anterior cerebral artery (ACA) A2

12.2 A subarachnoid haemorrhage.

12.3 A berry aneurysm is the usual cause. This most commonly occurs in the anterior communicating artery (followed in frequency by the posterior communicating artery).

12.4 Up to one-third of patients who have autosomal dominant polycystic kidneys are thought develop intracranial berry aneurysms over the course of their lives.

12.5 To diagnose a subarachnoid haemorrhage the initial investigation of choice is CT imaging of the brain without intravenous contrast. If this proves to be negative then a lumbar puncture should be performed no sooner than 12 hours from the onset of the clinical symptoms to identify xanthochromia.

12.6 The blood brain barrier (BBB) consists of endothelial cells that line the capillaries of the brain. They differ from other endothelial capillary cells by the tight junctions they form that repel molecules from passing through the capillary walls. The function of the BBB is to maintain homeostasis and only allow the entrance of essential nutrients from the blood whilst preventing toxins from being transmitted. Water-soluble substances are impermeable, whereas those that are lipid soluble are permeable.

12.7 The areas of the brain that lie outside the BBB (and are therefore at risk of exposure to toxins from the bloodstream) include the area postrema (the chemoreceptor trigger zone within the medulla) and the posterior pituitary gland. The capillaries in these regions are different in that they are fenestrated and more similar to those seen in peripheral tissues than to the other regions of the brain.

Station 13

13.1 The sphenoid bone. This is located in the midline within the base of the skull. It has a very characteristic shape that makes it easily recognisable and resembles 'bat wings' (**Figure 4.13**).

13.2 A Right greater wing of the sphenoid bone

    B Right foramen ovale

    C Sella turcica

    D Left lesser wing of the sphenoid bone

    E Left lateral pterygoid plate

13.3 X Foramen rotundum. This transmits the maxillary nerve (CN V2), a branch of the trigeminal nerve (CN V).

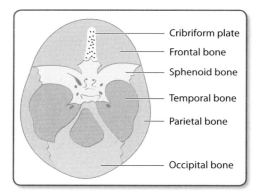

Figure 4.13 The position of the sphenoid bone viewed from the interior aspect of the base of the skull.

Y The superior orbital fissure. This transmits the oculomotor (CN III), trochlear (CN IV), ophthalmic (CN V1) and abducens (CN VI) nerves.

13.4 The structure labelled Q, the anterior clinoid process, gives rise to the attachment of the tentorium cerebelli along its medial aspect.

13.5 There are 12 bones that the sphenoid bone articulates with (**Table 4.6**).

Table 4.6 Paired and unpaired bones articulating with the sphenoid bone	
Paired bones	**Unpaired bones**
Parietal	Vomer
Temporal	Ethmoid
Zygomatic	Frontal
Palatine	Occipital

13.6 Middle cranial fossa.

13.7 The pituitary gland sits within a space in the sphenoid bone known as the sella turcica (the Latin translation of this is 'Turkish saddle', named after its resemblance [**Figure 4.14**]). The anterior boundaries of this region are the middle clinoid processes and the posterior boundary is formed by the dorsum sellae, a rectangular shaped part of the sphenoid bone that juts vertically upwards.

13.8 Upon the superior aspect of the lesser wings of the sphenoid sit the inferior aspect of the frontal lobes of the brain.

Station 14

14.1 A Posterior cerebellar lobe

  B Anterior cerebellar lobe

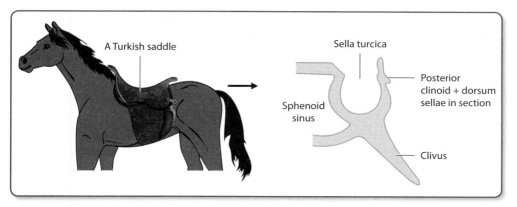

Figure 4.14 The sagittal view of the sella turcica and its resemblance to a Turkish saddle.

  C Cerebellar tonsil

  D Pons

  E Medulla

  F Optic chiasm

  G Pons

  H Right cerebellar hemisphere

  I Mamillary bodies

14.2 The cerebellum is located within the posterior cranial fossa. The posterior cranial fossa is the area of the base of the brain formed by the occipital and petrous temporal bones. Its anterior border is formed by the clivus, amongst many other structures; it contains the cerebellum and brainstem.

14.3 The cerebellum is connected to the brainstem via three pairs of thick fibrous bundles known as peduncles. **Table 4.7** outlines where the peduncles of the cerebellum attach.

14.4 The fourth ventricle and Aqueduct of Sylvius lie in-between the cerebellum and the pons. Masses that occupy the vermis of the cerebellum may grow to encroach on the fourth ventricle anteriorly, causing a non-communicating hydrocephalus as a result.

14.5 The main functions of the cerebellum include:
- maintenance of balance
- co-ordination of movement
- contribution to maintenance of posture and muscle tone.

14.6 The cerebellum contributes only to motor function and does not have any sensory function at all, although it does receive sensory information from the body.

14.7 Right-sided cerebellar lesions produce right-sided signs and symptoms, unlike lesions within the cerebral cortices that produce contralateral signs. The reason for this finding is due to the nature of the descending and decussating pathways

Table 4.7 The cerebellar peduncles and their relation to the structures of the midbrain

Cerebellar peduncle	Connects the cerebellum to which brainstem area	Comments
Superior (superior brachium con-junctivum)	Midbrain	This peduncle contains efferent fibres from the dentate, emboliform and globose nuclei. The afferent fibres provide the cerebellum with information of proprioception of the lower limbs ascending via the ventrospino-cerebellar tract.
Middle (middle brachium pontis)	Pons	Largest of the three peduncles and related to muscle movement.
Inferior (restiform bodies)	Medulla	The afferent fibres from this peduncle provide the cerebellum on proprioceptive information of the upper limbs via the dorso-spinocerebellar tract.

of the cerebellar tracts. The knowledge of these pathways are rather detailed and complex and not required for the MRCS Part B examination.

14.8 The features of cerebellar dysfunction can be remembered by the mnemonic 'DANISH':

- **D**ysdiadokokinesia (inability to perform rapid alternating movements)
- **A**taxia (lack of co-ordination and muscle movements)
- **N**ystagmus (impaired co-ordination of eye movements)
- **I**ntention tremor (ipsilateral mal-coordination)
- **S**lurred/staccato/scanning speech pattern
- **H**ypotonia.

In a right-sided lesion of the cerebellum, as described in the clinical scenario, the clinical findings would be ipsilateral. Nystagmus would demonstrate greatest amplitude with the patient looking towards the affected side and altered postural control would lead the patient to tilt towards the side of the lesion.

14.9 If a cerebellar abnormality were located in the midline without a predilection for either lobe then the signs would not localise to either side. A midline lesion would generally lead to loss of postural control whereby the subject would not be able to stand without falling despite preserved co-ordination of their limbs. Patients would also generally not present with nystagmus or features of dysarthria.

Station 15

15.1 **A** Right ethmoid sinus

B Right sphenoid sinus

C Right dentate nucleus

D Aqueduct of Sylvius

E Left cerebellar hemisphere

15.2 The cerebellum can be classified into the right and left cerebellar hemispheres (each consisting of an anterior and posterior lobe separated by the primary fissure), the vermis (in the midline) and the flocculonodular lobe (consisting of a small area of each cerebellar hemisphere and the vermis). Note that the vermis is part of the flocculonodular lobe, but is also sometimes described on its own as the midline portion of the cerebellum.

15.3 Another way of classifying the cerebellum is by function (**Table 4.8**).

15.5 The four paired nuclei in the cerebellum are called:
- the dentate nuclei (the only nucleus visible to the naked eye)
- the emboliform nucleus
- the globose nucleus
- the fastigial nucleus.

The dentate nucleus is the most laterally located of the four nuclei within the deep white matter of each cerebellar hemisphere forming part of the cerebrocerebellum. The remaining three paired nuclei are located adjacent to the dentate in the following order (from most lateral to medial): emboliform, globose and fastigial (**Figure 4.15**). The fastigial nuclei are located immediately over the room of the

Table 4.8 The functional regions of the cerebellum		
Functional cerebellar region	**Gross anatomical area**	**Function**
Vestibulocerebellum (archicerebellum)	Flocculonodular lobe	Regulates the maintenance of balance. The influence of this region on the lower limbs is bilateral and disturbances of this region lead to problems with gait and balance.
Spinocerebellum (paleocerebellum)	Vermis and the medial aspects of the cerebellar hemispheres	Regulates muscle tone and posture. It receives information on the proprioception of the body from the dorsal spinal column, trigeminal nerve and visual and auditory systems.
Cerebrocerebellum (neocerebellum)	Lateral hemispheres	Muscle coordination including the planning of certain movements such as the speed, force, and direction of movements. It only receives input from the cerebral cortices and helps with the fine-tuning of anticipated movements.

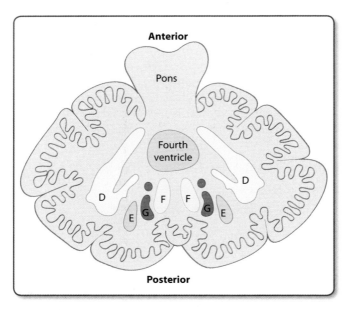

Figure 4.15 The location of the various cerebellar nuclei. D, dentate nuclei; E, emboliform nuclei; F, fastigial nuclei; G globose nuclei.

fourth ventricle in the midline. A mnemonic which can help you remember the position and names of these four nuclei is: **D**on't (**d**entate) **E**at (**e**mboliform) **G**reen (**g**lobose) **F**ish (**f**astigial).

15.6 The foramen magnum.

15.7 Clinical signs of raised intracranial pressure include papilloedema, decreased levels of consciousness and altered visual acuity and ocular palsies. Clinical symptoms include headache (worse on straining), vomiting (without necessarily symptoms of nausea), and occasionally backache. Note that although imaging of the brain is usually requested to determine whether there is the presence of raised intracranial pressure, it is actually a very poor investigation for ruling this out unless there is herniation of the cerebellar tonsils or gross hydrocephalus present.

15.8 The line joining the basion to the opisthion (also known as 'McRae's Line' – **Figure 4.16**) defines the lower limit of the cerebellar tonsils within the posterior fossa. If the cerebellar tonsils are seen to lie significantly below this level then there is the suggestion that cerebellar tonsillar herniation is occurring.

15.9 An Arnold–Chiari (I) malformation.

Station 16

16.1 The anterior circulation is being examined. Although the catheter is placed within the internal carotid artery, it is demonstrating the branches of the anterior cerebral artery. **Figure 4.17** demonstrates the branches of this artery in more detail.

16.2 The anterior cerebral artery supplies the medial surface of the frontal and parietal lobes, anterior portions of the basal ganglia and anterior limb of the internal capsule as well as the majority of the corpus callosum.

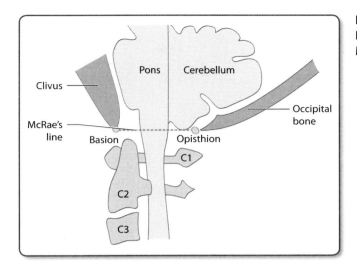

Figure 4.16
Demonstration of
McRae's line.

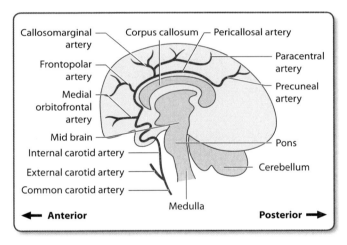

Figure 4.17 The
branches of the
anterior cerebral
artery.

16.3 Complete proximal obstruction of the anterior cerebral arteries is rare due
to the anastomosis between the two arteries by the anterior communicating
artery. Nevertheless, those that are distal to the anterior communicating
artery can cause a variety of effects. Unilateral occlusion distal to the anterior
communicating artery can result in contralateral sensorimotor deficits
mainly affecting the lower limb (as the part of the cortex supplied by the
anterior cerebral artery represents the lower limbs on the motor and sensory
homunculus). Bilateral occlusion of the anterior cerebral arteries is rare but if
this occurs at their origins, the result will be infarction of both anteromedial
cerebral hemispheres leading to paraplegia of both lower limbs (sparing the
face and upper limbs), incontinence, potential change in personality and
decision making (due to frontal lobe symptoms).

16.4 The anterior communicating artery connects the right anterior cerebral artery with the left anterior cerebral artery.

16.5 **A** Ophthalmic artery

   B Internal carotid siphon (right) – cavernous portion

   C Internal carotid artery (right)

   D Pericallosal branch of the anterior cerebral artery (right)

   E Internal carotid artery (petrous portion)

16.6 There are seven parts to the internal carotid artery, detailed in **Figure 4.18** and **Table 4.9**.

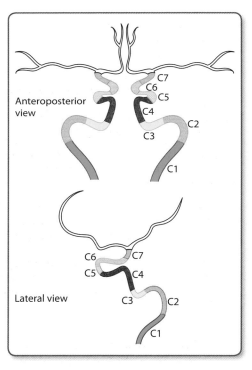

Figure 4.18 The segments of the internal carotid artery.

Knowing the seven segments of the internal carotid artery is useful not only in the description of the arterial anatomy but also because it helps to remember its course.

16.7 Given the presenting symptoms in the clinical scenario, the ophthalmic artery (vessel labelled A and a branch of the ophthalmic segment of the internal carotid artery) is the most likely affected vessel. This artery supplies all the structures in the orbit.

16.8 **A** Ophthalmic artery

Table 4.9 The segments of the internal carotid artery

Number of segment	Name of segment	Notes
C1	Cervical	• Runs from where the common carotid artery bifurcates up to the level where the internal carotid artery enters the carotid canal in the skull base • The internal carotid canal has no branches within the neck
C2	Petrous	• Extends from the base of the skull, running within the petrous portion of the temporal bone to the foramen lacerum
C3	Lacerum	• Continues from the petrous segment originating above the foramen lacerum and continuing until the apex of the sphenoid bone • It does not actually travel through the foramen lacerum
C4	Cavernous	• Passes through the cavernous sinus adjacent to the abducens (CN VI) nerve • Branches given off by this section supply the posterior aspect of the pituitary gland
C5	Clinoid (or supraclinoid)	• Continues from where the artery exits the cavernous sinus to where it enters the subarachnoid space • Segment is very short
C6	Ophthalmic	• Extends from the distal dural ring (where the clinoid segment first becomes intradural) and terminates at the level where the posterior communicating artery is given off • Gives off the 'ophthalmic artery' branch that supplies all the structures in the orbit, frontal and ethmoidal sinuses, and a part of the scalp covering the frontal bone
C7	Communicating	• The terminal segment • Continues from the ophthalmic segment up to where the artery bifurcates into the anterior cerebral and middle cerebral arteries

Station 17

17.1 A Septum pellucidum

B External capsule

C Lentiform nucleus

D Third ventricle

E Head of caudate nucleus

F Internal capsule

G Thalamus

17.2 The basal ganglia is composed of the following structures:
- claustrum
- caudate nucleus
- globus Pallidus
- putamen

17.3 There are a multitude of functions provided by the basal ganglia. In general, it is responsible for the co-ordination of movements, behaviour and also the inhibition of unwanted movements. It does not cause the movements to happen but manages the way in which they occur. The pathways involved are rather complex and their detailed knowledge is not required for the examination.

17.4 A right-sided basal ganglia lesion would give symptoms on the contralateral (i.e. left) side of the body. As touched upon earlier, a deficit within the basal ganglia would not cause paralysis of a movement as its function is not concerned with the production of the movement. However, it would result in abnormal motor control of the limb (including reduced or slow movements, tremors, athetosis, and choreas) and alteration in the muscle tone (which can either be increased leading to rigidity or reduced resulting in hypotonia).

17.5 The amygdala is closely located to the structures of the basal ganglia and shares a similar embryological derivation, however it is actually part of the limbic system and concerned with aspects of memory and emotion.

17.6 The corpus striatum is composed of the following structures:
- caudate nucleus
- putamen

17.7 The lentiform nucleus is composed of the following structures:
- putamen
- globus pallidus

An easy way of visualizing the structures that make up the striatum, lentiform nucleus, and basal ganglia is displayed in the Venn diagram (**Figure 4.19**) below.

17.8 The globus pallidus is the portion of the lentiform nucleus that has an extension to the midbrain, specifically the substantia nigra.

17.9 **E** Caudate nucleus. This is a 'C' shaped structure and is anatomically closely associated with the lateral ventricle (**Figure 4.20**). The different anatomical regions of the caudate nucleus are the head, body, and tail. The head and the body of the caudate nucleus both form part of the floor of the anterior horn of the lateral ventricle. The tail of the caudate nucleus forms part of the roof of the temporal horn of the lateral ventricle.

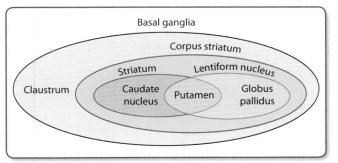

Figure 4.19 Venn diagram demon-strating the components of the basal ganglia.

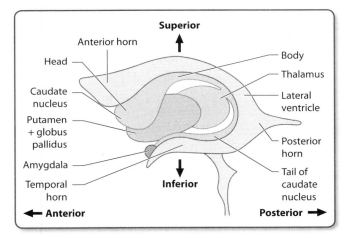

Figure 4.20 The caudate nucleus.

Station 18

18.1 A Left frontal lobe

B Midbrain

C Red nucleus

D Substantia nigra

E Cerebral aqueduct

F Nucleus of the oculomotor nerve (CN III)

G Medial longitudinal fasciculus

The regions of the midbrain are more easily identified and demonstrated in **Figure 4.21**.

18.2 The medial longitudinal fasciculi are a pair of white matter tracts within the brainstem. Their primary role is in the co-ordination of conjugate eye movements, in particular the vertical eye movements.

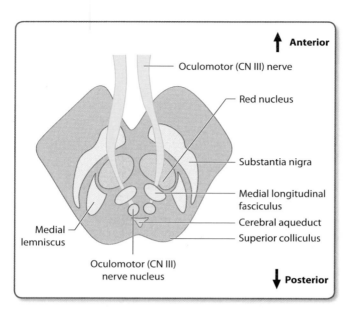

Figure 4.21 The regions within the midbrain.

18.3 A deficit in the function of the medial longitudinal fasciculus results in abnormal (predominantly vertical) eye movements. Clinical signs include vertical gaze nystagmus, decreased vertical smooth pursuit, and diminished vertical gaze holding. Clinical symptoms may include diplopia, blurred vision, or even the impression that the environment is moving around them. This deficit is known as 'internuclear ophthalmoplegia' (INO) and it tends to be bilateral in multiple sclerosis or unilateral when the cause is due to cerebrovascular disease. In order to test for the signs, a thorough cranial nerve examination must be carried out, including testing the full range of eye movements with an assessment of how long the patient is able to hold their gaze in all directions, and examination of horizontal and vertical nystagmus (**Figure 4.22**).

18.4 The term brainstem refers to the midbrain, pons and medulla

18.5 The majority of the cranial nerves originate from the brain stem. These include the CN III–XII, namely the oculomotor, trochlear, trigeminal, abducens, facial, vestibulocochlear, glossopharyngeal, vagus, accessory, and hypoglossal nerves.

18.6 The corticospinal tract fibres decussate within the medulla before entering the spinal cord.

18.7 The dorsal column transmits information on proprioception and vibration sense. The first order dorsal column proprioceptive fibres transmit their sensory signals within the ipsilateral dorsal column of the spinal cord until reaching the brainstem where they relay to the dorsal nuclei within the medulla. Here the second order fibres decussate to form the medial lemniscus and with sensory input from the trigeminal nerve (CN V) which offers sensory information from the face the fibres continue to the thalamus where they relay to the third order fibres. The third order fibres start at the thalamus and eventually synapse with the primary somatosensory cortex. This pathway is demonstrated in **Figure 4.23**:

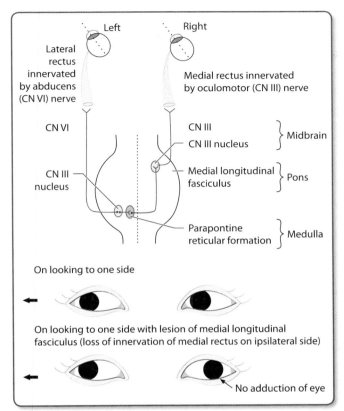

Figure 4.22 The medial longitudinal fasciculus and resultant clinical effects during an abnormality of this region.

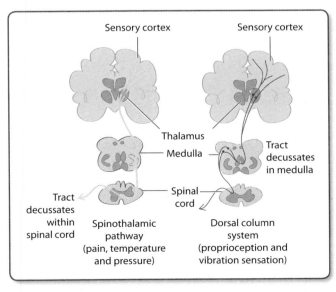

Figure 4.23 The dorsal column and lateral spinothalamic pathways.

18.8 The lateral spinothalamic tract transmits pain, temperature, and crude touch. The first order neurones transmit sensory information by entering the ipsilateral dorsal horn of the spinal cord and synapsing with the second order neurones within this region. The second order axons then decussate via the 'ventral white commissure' lying anterior to the central canal of the cord. The decussation usually occurs within one or two vertebral levels from the original vertebral level at which the first order neurons enter the spinal cord. From the contralateral dorsal horn, the second order axons run towards the brainstem adjacent to the medial lemniscus of the dorsal column fibres (mentioned above) where they are termed the 'spinal lemniscus'. These fibres terminate in the thalamus synapsing with the third order neurons that project to the somatosensory cortex (**Figure 4.23**).

18.9 This information helps us to predict the clinical signs that would result from a transected cord. Conversely, if a patient presents with a collection of signs and symptoms we can also predict where a potential transection could have occurred.

18.10 Ipsilateral cranial nerve dysfunction, contralateral spastic hemiparesis, hyperreflexia and an contralateral hemisensory loss and ipsilateral mal co-ordination.

18.11 Bilateral brain stem lesions are rarely compatible with life. Commonly patients who present with this pathology have severely decreased conscious levels and eventually succumb to respiratory depression.

Station 19

19.1 **A** Right basal ganglia

   B Right head of caudate nucleus

   C Interhemispheric fissure

   D Corpus callosum

   E Left Sylvian fissure

   F Left hippocampus

19.2 The blood supply to the basal ganglia is primarily via end branches, the lenticulostriate branches, of the middle cerebral artery (MCA). These vessels are very narrow and easily damaged either by haemorrhage in patients with uncontrolled hypertension or blocked by thrombus leading to tiny infarcts known as lacunar infarcts.

19.3 The knowledge that the lenticulostriate branches are end branches is significant because in a proximal MCA infarct the basal ganglia are at risk of early ischaemic damage. The cortex supplied by the MCA is conversely at less risk of early ischaemia because the contralateral MCA also provides some crossover supply. Early thrombolysis can help to restore the original blood supply to the cortex before substantial damage to the cortex has occurred, however early damage to the basal ganglia is less successful and may lead to movement disorders.

19.4 The middle cerebral artery lies in the Sylvian fissure.

19.5 The hippocampus serves us primarily in the function of memory. Patients with Alzheimer's disease typically demonstrate atrophy in this region.

19.6 The massa intermedia is the part of the medial surface of the two thalami (one in each cerebral hemisphere) that fuse together in the midline. It is also known as the 'interthalamic adhesion' and does not appear to perform any unique function, as patients who lack this adhesion are asymptomatic, unlike those that lack a corpus callosum.

19.7 Within the region labelled G, one would expect the midbrain to be situated.

19.8 The trigeminal, abducens, facial and vestibulocochlear nerves (CN V, VI, VII and VIII respectively) arise from this level.

19.9 There are numerous parts of the brainstem and cortex that exert control on respiration. Within the pons, two areas influence the pattern of breathing but are not essential for breathing. The areas include the apneustic centre (which prolongs inspiration) and the pneumotaxic centre (which inhibits the inspiratory neurons resulting in shorter inspirations and longer expirations).

Station 20

20.1 A Basilar artery

　　　B Vertebral artery

　　　C Muscular branches of the vertebral artery

　　　D Superior cerebellar artery

　　　E Anterior inferior cerebellar artery

20.2 There are four parts to the vertebral artery (B), named V1–V4. The origin and transition points between the segments have been discussed previously.

20.3 The branches of vertebral artery can be thought of as those that originate within the neck and those that originate in the skull (**Figure 4.24**). Those that are given off in the neck include: the muscular branches that supply the deep muscles of the neck and the lateral spinal arteries, which travel within the intervertebral foramina of the cervical vertebra and supply the spinal cord, meninges and vertebral bodies.

Those that are given off in the skull include the:

- posterior inferior cerebellar artery that partly supplies the cerebellum, fourth ventricle and choroid plexus
- anterior spinal artery that supplies the anterior portion of the spinal cord.

20.4 The origin of the basilar artery (A) is at the confluence of the two vertebral arteries just inferior and anterior to the pons.

20.5 After the origin of the basilar artery it ascends within the 'sulcus basilaris', a straight midline groove on the ventral surface of the pons, before terminating at a level just inferior to the optic chiasm and pituitary infundibulum by dividing into two posterior cerebral arteries.

20.6 The cerebellum is supplied by three main arteries (**Figure 4.25** and **Table 4.10**).

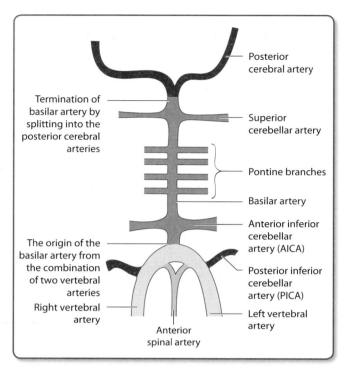

Figure 4.24 The branches of the vertebral and basilar artery.

Posterior cerebral artery

Termination of basilar artery by splitting into the posterior cerebral arteries

Superior cerebellar artery

Pontine branches

Basilar artery

Anterior inferior cerebellar artery (AICA)

The origin of the basilar artery from the combination of two vertebral arteries

Posterior inferior cerebellar artery (PICA)

Right vertebral artery

Left vertebral artery

Anterior spinal artery

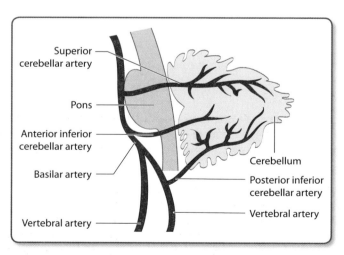

Figure 4.25 The arterial blood supply to the cerebellum.

Superior cerebellar artery

Pons

Anterior inferior cerebellar artery

Basilar artery

Cerebellum

Posterior inferior cerebellar artery

Vertebral artery

Vertebral artery

Table 4.10 The arterial blood supply of the cerebellum

Artery	Branch of vessel	Part of cerebellum supplied	Comments
Posterior inferior cerebellar artery	Vertebral artery	Inferior surface of the cerebellum (and the dorsolateral aspect of the medulla oblongata)	Occlusion of this artery results in the 'lateral medullary syndrome' or 'locked-in syndrome'
Anterior inferior cerebellar artery	Basilar artery	A very small anterior inferior aspect of the cerebellum, the cerebellar flocculus (also the dorsolateral pons and middle cerebral peduncle)	Its origin is variable, but in the majority of cases it arises from the inferior third of the basilar artery
Superior cerebellar artery	Basilar artery	The whole superior aspect of the cerebellum, most of the cerebellar white matter and the dentate nuclei (also the dorsolateral aspect of the midbrain)	

Station 21

21.1 **A** Right olfactory (CN I) nerve

   B Optic chiasm

   C Infundibulum (pituitary stalk)

   D Left optic tract

   E Medulla oblongata

21.2 In this state a patient is permanently unconscious and lacks brainstem reflexes. Declaring a patient 'brainstem dead' or 'brain dead' consists of a set of criterion to confirm death by neurological grounds. This criterion has been in use in the United Kingdom since the late 1970s.

21.3 In a persistent vegetative state, the patient still maintains some level of their consciousness and has preserved sleep wake cycles, breathing, brainstem, and some primitive reflexes. Nevertheless, they do not necessarily interact in any meaningful manner to their environment and may not possess any awareness of their own state or of the stimuli around them. They do not produce any voluntary movements and their gestures and sounds are usually without purpose and inconsistent.

	Reflex	Afferent nerve	Efferent nerve
A	Pupillary light reflex	Optic (CN II) nerve detects the light stimulus reaching the retina	Oculomotor (CN III) nerve acts to constrict the pupil in response to light stimulus
B	Corneal reflex	Trigeminal (CN V) nerve detects light touch stimulus on the surface of the cornea	Facial (CN VII) nerve acts to shut the eye in response to the corneal irritation
C	Gag reflex	Glossopharyngeal (CN IX) nerve detects sensation at the soft palate at the back of the throat	Vagus (CN X) nerve acts to prevent any foreign object from entering the respiratory tract by elevating the uvula and constricting the cricopharyngeus muscle, thereby creating the 'gagging' sensation that gives this reflex its name

Table 4.11 The afferent and efferent limbs of brainstem reflexes

21.4 There are several preconditions and an awareness of them is important. Some of the important preconditions are listed below:
   - An irreversible pathology must be identified.
   - Exclusion of causes for decreased consciousness must be made (e.g. exclusion of the effects of hypothermia, narcotics or other sedative drugs).
   - There must be correction of other potentially reversible physiological causes for the decreased conscious level such as circulatory and biochemical disturbances.
   - The patient must be reliant on the aid of mechanical ventilation and not able to breathe unassisted.

21.5 **Table 4.11** demonstrates the efferent and afferent cranial nerves for each reflex.

21.6 Other tests for brainstem death (in addition to those outlined in the 21.4) must include the following:
   - Absence of any respiratory effort or movement during the disconnection of a mechanical ventilator machine (despite pre-oxygenation).
   - No motor response to pain stimulus (this is commonly inflicted by pressure over the supraorbital ridge).
   - Vestibulo-ocular reflexes should be absent, which is usually tested by instilling ice-cold water into each external acoustic meatus slowly and repeating the test for both sides; a normal reflex is to observe eye movements away from the stimulus.

Index